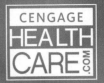

T0131190

ECG
ESSENTIALS OF
Electrocardiography

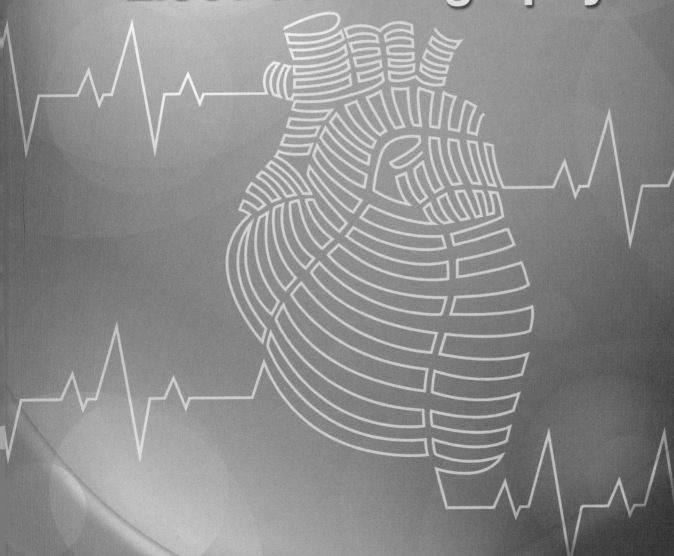

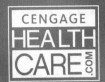

Access. Engage. Learn.

ECG
ESSENTIALS OF
Electrocardiography

Cathy D. **SOTO** PhD

CENGAGE

Australia • Brazil • Mexico • Singapore • United Kingdom • United States

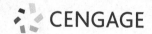

ECG: Essentials of Electrocardiography,
Cathy D. Soto, PhD

SVP, GM Skills & Global Product
Management: Dawn Gerrain

Product Director: Matthew Seeley

Product Manager: Laura Stewart

Senior Director, Development: Marah Bellegarde

Product Development Manager: Juliet Steiner

Associate Content Developer: Kaitlin Schlicht

Product Assistant: Deborah Handy

Vice President, Marketing Services: Jennifer
Ann Baker

Marketing Manager: Jonathan Sheehan

Senior Production Director: Wendy Troeger

Production Director: Andrew Crouth

Senior Content Project Manager: Kenneth
McGrath

Senior Art Director: Jack Pendleton

For product information and technology assistance, contact us at
**Cengage Customer & Sales Support, 1-800-354-9706
or support.cengage.com.**

For permission to use material from this text or product, submit all
requests online at **www.cengage.com/permissions.**

Library of Congress Control Number: 2015956900
ISBN: 978-1-285-18098-4

Cengage
20 Channel Street
Boston, MA 02210
USA

Cengage is a leading provider of customized learning solutions
with employees residing in nearly 40 different countries and sales in more
than 125 countries around the world. Find your local representative at:
www.cengage.com.

Cengage products are represented in Canada by
Nelson Education, Ltd.

To learn more about Cengage platforms and services, register or access
your online learning solution, or purchase materials for your course,
visit **www.cengage.com.**

Notice to the Reader

Printed at CLDPC, USA, 06-24

Dedication

I sincerely appreciate and dedicate this first edition to my spouse of 40 years, Jose Soto III. Thank you for all your patience, especially as we traveled—and I just needed to "write one more section"—for all the meals you shopped for and prepared, and for being a positive influence when I became discouraged. I couldn't have done it without you, Joe!

Table of Contents

CHAPTER 3

Heart Electrical Physiology

CHAPTER 7
Waveforms, Rate, Rhythm, and Artifacts 185

Preface

For years, while teaching ECGs as a standalone course embedded within a medical assisting program, I could not find an introductory book that included the basics in detail. So I had to develop much of my own material and used books only as a supplemental part of the class. Most books that were on the market skipped the building blocks of knowledge needed to be successful when learning the core information by not answering the question of why the student needed to learn particular information, or what the information being studied has to do with taking an ECG. Also, I found that too many books on the market assumed that the student had already mastered all of the basics because most books started with arrhythmia interpretation, with little emphasis on the other aspects of administration of the electrocardiogram (ECG), such as Holter testing, stress testing, documentation of the procedures completed, HIPAA requirements, and when to seek immediate attention by a licensed practitioner for abnormal test results.

Thus, the goal of *ECG: Essentials of Electrocardiography* is to present clear and concise introductory material for entry-level college students in the field of electrocardiography. This book is especially intended for students who have had no previous coursework in the field of ECGs. My vision in writing a basic ECG book is to ensure that students do not have gaps in their knowledge of anatomy of the heart, electrophysiology, and basic ECG administration and interpretation. This book is ideal for use in a standalone ECG course, as part of the curriculum of various college technology programs, as a good book for a review course, or as a supplemental text to strengthen foundational skills for students in advanced ECG courses. To prepare students for completing ECGs in the field, this book provides students with a combination of introductory cardiovascular anatomy, relationships of other body systems to heart health, legal and ethical considerations, patient assessment techniques, instructions on how to complete and document ECGs, and basic interpretation of ECG tracings. Objectives that students must master to be qualified to sit for the National Healthcareer Association's (NHA's) EKG Technician Certification exam are addressed throughout the text. The NHA Certified EKG Technician (CET) Detailed Test Plan can be found on NHA's website (www.nhanow.com).

TEXT ORGANIZATION

ECG: Essentials of Electrocardiography, written as a short, eight-chapter book, is organized in such a way that students can learn the material in a timely manner. The book presents the basics of electrocardiography, with each concept building off prior concepts, and with a focus on mastery learning. Chapters 1 through 4 focus on the cardiovascular system, electrophysiology of the heart, and cardiovascular medications. This helps students build the foundation that they will need to interpret an ECG and relate their findings to what is happening in the heart. Chapters 5 through 8 walk students through patient assessment, completing and documenting an ECG, and basic ECG interpretation. After completion of these chapters, students will be able to perform ECGs and identify artifacts and basic arrhythmias, allowing them to understand when they need to readminister an ECG and when patients may need immediate medical attention.

The step-by-step approach of the book, which incorporates "Quick Checks" for students to test their knowledge of important concepts, allows students to master objectives with minimal instructor-led teaching needed. With the 290 "Quick Check" questions, if students do not master a particular concept, they will know exactly what to reread in each chapter and where it is located. All of the answers to the "Quick Check" problems are included at the end of each chapter for student reference and confirmation of student learning.

The chapters are rich in visual aids, and include over 150 figures. More than 50 realistic ECG tracings appear in Chapters 7 and 8. The wavelength figures and electrode placement figures are color coded as they are introduced in Chapter 6 so that students can identify the concepts faster than they would if black-and-white figures were used. Through the use of both text and visuals, learners are presented with different opportunities to learn and review the material, and they can focus on their learning style preference.

Moving to the end of each chapter, students will find a bulleted summary that directly correlates to the objectives found on the first page of the chapter. After the summary, there are three critical thinking problems, many of which are composed of multiple parts or tables that students can fill in for future review. More review activities follow the critical thinking problems. The review activities are often matching or terminology reviews, as well as other activities that will appeal to the tactile learner. Each chapter concludes with a test that highlights the important concepts presented. This activity-driven approach ensures that students have ample opportunity to practice what they learn.

FEATURES

Each chapter includes the following features:

Key terms appear boldfaced within the chapter text and are defined in the margin on the page where the terms first appear. All key terms also appear in the student-friendly glossary, which includes the chapter number where each term is first defined so that students may quickly reference the key term in context within the chapter.

Learning objectives are included at the start of each chapter and address the knowledge and skills that students must master.

Spotlight Call-outs appear throughout the text. These are short, to-the-point references to material that the student should memorize.

Boxes highlight important information that students do not necessarily need to memorize, but with which they should become very familiar. For example, arrhythmia rules that distinguish variances from a normal sinus rhythm are shown as boxes in Chapter 7. Over 30 boxes highlight key information throughout the text.

Quick Checks are short, 5-question quizzes sprinkled throughout each chapter that students can use to immediately test themselves on the material they just read. Answers to the Quick Checks are at the end of each chapter.

A **summary** provides a brief, bulleted list that captures the main points of the chapter. Each summary directly correlates to the objectives listed at the beginning of the chapter.

Critical Thinking Challenges and **Review Activities** provide the student with additional practice activities. Answers are not included in the book, allowing these activities to be assignable and gradable.

A **Chapter Test** concludes each chapter by testing the student on key learning objectives.

SUPPLEMENTS

The following supplements accompany this text:

- **Instructor Companion Website**
- **MindTap**

Instructor Companion Website

(ISBN 978-1-305-39385-1)

Spend less time planning and more time teaching with Cengage Learning's Instructor Companion Website to Accompany *ECG: Essentials of Electrocardiography*. As an instructor, you will have access to all of your resources online, anywhere and at any time. All the instructor resources can be accessed by going to http://www.cengagebrain.com to create a unique user login. The password-protected instructor resources include the following:

- An electronic *Instructor's Manual* for access at any time. The *Instructor's Manual* that accompanies the text includes a sample syllabus, a lesson plan guide for each chapter, additional activities including projects and online activities, a "find-it-fast" chapter outline, and the answers for all end-of-chapter activities and tests.
- Customizable Microsoft PowerPoint® slides for each chapter.
- *Cengage Learning Testing Powered by Cognero*, which is a flexible, online system that allows you to write, edit, and manage test bank content from multiple Cengage Learning solutions; you can also create multiple test versions in an instant and deliver tests from your learning management system (LMS), your classroom, or elsewhere.

MindTap

(Printed Access Code ISBN 978-1-305-11901-7)

(Instant Access Code ISBN 978-1-305-11900-0)

ECG: Essentials of Electrocardiography on MindTap is the first of its kind in an entirely new category: the Personal Learning Experience (PLE). This personalized program of digital products and services uses interactivity and customization to engage students, while offering instructors a wide range of choice in content, platforms, devices, and learning tools. MindTap is device agnostic, meaning that it will work with any platform or LMS and will be accessible anytime, anywhere: on desktops, laptops, tablets, mobile phones, and other Internet-enabled devices.

This MindTap includes the following:

- **An interactive eBook with highlighting, note-taking, and more**
- **Flashcards for practicing chapter terms**
- **Computer-graded activities and exercises**
- **Self-check and application activities, integrated with the eBook**
- **Easy submission tools for instructor-graded exercises**

Activities in the book also appear on MindTap, allowing students to complete and submit the activities online. Some of the activities in the book may appear differently on MindTap, but they will assess the same content. Each activity has been optimized for print or digital use.

ACKNOWLEDGMENTS

I would like to acknowledge Kaitlin Schlicht, Associate Content Developer, Health Care, at Cengage Learning, for working diligently to bring this book to a conclusion and for presenting editing suggestions to make the book a stronger product. Early on, I worked with Elisabeth Williams, Senior Content Developer at Cengage Learning, whom I would like to thank for her patience and for getting early reviews out. I would also like to thank Matthew Seeley, Product Director at Cengage Learning, who was my initial contact to begin this book. Finally, I would like to thank Kenneth McGrath, Senior Content Project Manager, Higher Education Content Production, for his help during the copyediting process.

REVIEWERS

Cengage Learning and the author would like to thank the following individuals for their valuable input:

DONNA M. CATALDO, PhD
Clinical Associate Professor
Arizona State University
Tempe, AZ

SUJANALATHA DE ALMEIDA, RMA, RPT (AMT), A.S. AHI, CPT1
Educator
San Joaquin Valley College
Temecula, CA

JULIE MORRIS, RN, BSN, CBCS, CCMA, CMAA
Director of Career Services
Medtech College
Atlanta, GA

JOHN PERI-OKONNY, MD
Adjunct Instructor
The Fieldstone School
Worcester, MA

NICKOLAS RAY, BS, RN, NRP
Instructor
Southern Union State Community College
Opelika, AL

SUZANNE WAMBOLD, RN, PhD
Professor
Department of Kinesiology
The University of Toledo
Toledo, OH

LISA WRIGHT, CMA (AAMA), MT, SH
Medical Assisting Program Coordinator,
Medical Support Programs Department Chair
Bristol Community College
Fall River, MA

VIRGINIA V. YORK, MD
MA Program Director
Ohio Business College – Hilliard
Hilliard, OH

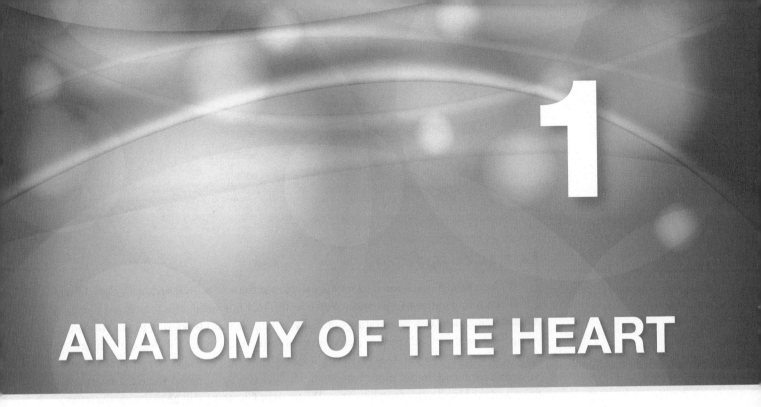

1

ANATOMY OF THE HEART

OBJECTIVES

After reading the chapter and completing all Quick Check activities, the student should be able to:

1. Explain the heart's directional positions.
2. Recognize the heart's anatomy.
3. Contrast three types of cardiac cells.
4. Identify four differences between arteries and veins.
5. Diagram the path of oxygenated and deoxygenated blood flow.

KEY TERMS

aorta

aortic valve

artery

arterioles

atrioventricular (AV) node

atrium {atria (plural)}

bicuspid valve

capillary

cardiac output (CO)

chorda tendinea {chordae tendineae (plural)}

coronary arteries (CA)

coronary sinus

coronary sulcus

endocardium tissue

epicardium tissue

great coronary vein

His-Purkinje system

inferior vena cava

myocardium tissue

papillary muscle

pulmonary artery

pulmonary circulation

pulmonic valve

sinoatrial (SA) node
septum
superior vena cava
systemic circulation

total peripheral resistance (TPR)
tricuspid valve
vasoconstriction
vasodilatation

vein
ventricles
venules

INTRODUCTION

Even though the human heart is small (about the size of an individual's closed fist), it is imperative to a person's overall health that this small, muscular organ is maintained and always operating optimally. Often, the heart is referred to as a two-sided pump because the blood is either rich in oxygen (saturated) on the left side of the heart, or in need of oxygen (desaturated) on the right side of the heart. In healthy hearts, both pumps work in unison and do not mix oxygenated with deoxygenated blood when the heart contracts and the blood moves to a new area. The focus of Chapter 1 will be to review the heart's anatomy from both the pulmonary and systemic circulation processes.

ANATOMICAL ORGANIZATION

The heart is surrounded by a protective, fibrous membrane called the pericardium. The pericardium is composed of a closed, double-layered sac called the pericardial sac, which contains a small amount (10–20 mL) of pericardial fluid. The pericardial fluid acts as a lubricant and plays an important role in preventing friction during the normal movement of the heart during contractions. The pericardial sac contains a tough, inelastic outer surface known as the parietal pericardium, which prevents the heart from overexpanding during a contraction, and an inner, smooth surface called the visceral pericardium, which is also known as the epicardium.

A typical adult male heart weighs approximately 10–12 ounces (283–340 g) and an adult female heart is slightly smaller, weighing approximately 8–10 ounces (226–283 g). The approximate dimensions of the heart are 2 ½–3 ½ in. (6–9 cm) wide and approximately 5 in. (12–13 cm) long.

Directional Positions

Often when the heart is shown in books, it is shown as a cross section (that is, a sliced section) of a one-dimensional frontal view (also called the coronal plane), but it might be easier to think of the heart as being multidimensional. Understanding directional references is an important starting point to understanding exactly what one is looking at.

The heart is usually shown in pictures from the anterior (front), also called the coronal or ventral view; the posterior (rear), or dorsal view; the lateral (side) view; or the inferior view vertically on the midsagittal plane; or on a horizontal transverse plane. **Figure 1-1** identifies the heart in anterior and posterior views.

The heart is not on an actual vertical plane in the body, it is normally tilted to the left in most people, but it can also be tilted to the right in a minor portion of the human population. **Figure 1-2** shows the heart planes of orientation as the heart would be typically found in the human body.

Anterior View **Posterior View**

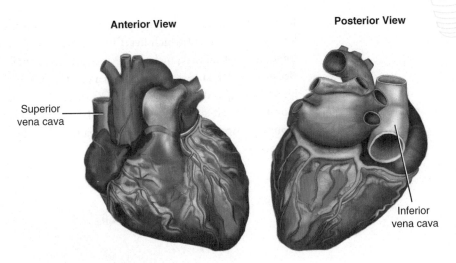

Superior
vena cava

Inferior
vena cava

Figure 1-1 Heart anatomical views

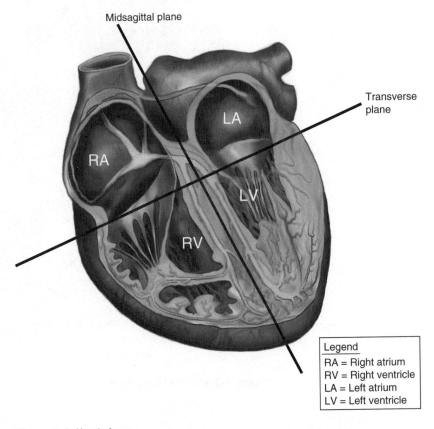

Midsagittal plane

Transverse
plane

LA

RA

LV

RV

Legend
RA = Right atrium
RV = Right ventricle
LA = Left atrium
LV = Left ventricle

Figure 1-2 Heart planes

septum
A dividing wall in the heart made of thick muscle, which separates the right side of the heart from the left side.

In the heart, the midsagittal plane is often divided along a vertical wall called the **septum**. With the anterior view of the heart, the right atrium and right ventricle are shown on the left side of the midsagittal plane and the left atrium and left ventricle are shown on the right side. It is important to note that the left side of the heart is actually larger than the right side because the purpose of the left side is to pump blood to the rest of the body, whereas the purpose of the right side is to pump blood only to the lungs. The transverse plane division is often sectioned between the atria and ventricles.

Important landmarks necessary to complete an electrocardiogram (ECG) are usually referred to in terms of which heart wall is being monitored. The heart walls that are monitored in a 12-lead ECG include the anterior wall, septal wall, left lateral wall, and apical wall. Because the left side of the heart has a greater number of major blood vessels to pump the blood throughout the body, most ECG machines record heart activity from leads placed to monitor the left side of the heart. **Figure 1-3** identifies the main heart walls that an ECG monitors. More discussion on the 12-lead ECG and placement of leads will be provided in Chapter 6.

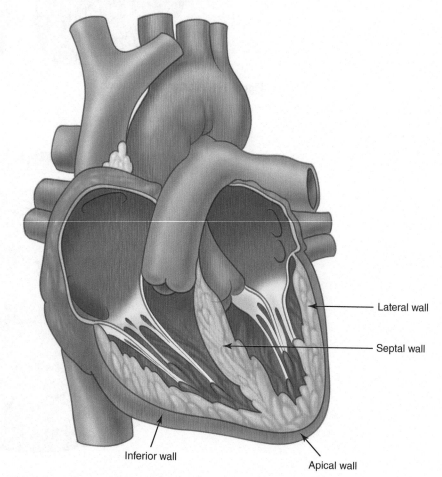

Lateral wall

Septal wall

Inferior wall

Apical wall

Figure 1-3 ECG heart walls monitored

Heart Location and Surrounding Structures

The heart is located in the thoracic cavity, in the anterior mediastinum region between the two pleural cavities (lungs). The base (top) of the heart holds the great vessels, where blood enters and leaves the heart. The base is approximately level with the third rib and is broader than the apex (bottom) of the heart. The apex is cone shaped and projects downward and normally to the left, just above the diaphragm. The heart is moderately protected by the sternum and rib cage ventrally and spinal column dorsally. **Figure 1-4** identifies the location of a normal heart within the chest cavity.

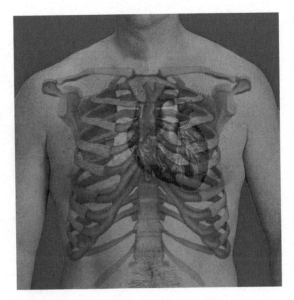

Figure 1-4 Heart location in the human body

Quick Check 1-1

Fill in the blanks.

1. Pericardial fluid acts as a(n) _____ to the heart during contractions.

2. The _____ view of the heart is also called the frontal view, whereas the posterior view is also called the _____ view.

3. The purpose of the _____ side of the heart is to pump blood throughout the body.

4. The 12-lead ECG views the heart from the _____ wall, _____ wall, _____ wall, and the _____ wall.

5. The heart is located in the _____ cavity between the two _____.

HEART CHAMBERS AND VALVES

The largest part of the human heart is composed of four hollow cavities (like four quadrants) often referred to as the heart chambers. A muscular membrane called a septum separates the heart chambers medially into right and left sides. Starting with the four heart chambers, the **atria** are upper (or superior) right and left chambers, and the **ventricles** are lower (or inferior) right and left chambers. Refer to **Figure 1-5** to compare the heart chambers. Notice that the atria are smaller than the ventricles. The standard abbreviations (RA, LA, RV, and LV) identify whether it is right or left and whether it is an atrium or ventricle.

The blood in the four chambers should never mix because each chamber has a specific purpose of either moving oxygen-poor or oxygen-rich blood through a particular chamber. The purpose of the heart septal wall is to prevent the blood from mixing. Because the blood should never mix, many texts refer to the heart as being a "two-sided pump."

atrium {atria (plural)}
One of the upper chambers of the heart, primarily functions as a reservoir for incoming blood.

ventricles
The lower chambers of the heart.

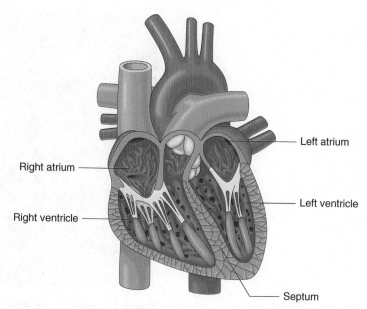

Right atrium

Right ventricle

Left atrium

Left ventricle

Septum

Figure 1-5 Heart chambers

tricuspid valve
A valve located between the right atrium and right ventricle which prevents the backflow of blood into the right atrium during ventricular systole.

bicuspid valve
Also called mitral valve, a valve that separates the left atrium from the left ventricle and prevents the backflow of blood into the left atrium during ventricular systole.

chorda tendinea {chordae tendineae (plural)}
Fibrous connective tissue that attaches the tips of the mitral and tricuspid valves to the papillary muscles of the ventricles, thus preventing the AV valves from being pushed backward into the atria during ventricular contractions.

pulmonic valve
Also called the pulmonary semilunar valve, a valve located between the right ventricle and the pulmonary arteries.

aortic valve
Also called aortic semilunar valve, a valve located between the left ventricle and the ascending aorta which prevents the backflow of blood into the left ventricle.

The heart also consists of four valves. Each of the four valves have cusps (also called leaflets) which are flaps designed to open and close the valve so that blood can flow in only one direction. Two of the heart valves, collectively called the atrioventricular (AV) valves, separate the atria from the ventricles. One AV valve is located between the right atrium and right ventricle and is called the **tricuspid valve**. The second AV valve, the **bicuspid valve**, separates the left atrium from the left ventricle. The bicuspid valve has two cusps, whereas the other three valves normally have three cusps each, although the tricuspid valve has been observed to have between two and six cusps. When the AV valves are working correctly, the heart is in a state of relaxation, and the valves will close completely at nearly the same time to allow blood to fill the right and left atria.

The AV valves are very different from the remaining two valves because the AV valve structure includes **chordae tendineae**, which are fibrous strands of connective tissue designed to hold the AV valves in place. A third valve, called the **pulmonic valve** or pulmonary semilunar valve, is located between the right ventricle and the main pulmonary artery. From the right ventricle, the deoxygenated blood is pushed through the pulmonic valve into the pulmonic trunk, where the pulmonary artery then divides into the right and left pulmonary arteries and into the right and left lung. When the pulmonic valve is working correctly, as the ventricles contract, the valve helps to maintain the blood's pressure as blood goes toward the lungs. The fourth heart valve is the **aortic valve** or aortic semilunar valve, which is located between the left ventricle and the ascending aorta. **Figure 1-6** maps the directional flow of blood through the heart's pulmonary circulation. The blue areas signify blood returning to the heart via the venae cavae, in need of oxygen. The red areas signify blood returning from the lungs, full of oxygen.

When all four valves are operating correctly, the valves should open and close completely once each cardiac cycle. It is critical for a healthy heart that all four valves are working in a sequential manner. The tricuspid valve, when closed, holds blood in the right atrium and prevents backflow of blood from the right ventricle back into the right atrium when the

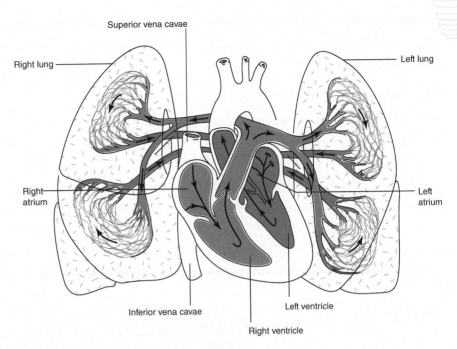

Figure 1-6 Pulmonary circulation blood flow

ventricles contract. When open, the tricuspid valve dumps blood into the right ventricle. The bicuspid (also called the mitral valve) holds blood in the left atrium, preventing blood in the left ventricle to flow back into the left atrium when the ventricles contract. When open, the mitral valve dumps blood into the left ventricle. The pulmonic valve, when closed, holds blood in the right ventricle until a contraction opens the valve and allows the blood to be pumped into the lungs. The aortic valve, when closed, holds the blood in the left ventricle. A contraction of the ventricles causes the aortic valve to open and release blood into the aorta and then into the body. A summary of the valve positions and actions they control is shown in **Table 1-1**.

Table 1-1 Valve Position and Control

Valve	Position	Control
Tricuspid	Open	Releases blood from the right atrium into the right ventricle
Tricuspid	Closed	Holds blood in the right atrium
Mitral	Open	Releases blood from the left atrium into the left ventricle
Mitral	Closed	Holds blood in the left atrium
Pulmonic	Open	Releases blood from the right ventricle into the lungs
Pulmonic	Closed	Holds blood in the right ventricle
Aortic	Open	Releases blood from the left ventricle into the body
Aortic	Closed	Holds blood in the left ventricle

Quick Check 1-2

Fill in the blanks.

1. The heart consists of two upper chambers, called the right and left _____, and two lower chambers, called the right and left _____.

2. The _____ (AV) valves separate the _____ from the _____.

3. The _____ valve has two cusps, whereas the other three valves have three cusps each.

4. In a state of heart relaxation, the _____ valves are closed to allow the right and left _____ to fill with blood.

5. As the ventricles contract, the _____ valve opens to allow blood to enter the _____.

CARDIAC CELLS

Several different types of cell tissue are found in the human heart. Cell tissues can be broken down into three main categories: endothelial cells, smooth muscle cells, and cardiomyocytes. Cardiac muscle cells must have a rich supply of oxygen continuously or they will begin to die.

Endothelial Cells

The prefix *endo* means "inside"; therefore, endothelial cells line the inside of the circulatory system, which includes the blood vessels and the valves of the heart. They form the endocardium and also line the inside of many body cavities. Endothelial cells are metabolically active in producing the compounds needed for platelets by allowing nutrients to be released into the blood. Endothelial cells are of epithelial origin. Epithelial cells are also found in the heart, blood, and lung alveoli (air sacs). Epi means "outside," as in the outside layer of cells of a blood vessel, gland, or organ, and provide protection from microbial invasions, selective absorption, and transcellular transportation. The cells are densely packed, flat, and irregularly shaped and correctly noted as being squamous epithelial cells. Squama means a formation that is platelike or consisting of scales, as shown in **Figure 1-7**. An easy way to remember the difference between endothelial and epithelial cells is that endothelial cells face the blood in the body and never are found on the outside of organs.

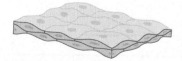

Figure 1-7 Squamous epithelial cells

A blood vessel is much like a "sandwich" of cell layers. Basically, in a sandwich, there are two pieces of bread with meat in between. The "outside" of the sandwich (the bread) would be the epithelial layer, and the inside of the bread, which faces the meat, would be the endothelial layer of cells.

Smooth Muscle Cells

Smooth muscle cells are found in blood vessels and provide the function of moving and controlling fluids through the blood vessels. **Figure 1-8** shows the components of smooth muscle.

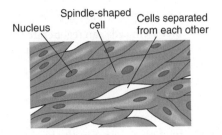

Figure 1-8 Smooth muscle

Smooth muscles are also located in the organs of the digestive and urinary systems. Smooth muscles in the blood vessels are responsible for causing the constriction and dilation of the blood vessels by changing the diameter of the blood vessels. These actions therefore cause changes in blood pressure. Smooth muscle cells move involuntarily, meaning a person cannot control the movements because they are controlled through the autonomic nervous system. **Figure 1-9** shows how the smooth muscle wraps around the lumen (hollow tube) of an artery.

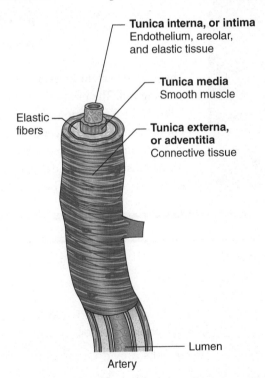

Figure 1-9 Smooth muscle wrapped around an artery

Cardiomyocytes

A heart is more than just a structure. It also has mechanical and electrical properties and requires specialized cells to perform these functions. The conduction system of the heart is completed by specialized cardiomyocytes. It was thought 20 years ago that cardiomyocytes did not go through the normal cell cycle throughout the various stages of life, as other cells do. Instead, after birth, it was believed that cardiomyocytes mainly grew by enlarging in size, not by increasing in number. For this reason, once the cardiac myocytes had been injured or had been damaged, or were diseased, reversal of the damage or disease was not likely to occur. The paradigm has been switching over time though, as research is showing that primitive cells are present in the myocardium after birth, in the form of cardiac stem cells, and the cardiac stem cells can regenerate throughout a lifetime. These primitive cells can form smooth, endothelial, and myocyte cells, therefore maintaining the heart's homeostasis. Researchers are still developing theories of why the recovery after cardiac events is slow to show repair.

Cardiomyocytes are also very different than other cells in the body because only cardiac cells have the ability to produce and utilize an electrical current capable of creating a contraction to occur in the heart muscle. Cardiomyocytes are classified as branched, striated, involuntary muscles and are found only in the heart. **Figure 1-10** shows the composition of cardiomyocytes.

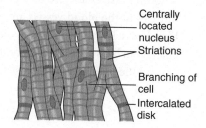

Centrally located nucleus
Striations
Branching of cell
Intercalated disk

Figure 1-10 Cardiac myocyte

There are two main types of cardiomyocytes. The first type of cell is called the myocardial working cell. The primary function of the cardiac working cell is to develop a contraction followed by a relaxation of the heart so that blood can be circulated throughout the body. For the contraction to occur, a second type of cell, called pacemaker cells, must generate an electrical impulse. The process of creating an electrical impulse can only occur in the pacemaker cells that are found in specific regions of the heart. The process by which the electrical current is generated will be discussed in detail in Chapter 3.

> Cardiomyocytes consist of cardiac working cells responsible for contractions and cardiac pacemaker cells responsible for electrical impulses.

Quick Check 1-3

Fill in the blanks.

1. The _____ cell layer is located next to the blood flow in blood vessels, whereas the _____ is the exterior cell layer.

2. _____ muscle cells provide for the movement of fluids through blood vessels.

3. Smooth muscle cells are responsible for the _____ and _____ of the diameter of blood vessels.

4. _____ have the ability to produce an electrical current, causing the heart muscle to _____ .

5. Cardiomyocytes are classified as _____, _____, and _____ muscles.

HEART MUSCLE

The human body has three major types of muscle: cardiac muscle, skeletal muscle, and smooth muscle. Cardiac muscle tissue has the ability to contract as well as to conduct electrical impulses. As mentioned earlier, the heart is composed of cardiomyocytes, which have a specific purpose of propelling blood by way of contractions either through the body or into the lungs. These cardiac muscle cells have some of the attributes of both skeletal muscle, which is striated voluntary muscle, and smooth muscle, which is involuntary and unstraited. Cardiac muscle is identified as involuntary striated muscle and is only found in the heart. Cardiac muscle is also different from other muscles in the body because cardiac muscle fibers form a network of crisscross patterns (or branches) and are not linear as other body muscle types are. This crisscross pattern branches in all directions, with each branch connected to the next through intercalated disks. The intercalated disks allow the muscle to create synchronized contractions.

papillary muscle
A muscle that holds the tricuspid and mitral valves in place along the heart wall.

Papillary muscles hold the tricuspid and mitral valves in place along the ventricle walls. There are five papillary muscles in the heart. Three of the papillary muscles connect to the chordae tendineae of the tricuspid valve, and the other two papillary muscles connect to the chordae tendineae of the bicuspid valve. **Figure 1-11** shows the papillary muscles and

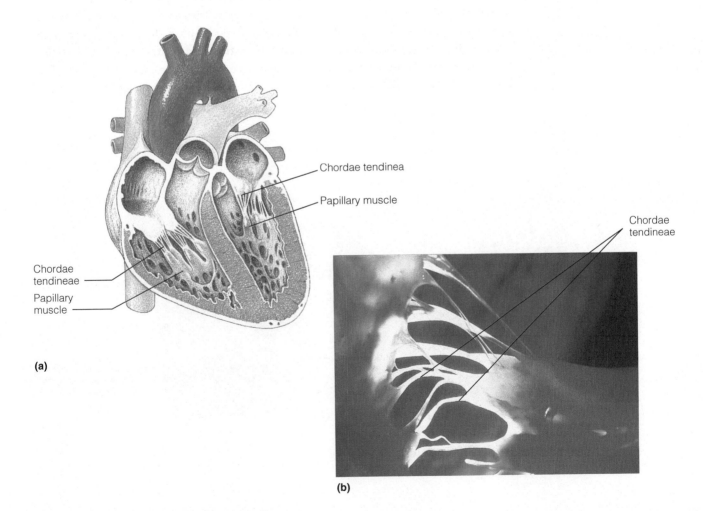

(a)

Chordae tendinea

Papillary muscle

Chordae tendineae

Papillary muscle

Chordae tendineae

(b)

Figure 1-11 Papillary muscles and chordae tendineae

chordae tendineae of the right and left atrioventricular valves. Think of the papillary muscles as the glue that holds the valves to the side walls of the ventricles so that the valves can act as a gate allowing blood to enter the ventricles or holding blood in the atrium; and to provide tension to the valve, which is needed to prevent regurgitation or prolapse of the valves from occurring when the ventricles contract.

The right and left ventricles are separated by a muscular wall called the intraventricular septum. The purpose of this septum is to keep the ventricles separated so the oxygenated blood in the left ventricle does not mix with the deoxygenated blood in the right ventricle during contractions.

HEART WALL

epicardium tissue
The smooth outer layer of the heart wall where the coronary arteries are located; also called visceral pericardium.

myocardium tissue
The thickest layer of muscle tissue in the heart wall.

endocardium tissue
The innermost layer of the heart wall, lines the chambers and the heart valves.

The heart wall is composed primarily of three layers of tissue. **Epicardium tissue** (also called visceral pericardium) is the smooth outer layer of the heart wall where the coronary arteries are located. The epicardium is composed of squamous epithelial tissue, and its purpose is protection of the heart. The middle layer of the heart wall is composed of **myocardium tissue**, which is composed of cardiac muscle and is the thickest layer of the heart wall. Myocardium tissue is thicker in the ventricles than in the atrium because the muscle is needed to push blood into the lungs or body with each contraction. The myocardium muscle tissue constantly contracts or relaxes to push the blood in a pumping motion; thus, myocardium tissue is responsible for the heart contractions. **Endocardium tissue** lines the chambers and the valves and is considered the innermost layer of the heart wall. **Figure 1-12** identifies and compares the different thicknesses of the tissues of

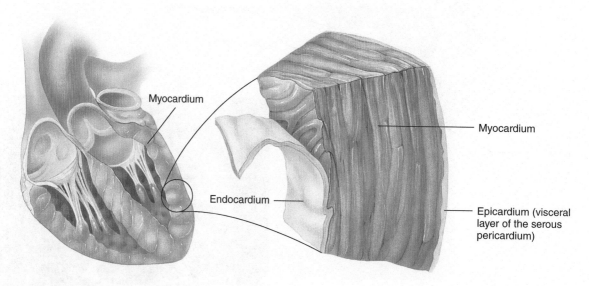

Figure 1-12 Tissue layers of the heart wall

the heart wall. Notice the thickness of the myocardium tissue compared to the thickness of the epicardium and endocardium tissues.

HEART CONDUCTION

When the heart is functioning correctly, the heart muscle is creating electrical stimulation for the movement that is necessary to maintain blood pressure and for oxygen to reach the cells of the body. The **sinoatrial (SA) node**, found in the upper wall of the right atria, is where electrical impulses are generated. Often the SA node is called the "heart's pacemaker." When the SA node is not working correctly, the heart has a backup pacemaker called the **atrioventricular (AV) node**. The AV node is also located in the right atrium, but it is located near the lower right side, on the interatrial septum. The electrical impulses continue to the **His-Purkinje system**, located in the ventricle walls. The His-Purkinje system consists of the bundle of His, the left and right bundle branches, and the Purkinje fibers. **Figure 1-13** identifies the names and location of the major electrical components of the heart. Chapter 3 will go into greater detail about how the heart's electrical system works.

atrioventricular (AV) node
The heart's secondary pacemaker, also part of the conduction system where electrical impulses are generated. Located in the lower right atrium.

His-Purkinje system
Consists of the bundle of His, the left and right bundle branches, and the Purkinje fibers, and is located surrounding the ventricles

sinoatrial (SA) node
The first site in the heart where electrical impulses are generated, often referred to as "the heart's pacemaker," located in the upper right atrium.

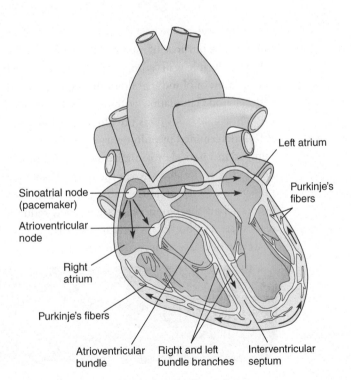

Figure 1-13 Heart electrical conduction system

Quick Check 1-4

Fill in the blanks.

1. The atrioventricular valves are held in place by _____ muscles.

2. Ventricular walls are separated by a muscular wall called the _____.

3. The heart wall is composed of three types of tissue. The innermost layer is composed of _____ tissue, the middle layer is composed of _____ tissue, and the outermost layer is composed of _____ tissue.

4. The thickest layer of heart wall tissue is the _____ layer.

5. Normal heart conduction begins in the _____, then travels to the _____, which is located near the lower right side of the _____, and finally travels into the _____ system.

pulmonary circulation
The process that takes place when deoxygenated blood leaves the heart to gather oxygen in the lungs and then returns to the heart as oxygenated blood.

cardiac output (CO)
A measure of pulmonary blood volume pumped by the left ventricle in 1 minute.

systemic circulation
The blood flow from the heart to the body *except* to the lungs; the process of oxygenated blood leaving the heart through the aorta and completing a loop throughout the body via the arteries and veins.

vasoconstriction
A process where blood vessels constrict, reducing in diameter, which causes blood pressure, vascular resistance, and body temperature to increase while blood flow and heart rate decrease.

vasodilatation
Blood vessels widen, increasing in diameter. Vasodilatation is the opposite of vasoconstriction, so blood pressure, vascular resistance, and body temperature decrease and blood flow and heart rate increase.

total peripheral resistance (TPR)
A change in blood pressure measured as blood completes the cycle from arterial blood leaving the heart to venous blood returning to the heart.

MAJOR BLOOD VESSELS AND BLOOD CIRCULATION

A blood vessel can be best described as a flexible, tubelike structure located throughout the body for the purpose of moving blood filled with oxygen and nutrients or waste. Blood vessels have flexible walls composed of smooth muscle that can adjust, to an extent, to the rate and amount of blood that flows through the vessels. The circulatory system consists of two distinct blood circulation systems in the body called the pulmonary and systemic circulation. **Pulmonary circulation** is the blood flow between the heart and the lungs. **Cardiac output (CO)** is determined by pulmonary circulation and is measured by the volume of blood that is pumped in a period of 1 minute by the right or left ventricle. **Systemic circulation** is blood flow to the entire body *except* the lungs. Vasoconstriction and vasodilatation control blood pressure, body temperature, and regulates and maintains arterial pressure. **Vasoconstriction** occurs when the blood vessels constrict, reducing in diameter. Blood pressure, vascular resistance, and body temperature increase when blood vessels constrict. Blood flow and heart rate decrease with vasoconstriction.

> Think of vasoconstriction as being like a garden hose with a nozzle attached, which restricts water flow.

Vasodilatation occurs when blood vessels widen, increasing in diameter. Vasodilatation is the opposite of vasoconstriction, so blood pressure, vascular resistance and body temperature are decreased and blood flow and heart rate are increased in vasodilatation. **Total peripheral resistance (TPR)** is determined by systemic circulation and is measured by the change in blood pressure as the blood completes the cycle from arterial blood leaving the heart to venous blood returning to the heart. Cardiac output and total peripheral resistance will be discussed in more detail in Chapter 3.

When Blood Vessels Change:

Effect on:	Vasodilation	Vasoconstriction
Blood pressure	↓	↑
Vascular resistance	↓	↑
Blood flow	↑	↓
Heart rate	↑	↓
Body temperature	↓	↑

Quick Check 1-5

Fill in the blanks.

1. _____ circulation is blood flow between the heart and the lungs, whereas _____ circulation is blood flow to the body (except the lungs).

2. The volume of blood that is pumped in one minute by either _____ determines cardiac _____.

3. _____ occurs when arterial pressure is forced to increase.

4. The change in blood pressure as the blood moves through the vessels of the body is known as _____.

5. Blood pressure decreases when the _____ and vascular resistance decreases.

artery
A blood vessel that is traveling away from the heart and is full of oxygen. The exception to oxygenated blood traveling away from the heart is found in the pulmonary artery, which carries deoxygenated blood to the lungs.

arterioles
The smallest arteries, control systemic blood flow and total peripheral resistance by contracting or relaxing.

vein
A blood vessel that carries deoxygenated blood back to the heart, except for the four pulmonary veins, which carry oxygenated blood from the lungs to the left atrium.

venules
The smallest veins.

Oxygenated and Deoxygenated Blood

The circulatory system consists of arteries, arterioles, capillaries, venules, and veins (as well as the lymphatic system, which is not discussed in detail in this book). There are two major types of blood vessels. The **artery** is a blood vessel that travels *away* from the heart and is full of oxygen (i.e., it carries oxygenated blood) and nutrients. **Arterioles** are the smallest arteries. They are very important in the cardiovascular system because they control systemic blood flow and determine total peripheral resistance. Arterioles constantly contract (vasoconstriction) or relax (vasodilatation) to adjust blood flow to the body's current metabolic condition.

A **vein** is the second type of blood vessel. Veins carry deoxygenated blood back to the heart to pick up oxygen so the cycle can repeat. **Venules** are the smallest veins. As noted earlier, the exception to arteries carrying oxygenated blood and veins carrying deoxygenated blood is the pulmonary artery.

Blood Flow in Arteries Versus Veins

Arteries = Away from the heart, is oxygenated; see EXCEPTION

Veins = Toward the heart, is deoxygenated

pulmonary artery
A blood vessel that carries deoxygenated blood to the lungs from the right ventricle.

The **pulmonary artery** carries deoxygenated blood and waste products such as carbon dioxide from the right ventricle to the lungs, where the lungs' capillary beds filter the blood and add oxygen before returning the blood to the left atrium via the pulmonary vein. It is in the capillaries of the lungs where the blood picks up oxygen.

Pulmonary Blood Flow EXCEPTION

Pulmonary Artery = Away from the heart *but* is deoxygenated

Pulmonary Vein = Toward the heart *but* is oxygenated

capillary
A very thin and fragile blood vessel, the smallest blood vessel in the body.

Capillaries are very thin, fragile blood vessels. They are located in the tissues of the body and play the important role of exchanging oxygen and nutrients or waste for the other vessels to transport. One could think of the capillaries as the blood's "turn-around" point from being oxygenated blood when it arrives to the capillary and being deoxygenated when leaving the capillary. **Figure 1-14** contrasts the terms and blood flow into and out of the capillaries. Recall that oxygenated, nutrient-enriched blood enters the capillaries through the arterioles and exits the capillaries deoxygenated, with waste products and gases through the venules.

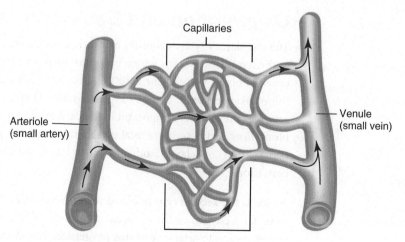

Capillaries

Arteriole
(small artery)

Venule
(small vein)

Figure 1-14 Capillary beds

Blood Flow: Arteries

Arteries have thicker walls than veins because the blood leaving the heart needs to be pushed with enough pressure to flow throughout the body. The artery carries blood that pulsates as it moves throughout the body. The largest blood vessel in the body is an artery called the **aorta**. The aorta is divided into two main sections, commonly called the ascending aorta and aortic arch. The ascending aorta originates at the base of the heart muscle beginning at the top of the left ventricle and is only approximately two inches long in an adult. The artery continues up and curves, creating the aortic arch before branching several times to supply oxygen and nutrients to the heart muscle itself and to the rest of the body. Two major **coronary arteries (CAs)** branch off the ascending aorta from a small opening in the aorta called the sinuses of Valsalva. There are left and right coronary arteries. The main branches of the left coronary artery include the left circumflex CA and the left anterior descending CA. When blood flows freely in these branches, the left atrium, left ventricle, and ventricular conduction system are nourished with oxygenated blood. The second major coronary artery, the right coronary artery, includes the right posterior descending CA. When blood flows freely, the right CA supplies rich, oxygenated blood to the right atrium, right ventricle, the inferior wall of the left ventricle and the posterior portion of the interventricular septum. In most people, the SA and AV nodes are also supplied by the right CA. A third major artery is called the pulmonary artery. Unlike the other two arteries, recall that the pulmonary artery does *not* carry oxygenated blood because the pulmonary artery carries deoxygenated blood *to* the lungs from the right ventricle.

aorta
The largest blood vessel in the body.

coronary arteries (CA)
Originating off the aorta, these arteries wrap around and are imbedded in the heart muscle to supply rich oxygenated blood to the atria and ventricles.

Blood Flow: Veins

Veins are not under the same pressure as arteries. Metabolic waste is returned to the heart via several major veins. Great veins in the body include the superior vena cava, inferior vena cava, and coronary sinus. The **superior vena cava** (also called the precava) drains deoxygenated blood from the upper body into the right atrium. The **inferior vena cava** (also called the postcava) drains deoxygenated blood from the body below the heart into the right atrium. Just as the heart muscle needs arteries to feed oxygen and nutrients to the organ itself, there must also be veins to carry away the waste. A major vein located within the heart is called the **great coronary vein**, and it begins along the anterior ventricles in the apex of the heart. As the veins of the heart come together to drain, they form a larger vessel called the **coronary sinus**, which is located between the inferior vena cava and the tricuspid valve in the posterior heart wall. Most of the veins of the heart muscle drain into the coronary sinus, which then empties the blood into the right atrium. Recall that the deoxygenated blood from the right atrium must flow into the pulmonary circulation and back into the heart through the left atrium before being pumped out of the heart systemically. In **Figure 1-15**, the major coronary arteries and veins responsible for pulmonary circulation are identified.

The study of the heart vessels cannot be complete without mentioning the coronary sulcus. Also known as the coronary groove, auriculoventricular groove, or atrioventricular (AV) groove, the **coronary sulcus** is a depression resembling a valley that surrounds the external surface of the heart muscle and separates the atria from the ventricles. The coronary arteries, coronary veins, and coronary sinus lie within this groove.

The systemic route of blood includes oxygenated blood leaving the aorta to the arteries, traveling toward the arterioles, emptying oxygen and nutrients into the capillary beds of the

superior vena cava
Also called precava, a vessel that drains deoxygenated blood from the upper body into the right atrium.

inferior vena cava
A vein that drains deoxygenated blood from the body below the heart into the right atrium.

great coronary vein
A blood vessel that carries waste from the heart muscle to the coronary sinus.

coronary sinus
The collection site for deoxygenated blood from the heart that will be drained into the right atrium.

coronary sulcus
A depression (resembling a valley) surrounding the external surface of the heart muscle, separates the atria from the ventricles.

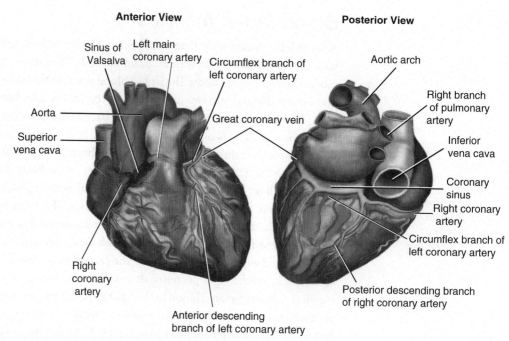

Anterior View

Sinus of Valsalva
Left main coronary artery
Circumflex branch of left coronary artery
Aorta
Great coronary vein
Superior vena cava
Right coronary artery
Anterior descending branch of left coronary artery

Posterior View

Aortic arch
Right branch of pulmonary artery
Inferior vena cava
Coronary sinus
Right coronary artery
Circumflex branch of left coronary artery
Posterior descending branch of right coronary artery

Figure 1-15 Major coronary arteries and veins

tissues, and returning waste and deoxygenated blood via venules that dump into the veins, which ends at the vena cava veins, returning deoxygenated blood to the heart so that the cycle can be repeated. The path of blood circulation is mapped in **Figure 1-16**.

Quick Check 1-6

Fill in the blanks.

1. Arterioles control _____ blood flow and determine _____ resistance.
2. Oxygenated blood flows _____ from the heart except for the pulmonary artery, which carries deoxygenated blood from the right ventricle to the _____.
3. The largest blood vessel in the body is called the _____.
4. The _____ is a vein that drains blood from the upper body into the _____ atrium.
5. The atrioventricular groove surrounds the _____ surface of the heart.

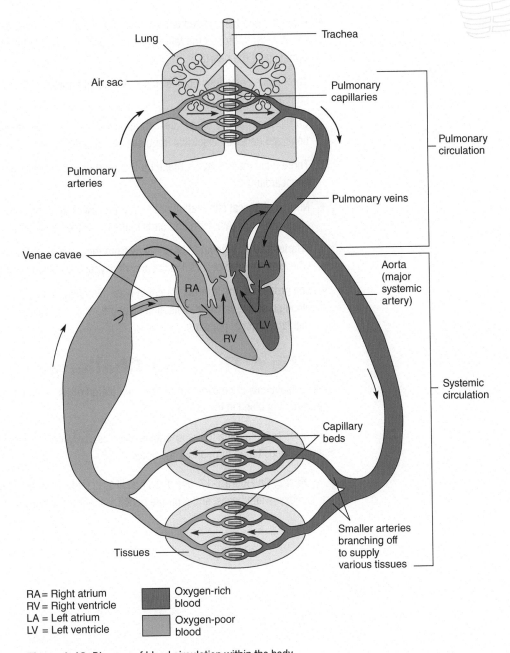

Figure 1-16 Diagram of blood circulation within the body

RA = Right atrium
RV = Right ventricle
LA = Left atrium
LV = Left ventricle

Oxygen-rich blood
Oxygen-poor blood

SUMMARY

- The heart is surrounded by a protective pericardial sac containing pericardial fluid.

- Adult human hearts weigh between 8 and 12 ounces and are approximately 3 inches wide by 5 inches long.

- ECG views of the heart are usually obtained from the anterior, septal, left lateral, and apical walls.

- There are four chambers in the heart, including a right and left atrium and a right and left ventricle.

- When the heart is operating correctly, four valves open and close in a sequential manner once each cardiac cycle. The valves include the tricuspid, bicuspid, pulmonary, and aortic valves.

- Often the heart is referred to as a "two-sided pump" because the blood is either rich in oxygen (saturated) on the left side of the heart or in need of oxygen (desaturated) on the right side of the heart.

- Three main categories of heart cells include endothelial cells, smooth muscle cells, and cardiomyocytes.

- Cardiomyocytes are unique cells in the body because they have the ability to develop contractions and generate electrical impulses and are only found in the heart.

- Three main muscle layers make up the heart wall: the epicardium, myocardium, and endocardium.

- Normal electrical stimulation of the heart follows a path from the sinoatrial (SA) node to the atrioventricular (AV) node and ends in the His-Purkinje system.

- Arteries carry oxygenated blood away from the heart, with the exception of the pulmonary artery, where the reverse occurs. Veins carry deoxygenated blood back to the heart.

- The process of the arteries widening (vasodilatation) or narrowing (vasoconstriction) changes blood pressure, vascular resistance, blood flow, heart rate, and body temperature, and also regulates arterial pressure.

Critical Thinking Challenges

1-1. Explain how the movement of the intercalated disks found in cardiac muscle relates to the movement of blood in the arteries.

1-2. Part 1: Explain the terms arterioles, venules, oxygenation, and deoxygenation in relation to the capillary beds found throughout the body.

> **Part 2:** On Figure 1-17, use a red pencil to identify oxygenated cells, a blue pencil to identify deoxygenated cells, and a purple pencil to identify the capillaries.

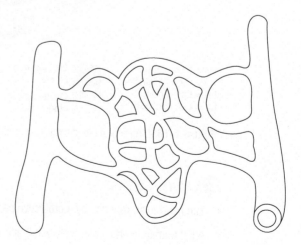

Figure 1-17

1-3. Part 1: On Figure 1-18, use arrows to identify and map the blood flow of the systemic circulation and pulmonary circulation.

Part 2: Using this same figure, color oxygenated blood with a red pencil and deoxygenated blood with a blue pencil.

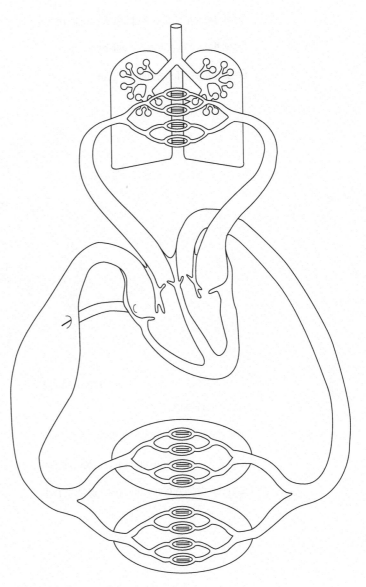

Figure 1-18

Review Activities

Directions: Color the figures as directed. Use colored pencils only.

1-1. Using Figure 1-19:

Color the right atrium and right ventricle blue.

Color the left atrium and left ventricle red.

Color the atrioventricular valves yellow.

Color the semilunar valves green.

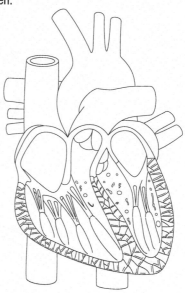

Figure 1-19

1-2. Using Figure 1-20:

Label the endocardium, and then color it pink.

Label the epicardium, and then color it brown.

Label the myocardium, and then color it red.

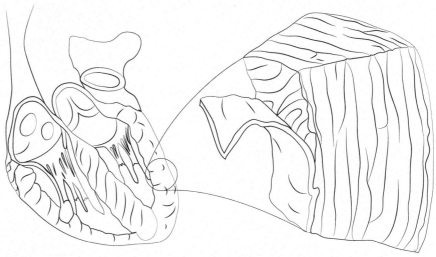

Figure 1-20

1-3. Using Figure 1-21:

Color the SA node orange.

Color the AV node red.

Color the His-Purkinje system yellow.

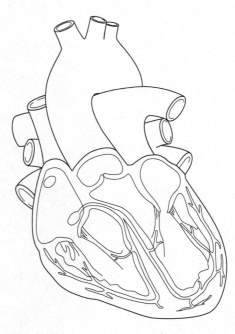

Figure 1-21

1-4. Fill in the table with the missing valve, position (open or closed), and control (where is the blood?)

Valve	Position	Control
Tricuspid		Releases blood from the right atrium into the right ventricle
	Closed	Holds blood in the right atrium
	Open	Releases blood from the left atrium into the left ventricle
Mitral	Closed	
Pulmonic		Releases blood from the right ventricle into the lungs
	Closed	Holds blood in the right ventricle
Aortic		
Aortic		Holds blood in the left ventricle

Chapter One Test

Part 1: Identify the parts of the heart by placing an answer on each line in Figure 1-22.

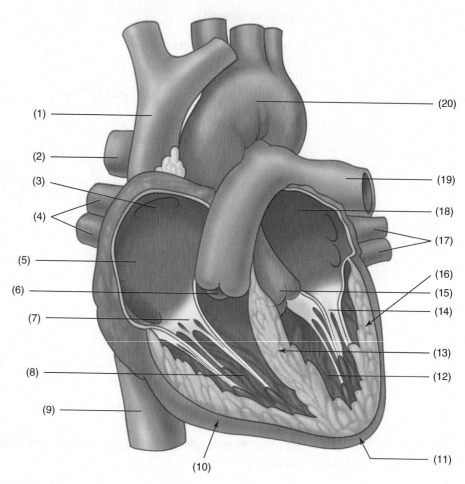

Figure 1-22

Part 2: Fill in the blanks.

1. The upper chambers of the heart are called _____.

2. The heart is located in the _____ cavity.

3. The heart has _____ valves.

4. _____ carry oxygenated blood.

5. Heart conduction begins with the _____ node.

6. Deoxygenated blood flows toward the heart in _____.

7. A protective fibrous membrane that covers the heart is called the _____.

8. _____ acts as a lubricant to prevent friction during ordinary contractions.

9. The _____ is located between the inferior vena cava and the tricuspid valve.

10. The thickest layer of tissue in the heart wall is called _____ tissue.

Chapter One Quick Check Answers

Answer order is important except where noted otherwise (shown in parentheses).

When two correct answers are possible, both answers are given, separated by the word *or*.

1-1:

1. lubricant
2. anterior, dorsal
3. left
4. anterior, septal, lateral, apical (any order)
5. thoracic, lungs

1-2:

1. atria or atrium, ventricles
2. atrioventricular, atria, ventricles
3. bicuspid or mitral
4. atrioventricular or AV, atria
5. pulmonic, lungs

1-3:

1. endothelial, epithelial
2. Smooth
3. constriction, dilation (either order)
4. Cardiomyocytes, contract
5. branched, striated, involuntary (any order)

1-4:

1. papillary
2. interventricular septum
3. endocardium, myocardium, epicardium
4. myocardium
5. SA node, AV node, right atrium, His-Purkinje

1-5:

1. Pulmonary, systemic
2. ventricle, output
3. Vasoconstriction
4. total peripheral resistance
5. body temperature, vascular resistance

1-6:

1. systemic, total peripheral
2. away, lungs
3. aorta
4. superior vena cava, right
5. external

2

BODY SYSTEMS AND HEART HEALTH

OBJECTIVES

After reading the chapter and completing all Quick Check activities, the student should be able to:

1. Identify the role that respiratory conditions may play in altering heart health.

2. Contrast the heart's response to stimuli between the sympathetic and parasympathetic nervous system.

3. Compare three types of cerebral vascular accidents.

4. List three functions of the integumentary system necessary for healthy heart maintenance.

5. Explain how homeostasis imbalance plays a role in body fluid retention.

6. Recognize the connection between heart health, the kidneys, and blood pressure.

7. Discuss how electrolytes produce electricity to make the heart beat.

8. Identify the endocrine glands that directly affect heart health.

9. Explain metabolic syndrome.

KEY TERMS

alveoli

autonomic nervous system (ANS)

bronchi

central nervous system (CNS)

cerebral vascular accident (CVA)

chronic obstructive pulmonary disease (COPD)

diaphoresis

diaphragm

dysautonomia

dyspnea

electrolytes

homeostasis

hyperkalemia

hypertension

infarct

metabolic syndrome

metabolism

nephrons

neurons

neurotransmitters

obstructive sleep apnea

parasympathetic nervous system (PSNS)

peripheral nervous system (PNS)

pH (potential of hydrogen)
renin

sympathetic nervous system (SNS)
thermoregulation

trachea
vagus nerve

INTRODUCTION

Think of the heart as the powerhouse of the body. If the heart is working inefficiently, there is usually a domino effect of increased disease processes to many major organs in the body. If the disease process is caught in the early stages, the damage caused by cardiovascular events might be corrected with lifestyle changes such as eating a healthier diet, adding daily exercise, or reducing stress; or with surgery along with the afore-mentioned lifestyle changes. More often, though, once heart damage has occurred, an individual will need to learn to live with continued physical and dietary limitations to maintain a previous good quality of life. This chapter will identify several important organs within five major body systems that directly affect heart health. Good health cannot be achieved or maintained within the body unless vital organs communicate and respond to the needs of the body's internal environment. Body organs react to deterioration, disease, or injury in different ways, but, as noted in Chapter 1, oxygen and nutrients from the cycle of the heart are vital to sustain life.

BODY SYSTEMS AND THE HEART

The heart affects every cell in the body, but some body systems play a more direct role in unison with the heart to control everyday heart function and body functions. The following body systems all play an important role to maintaining a well-functioning heart: respiratory system, nervous system, integumentary system, urinary system, and endocrine system. In the following sections, the function of each body system in relationship to the heart will be discussed. Discussion of each named body system is not inclusive, as the 5 body systems could each be a book in itself. Only the major organs of each system will be identified if they can add perspective to the study of the heart as an organ. When studying heart disease, understanding the interrelationship between the heart and underlying cause and effect of the various body systems through injury, disease, or deterioration will greatly enhance your ability to help educate patients so that they understand the scope of their condition.

RESPIRATORY SYSTEM

trachea
A tube that brings air to and from the lungs.

bronchi
A subdivision of the trachea that bring air into the lungs.

alveoli
Tiny air sacs located in the lungs at the end of the bronchi, where oxygen and carbon dioxide is exchanged.

Major organs in the respiratory system that can affect the heart's condition include the lungs, trachea, and bronchi. Filtered air is brought into the body through the **trachea** by inhaling. The trachea divides into two tubes called **bronchi**. There is left and right bronchi that take the filtered air into the right and left lung. Within the lungs, tiny sacs called **alveoli** act as the component responsible for the gas exchange of oxygen and carbon dioxide. Carbon dioxide is considered a waste product in the body, so the body expels it through exhaling.

Respiratory Organs and Functions

The primary function of the respiratory system is to deliver oxygen to the body while removing carbon dioxide from the cells. The heart places great importance in the oxygen/carbon dioxide gas exchange because with each cycle of the heartbeat, the carbon dioxide or oxygen is also exchanged within the capillaries to deliver oxygenated blood from the heart or to bring carbon dioxide back toward the lungs to be released. Every cell in the body needs the oxygen exchange in order to survive and maintain homeostasis within the body. The process of inhaling and exhaling by breathing is called external respiration, while the process of gas exchange within the systemic capillaries is called internal expiration. **Figure 2-1** shows the main organs and function of the respiratory system.

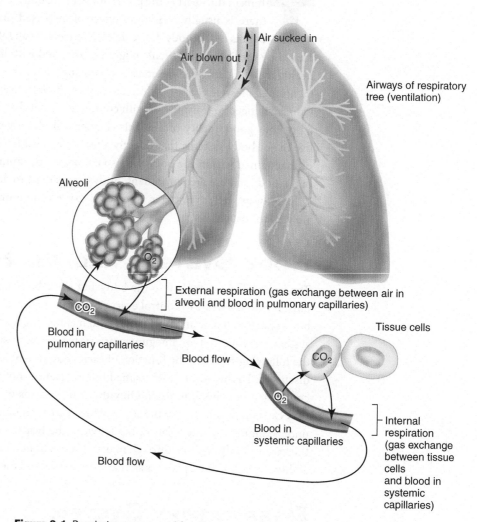

Figure 2-1 Respiratory organs and functions

diaphragm
The muscle that separates the thoracic cavity from the abdomen; its main purpose is to control breathing.

Carbon dioxide from the lungs is released from the body as the diaphragm expands. The **diaphragm** is composed of muscle and connective tissue and is located below the lungs separating the thoracic cavity from the abdominal cavity. **Figure 2-2** shows the diaphragm and the lungs. The diaphragm's main purpose is to control breathing. A diaphragm might be thought of as a balloon because breathing causes the air to expand and contract the diaphragm with each breath, therefore allowing the lungs to fill with fresh air and eliminate carbon dioxide.

Normal breathing can be defined as approximately 20 respirations per minute in an adult, but normal breathing is much faster in infants. Besides age, physical condition and heart health can also play an important role in the number of respirations per minute. Monitoring and recording a patients' respirations is one of the primary vital signs used to assess

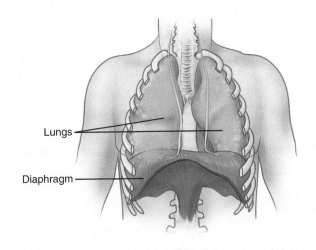

Figure 2-2 The diaphragm and the lungs

overall patient condition at a point in time. One complete cycle of respirations is usually recorded by observing a patient breathing (diaphragm rising and falling) over a period of 1 minute.

Respiratory Conditions and Heart Health

There are a vast number of respiratory conditions; however, this section will only identify three common ailments that originate within the respiratory system, which can eventually play a role in a person's deteriorating heart health. As with many disease processes, if the condition is not already a chronic condition and is identified and addressed early, the outcome to maintain overall health is easier to control. Many conditions are often only one sign or symptom on a list of symptoms that collectively may lead to a diagnosis or condition such as heart disease.

dyspnea
Shortness of breath.

It should be noted that many conditions, such as **dyspnea** (shortness of breath), does not, by itself, significantly lead to heart disease. There are many causes for dyspnea to occur, but if a person had been previously diagnosed with heart failure and presents with a chief complaint of dyspnea, the situation can become critical to heart health. With an underlying diagnosis of heart disease, dyspnea could indicate that blood is not able to enter the lungs and is backing up in the pulmonary veins, causing fluid retention in the lungs, which, if left untreated, could become congestive heart failure.

obstructive sleep apnea
A sleep disorder where the airway becomes blocked or collapses, preventing oxygen from reaching the lungs.

Obstructive sleep apnea is the most common type of chronic sleep disorder. It is a condition caused by the airway collapsing or becoming blocked during sleep, thereby preventing normal inhaling, so the lungs don't receive enough oxygen. This condition causes fragmented sleep and low oxygen levels. Many people are unaware that they have sleep apnea, so the condition is often underdiagnosed or not diagnosed until it becomes severe. Left untreated, sleep apnea can increase the risk of irregular heartbeats or, in cardiac compromised people, can increase or worsen the risk of heart failure due to oxygen starvation.

chronic obstructive pulmonary disease (COPD)
A progressive lung disease which, over time, prevents normal breathing due to damage of the alveoli or thickening of the bronchi.

Excluding accidents, one of the major causes of death in the United States is from **chronic obstructive pulmonary disease (COPD)**. COPD is a progressive lung disease that worsens over time, preventing a person from being able to breathe because of damage to the alveoli (emphysema) or thickening of the bronchi (chronic bronchitis). There are several causes of COPD, but smoking or inhaling secondhand smoke are the primary causes. Although there is no cure for COPD, oxygen therapy, bronchodilator medication, or a combination of both may slow the disease progression and prevent complications to organs such as the heart by opening the air passages and by allowing oxygen to be replenished in the capillary beds.

Quick Check 2-1

Fill in the blanks.

1. Two locations in the body where the oxygen/carbon dioxide gas exchange takes place are in the _____ and the _____.

2. The _____ controls breathing. Breathing causes a gas exchange to occur _____ from the body. Within the body at the systemic capillary level, _____ gas exchange occurs.

3. Normal breathing occurs approximately _____ times per minute in a healthy adult.

4. Left untreated, obstructive sleep apnea, a condition where the _____ do not receive enough oxygen during sleep due to the airway _____, can increase the risk of irregular heartbeats.

5. Chronic obstructive pulmonary disease (COPD) is a chronic, incurable disease thought to be primarily caused by _____.

NERVOUS SYSTEM

central nervous system (CNS)
Master controller, made up of the brain and the spinal cord.

peripheral nervous system (PNS)
Consists of 12 pairs of cranial nerves and 31 pairs of spinal nerves that utilizes three specialized types of nerve cells (autonomic, sensory, and somatic) to communicate from the CNS to the body.

Two main categories of the nervous system include the **central nervous system (CNS)**, which contains the brain and the spinal cord and is considered the master controller; and the **peripheral nervous system (PNS)**, which consists primarily of 12 pairs of cranial nerves and 31 pairs of spinal nerves.

Central Nervous System

The brain is the most complex organ in the body and is the center of the nervous system. The function of the brain is to exert centralized control over the body's other organs by generating muscle activity and by directing the secretion of hormones. The brain contains two types of cells: glial cells and neurons. Glial cells have several functions, including metabolic support and insulation. Glial cells play a major role in metabolism by controlling the chemical composition of fluid around a neuron and by maintaining the level of ions and nutrients. Neurons communicate signals to other cells through axons in a process called *action potential*. Axons send electrochemical pulses to other neurons by releasing a chemical neurotransmitter at specialized junctions called *synapses* when the action potential becomes activated. There are two main neurotransmitters, glutamate and gamma-aminobutyric (GABA), which attach to target cells and can affect the heart. Glutamate usually exerts excitability on target neurons, and GABA usually exerts inhibitory cell response. The main source of brain energy comes from glucose while the predominant energy consumption is to sustain the action potential of neurons.

Brain Hormone (BNP)

An important hormone found in the blood is called brain natriuretic peptide (BNP). It is secreted from the ventricles of the heart when the heart is under increased pressure and stress. Increased pressure in the heart can cause excessive stretching of cardiomyocytes, and the release of BNP decreases systemic vascular resistance and central venous pressure. These changes cause a decrease in blood volume, which will lower systemic blood pressure and increase cardiac output.

The clinical significance of the BNP hormone is that normal levels measured in a screening blood test can rule out acute heart failure, or the blood test may be used to diagnose or assess the severity of heart failure. However, an elevated level does not rule out other factors, such as renal disease.

Cerebral Vascular Accidents

A **cerebral vascular accident (CVA)**, in layman's terms, is called a stroke. A CVA can occur when the blood flow to the brain is blocked or greatly reduced (either by blood clots or plaque buildup), or by blood vessel hemorrhaging. Brain cells begin to die within a few minutes if they have been deprived of oxygen or nutrients. There are three major types of strokes—embolic, thrombotic, and hemorrhagic.

Embolic strokes are caused by a blood clot that forms somewhere in the body (many occur in the heart) and travels to the brain, where the clot then blocks blood flow. Fatty deposits (called plaque) and cholesterol can cause the arteries that lead to the brain to become blocked, causing a thrombotic stroke. A hemorrhagic stroke is caused by a breakage in a weak or thin spot on a blood vessel wall in the brain. The hemorrhagic stroke causes the tissue around the break to die due to the lack of blood. The localized dead tissue area is called an **infarct**.

Figure 2-3 shows a hemorrhagic CVA. Notice that the return of venous blood to the heart has been cut off from the point of the breakage. Uncontrolled high blood pressure is the usual reason for a hemorrhagic stroke to occur if the CVA is intracerebral, or by blood-contaminated fluid if the CVA is in the membrane surrounding the brain (subarachnoid hemorrhage). Although there have been many conditions related to increased risk factors of a stroke

BNP Heart Hormone

The BNP hormone is secreted in the blood by the ventricles when the heart is under increased pressure or stress.

cerebral vascular accident (CVA)
Blood flow to the brain is blocked or greatly reduced, either by blood clots or plaque buildup, or by blood vessel hemorrhage.

Causes of a Stroke

A stroke is caused by reduced or blocked blood flow to the brain.

infarct
Localized dead tissue area where a hemorrhagic event occurred.

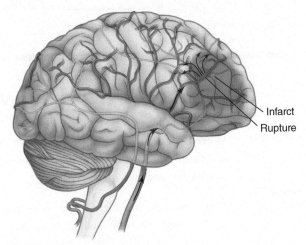

Infarct
Rupture

Figure 2-3 Hemorrhagic stroke

occurring, Box 2-1 identifies 10 common risk factors. The first 3 self-induced risk factors may be decreased with lifestyle changes, either with medical intervention or on their own.

Box 2-1 Ten Common Stroke Risk Factors

- Cigarette smoking
- Obesity
- Physical inactivity
- Hypertension
- Diabetes mellitus
- Hyperlipidemia
- Atherosclerosis
- Atrial fibrillation and flutter
- History of cerebral aneurysm
- Previous stroke or TIA (transient ischemic attack)

Quick Check 2-2

Fill in the blanks.

1. Two functions of the brain include generating _____ activity and directing the _____ of hormones.

2. Four functions of glial cells include controlling chemical composition of fluid around a neuron, maintaining the level of ions and nutrients, _____, and _____ support.

3. The process by which neurons communicate signals to other cells is called _____.

4. One particular hormone found in the brain that can be tested through blood work to diagnose or assess severity of heart failure is _____, or BNP.

5. Brain cells die within minutes when deprived of _____ or _____.

Autonomic Nervous System (ANS)

vagus nerve
The primary nerve between the brain and the heart.

autonomic nervous system (ANS)
The ANS's chief function is to act as a control system in the body through brain activity and nerve endings. Also called involuntary nervous system or visceral nervous system.

The remainder of this section will focus on the PNS, which is the communication link between the CNS and the body. The **vagus nerve** is the primary connector between the brain and the heart. The PNS consists of three types of nerve cells: autonomic nerve cells, sensory nerve cells, and somatic nerve cells.

More precisely, our focus will concentrate on a branch of the PNS called the **autonomic nervous system (ANS)**, which is also known as the involuntary nervous system or visceral nervous system. The ANS's chief function is to act as a control system in the body through brain activity and nerve endings. As shown in **Figure 2-4**, there are two major sections

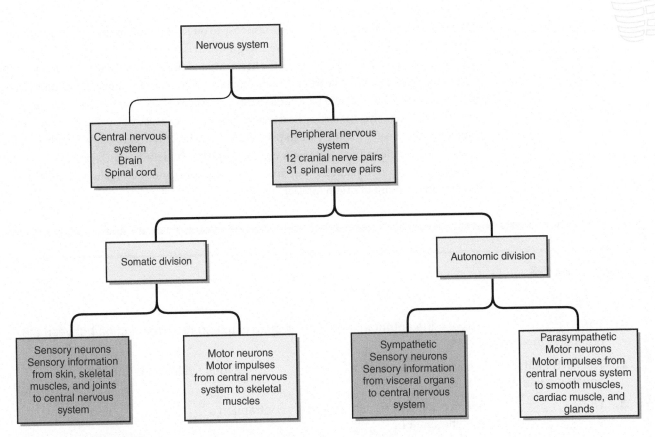

Figure 2-4 Branches of the nervous system

sympathetic nervous system (SNS)

A system that regulates the rate and force of a contraction through stimulation; often referred to as the heart's "fight-or-flight" response because the heart can respond by increasing the strength and rate of contractions very quickly in response to stress and other stimuli.

parasympathetic nervous system (PSNS)

The function of the PSNS is to conserve energy, which is done through sleep, resting, or lack of potential threats; often referred to as the heart's "rest-and-digest" response to outside stimuli or the lack of any stimuli.

of the ANS, the **sympathetic nervous system (SNS)** and the **parasympathetic nervous system (PSNS)**. The SNS and PSNS actually have opposite effects on the function they regulate. The SNS stimulates the heart to change its functioning and influences both the atria and ventricles, while the PSNS inhibits heart function changes and thus has no effect on the ventricles or the His-Purkinji system. The most important factor affected by the ANS is blood pressure (discussed in greater detail in Chapter 5).

Sympathetic Nervous System Function

The SNS nerve that serves the heart originates in the thoracic lumbar spinal cord region. In the heart, the function of the SNS is to regulate the rate and force of a contraction through stimulation. The SNS is often referred to as the heart's "fight-or-flight" response because the heart can respond by increasing the strength and rate of contractions very quickly in response to stress and other stimuli. The SNS prepares the body for anticipated intense physical activity and causes the heart rate to increase, increases blood pressure, increases the contractile forces of cardiac muscle which then causes vasoconstriction and increases oxygen to the brain. Brain response time to perceived threats is very fast so SNS stimuli usually receive immediate action.

Parasympathetic Nervous System Function

The PNS originates in the 10th cranial nerve (called the vagus nerve) for the heart and has both a sensory and motor function. The PSNS regulates the calmer functions of the heart, often referred to as the "rest-and-digest" response to outside stimuli or the lack of any stimuli. The function of the PSNS is to conserve energy, which is done through sleep, resting, or lack of potential threats. During this phase, the heart rate and the atrioventricular conduction rate both slow. With decreased heart rate, body functions will return to a normalized state if they had previously been activated by stimuli to the SNS. Vagus nerve function has been linked to mortality in the analysis of resting heart rate performance because the higher the vagus nerve activity is, the greater the increase in parasympathetic heart rate variability. Simply put, the heart must be able to relax to remain healthy. **Figure 2-5** identifies the sympathetic "fight-or-flight" and parasympathetic "rest-and-digest" divisions and the organs that are affected, along with the point of origin for each division.

Quick Check 2-3

Fill in the blanks.

1. The _____ nerve in the autonomic nervous system is the primary connection between the brain and the heart.

2. The ANS splits into two major sections, the _____ nervous system and the _____ nervous system.

3. The _____ nervous system regulates a heart contraction's _____ and _____ through stimulation.

4. Increases in blood pressure and heart rate can be attributed to the SNS in anticipation of intense _____ caused by increased _____ forces caused when the cardiac muscle contracts.

5. Sleep and resting help to conserve energy in the _____ nervous system.

Cardiac Performance and the Nervous System

neurons
Basic nerve cells that carry signals along electrochemical waves for communication.

The primary function of the nervous system is to coordinate and transmit signals throughout the body through nerve cells. This occurs at the cellular level through **neurons**, which are nerve cells that carry the signals along electrochemical waves. In order for the signal to travel between the neuron and the target receptor or between two neurons, neurotransmitters are needed.

neurotransmitters
Chemicals that transmit signals to the adrenal glands.

Neurotransmitters are actually chemicals that transmit signals to the adrenal glands, which then release chemicals into the bloodstream. The SNS nerve endings are called adrenergic, with the major chemical neurotransmitter being norepinephrine, also called epinephrine or adrenalin. Norepinephrine is an important neurotransmitter to remember when learning about the heart because it releases and stores glucose in response to stress. Stress can increase blood pressure and heart rate. The PSNS nerve endings are called cholinergic, with the major chemical neurotransmitter called acetylcholine, and to a lesser extent, peptides may act as neurotransmitters as well.

Acetylcholine is an important neurotransmitter to remember when learning about the heart because acetylcholine influences heart muscle action. Cardiac performance is directly

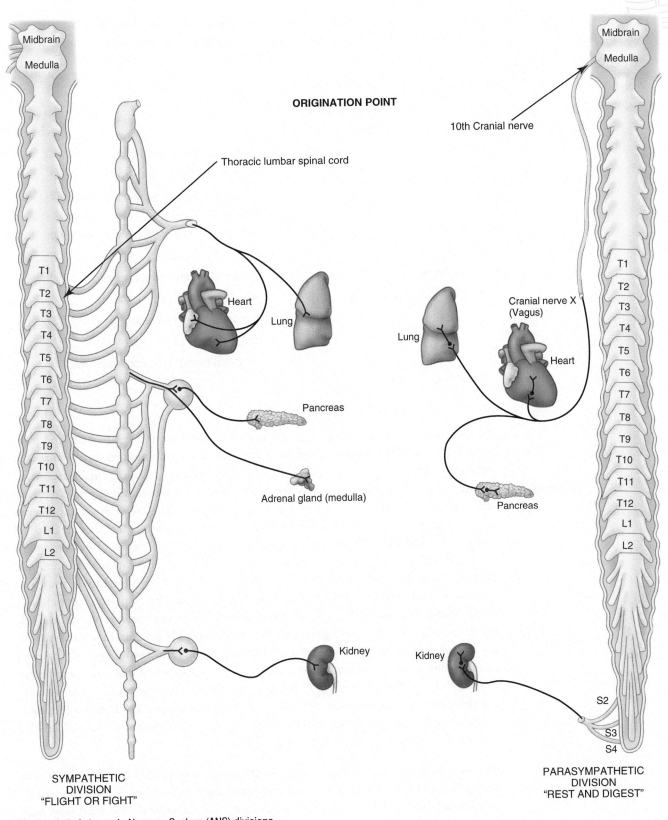

Figure 2-5 Autonomic Nervous System (ANS) divisions

related to the activity of neurotransmitters in the heart, telling the heart how fast or slow to beat. **Table 2-1** compares the sympathetic and parasympathetic neurotransmitter functions.

Table 2-1 Neurotransmitter Functions

System	Major Chemical Neurotransmitters	Functions
Sympathetic nervous system	Norepinephrine, adrenalin, epinephrine	Nerve endings are called *adrenergic*
		Releases and stores glucose
		Increases blood pressure and heart rate in response to stress
		Regulates the rate and force of a heart contraction
		Fight-or-flight response to stimulus
Parasympathetic nervous system	Acetylcholine	Nerve endings are called *cholinergic*
		Influences heart muscle action
		Function is to conserve energy
		Modifies heart rate
		"Rest-and-digest" response to stimulus

Autonomic Dysfunction

dysautonomia
Conditions, malfunctions, or diseases of the Autonomic Nervous System.

Most of the time, an autonomic disorder will consist of both the sympathetic and parasympathetic nervous systems. In addition, more than one symptom will usually appear at the same time, causing multiple problems. The term given to conditions, malfunctions, or diseases of the autonomic nervous system is **dysautonomia**. Dysautonomia does not only affect the heart; rather, it is a systemic condition. People affected with dysautonomia can have very mild symptoms, while others may have symptoms so severe that they are disabled and possibly bedridden. There are many causes, signs, and symptoms of dysautonomia, but the one that is important to remember is postural orthostatic tachycardia syndrome (POTS). With the condition of POTS, the primary symptom is an increase in heart rate of more than 30 bpm, or a heart rate of more than 120 bpm when a person moves from a supine position to an upright position. Autonomic disorders can also be an undesired side effect of medications that were given for other conditions. Medications may interfere with the normal transmission of the chemicals from the autonomic nervous system. The most common disease associated with autonomic nerve damage or autonomic failure is diabetes. Diabetes is one of the fastest-growing diseases in the world. In the past, it affected mostly the elderly, but nowadays it shows much less of an age preference, especially in the United States. A small percentage (10 percent or less) of people diagnosed with diabetes will develop peripheral nerve disease, commonly called neuropathy.

As a starting point toward diagnosis, the electrocardiogram (ECG), blood pressure readings, pulse oximeter readings, and timed deep breathing tests are administered to determine autonomic function. Practitioners look for changes in blood pressure and short-term heart rate fluctuations to measure how well the involuntary nervous system is working. One of the more common clinical physiological tests used to diagnose autonomic dysfunction is called the Valsalva maneuver. This test is performed via resistance breathing to manipulate the blood vessels in the heart. During testing, blood pressure is altered, but it should rebound to normal within a few heartbeats after resting. In people with autonomic dysfunction, the blood vessels do not constrict reflexively when norepinephrine is released under the pressured breathing; therefore, blood pressure falls and will not rapidly rebound when the heart is at rest. Instead, the blood pressure slowly increases, returning to the baseline.

Quick Check 2-4

Fill in the blanks.

1. _____ are nerve cells that use neurotransmitters to move chemical signals to the _____ glands.

2. Norepinephrine is a major neurotransmitter, more commonly called _____ or _____.

3. Cardiac performance is directly related to neurotransmitters because the neurotransmitters control how _____ or _____ the heart beats.

4. The most common disease associated with autonomic nerve damage or autonomic failure is _____.

5. The Valsalva maneuver uses _____ breathing to manipulate _____ to measure how well the autonomic nervous system is working.

INTEGUMENTARY SYSTEM

Many students do not relate the functions of the integumentary system with heart function; however, the integumentary system is the largest organ system in the body and it has several primary functions necessary for healthy heart maintenance. These functions include removal of waste, retaining body fluids, and thermoregulation. The major sections of the integumentary system include the skin, hair, glands, and sensory nerve endings. **Figure 2-6** shows a cross section of skin with the major features identified.

Waste Removal

diaphoresis
Excessive sweating.

Dead cells, salts, and water are removed through the skin through perspiration (also called sweating). Normal sweating originates in the SNS when the nerve cells activate sweat glands. Most humans experience normal perspiration that will increase with physical activity, but excessive perspiration is usually not normal; this is called **diaphoresis**. Diaphoresis can be one of the symptoms of an acute myocardial infarction (heart attack), but it also can be a symptom of many additional abnormal conditions, including various drug reactions, anxiety, and some bacterial infections. Substances used every day, such as caffeine found in energy drinks, coffee, teas, and soda, can also cause diaphoresis; therefore, diaphoresis is usually only considered a nonspecific symptom of some other medical condition.

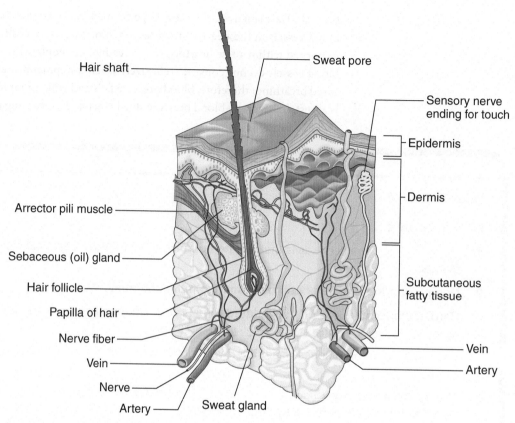

Hair shaft

Sweat pore

Sensory nerve ending for touch

Epidermis

Dermis

Arrector pili muscle

Sebaceous (oil) gland

Hair follicle

Papilla of hair

Nerve fiber

Vein

Nerve

Artery

Sweat gland

Subcutaneous fatty tissue

Vein

Artery

Figure 2-6 Cross section of skin

Fluid Retention

The human body is composed of approximately 60 percent water. Water is a necessary nutrient to every cell in the body and helps the body maintain a healthy metabolism. **Metabolism** is the process of using water, oxygen, ions, and other components of blood to grow, heal, and create energy. Water is also the major component of blood volume. The body loses water through sweat, respiration, or expelled waste (i.e., urine). Retaining proper body fluids is important for homeostasis. **Homeostasis** is the process of stabilizing the body's internal environment so that all of the body's organs work optimally. The most important properties the body keeps stable include temperature, glucose, and body **pH** (which stands for "potential of hydrogen" and means the amount of acidity or alkalinity in the body). Homeostatic imbalance is the root cause of many illnesses such as heart disease, diabetes, chronic hypoglycemia and hyperglycemia, chronic dehydration, and other conditions caused by blood toxins.

Thermoregulation

Thermoregulation means regulation of the body's core temperature. A healthy person has the ability to self-regulate internal body temperature, but a person with cardiovascular disease may have difficulty with blood pressure or heart rate if the body core temperature fluctuates for any period of time. The body's temperature is regulated in the hypothalamus region of the brain. **Figure 2-7** shows the location of the hypothalamus. Some additional hypothalamus regulation activities include controlling the autonomic nervous system functions, including heart rate, blood pressure, and the rate of respiration.

Quick Check 2-5

Fill in the blanks.

1. Three main functions of the integumentary system include _____, retaining body fluids, and _____.

2. Excessive sweating, medically called _____, can be one of the symptoms of an acute myocardial infarction. This condition can also be a symptom of excessive caffeine.

3. _____ is obtained when all the body's organs are operating optimally.

4. Important body properties to maintain in optimum condition include body _____, blood _____, and _____.

5. Metabolism is easiest to maintain when the body receives sufficient _____, _____, ions, and nutrients in blood.

Thermoregulation is a part of homeostasis. The body has many methods of reacting to varying external conditions that could change the core temperature. For example, when the internal temperature rises, the body will try to react by sweating or by arterial vasodilatation. When the internal temperature has fallen, tiny arrector pili muscles will raise hair on the body's surface to trap warmth and allow capillaries to open, causing flushing and warmth. Blood vessels will begin to constrict so that warmer blood is closer to the vital organs. The body can gain heat through conduction or radiation. An example of gaining heat through conduction would be the use of an electric blanket or heating pad near the skin. An example

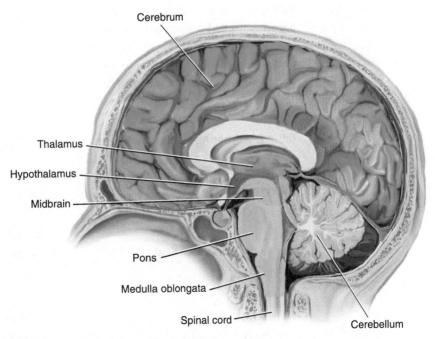

Figure 2-7 Hypothalamus region in the brain

of heat gain through radiation would be getting warm by sitting in the sun (sunbathing). Three main body organs (the liver, heart, and brain) generate most of the body's heat. Heat can also be generated in the body through exercising when muscles contract. Thermoregulation within the body is considered neutral, and the skin receives about 5 to 10 percent of resting cardiac output when the body is at normal body temperature (98° F or 37°C). However, when the whole body is overheated, the skin blood flow can reach 50 to 70 percent of cardiac output, which becomes critical if blood pressure is not able to adjust by increasing enough to maintain cardiac output.

Hyperthermia

A condition called heat stress is caused by hyperthermic conditions. When the whole body becomes overheated, cardiac output must increase to offset a decrease in vascular resistance that is caused when the arterioles dilate. People who already suffer from cardiovascular disease are more prone to experience adverse cardiac events when the body temperature rises above normal because their hearts have less thermal tolerance due to limited cardiac output reserve (vasodilatation) ability. Besides atmospheric temperatures being high, other causes of hyperthermia can include illness, infection, fever, exercise, digestion issues, and dehydration. Too high a temperature in the body can stress the body enough to cause brain damage, severe dehydration, heat stroke, or death.

Body heat can be reduced in four ways: conduction, convection, evaporation, and radiation. Conduction heat loss is loss through physical contact from one body to another or to an object. An example would be using an ice pack on the skin. In convection heat loss, air or water molecules move across the skin, cooling it. An example of convection loss would be taking a tepid shower after getting a mild sunburn or sitting in front of a fan blowing cool air. Evaporation heat loss is body heat lost through sweating, which causes the body to lose both water and electrolytes. Humidity limits sweating, therefore limiting body heat loss. Evaporation is the only physiological way the body can lose heat. The final way that the body loses heat is through radiation, which is heat transfer without physical contact. An example of radiated heat loss would be when many people come inside a cool room from being out in the hot sun, causing the room temperature to increase, yet the people themselves feel cooler because they have transferred their heat to the room's atmosphere. **Table 2-2** shows two ways that the body gains heat and four ways that body heat can be reduced.

Table 2-2 Thermoregulation

Ways the Body Gains Heat	Example
Conduction	Using a heating pad or blanket to warm the skin
Radiation	Being in direct sunlight
Ways the Body Loses Heat	**Example**
Conduction	Using an ice pack on the skin
Convection	Taking a cold shower
Evaporation	Sweating
Radiation	Running a fever

Hypothermia

Hypothermia occurs when the body's core temperature is reduced below normal. A total body heat loss of just 3° (95°F or 35°C) can cause cardiac arrest, stroke, or death. Typical causes of hypothermia include cold atmospheric temperature exposure, drugs, alcohol, or metabolic conditions such as diabetes. Whole-body cooling causes the blood vessels near the skin to constrict, drawing the blood deeper into the body to protect the internal organs. The body will try to compensate for the cold and produce heat. One internal example is the thyroid gland, which becomes activated if the core temperature decreases in an effort to increase metabolism, which in turn will increase body energy. Another example of the body trying to create heat is the process of thermogenesis and shivering.

Quick Check 2-6

Fill in the blanks.

1. People with cardiovascular diseases may have difficulty with _____ or _____ when their body temperature fluctuates.

2. Body temperature is regulated in the _____ region of the brain.

3. Arterial vasodilation may occur when the internal body temperature is _____, whereas tiny _____ muscles trap warmth and allow capillaries to open.

4. The only physiological way that the body can lose heat is through _____.

5. The thyroid gland tries to maintain internal body heat by increasing _____.

URINARY SYSTEM

The main organs in the urinary system that affects the heart are the kidneys. Humans are born with two kidneys, located on either side of the spinal cord in the superior lumbar region. **Figure 2-8** identifies where the kidneys, as well as the surrounding structures, are located.

The kidneys have four major functions: to eliminate waste, excess electrolytes, and toxins from the body; to control sodium (Na) and maintain water balance (pH); to regulate blood volume and blood chemistry; and to secrete renin.

Electrolytes

electrolytes
Compounds that are soluble in water and form free ions, which then conduct electricity.

Understanding the movement of ions into and out of the heart is an important step in understanding heart health because this movement produces the "electricity" that the heart needs to create blood flow through heartbeats. The ions, often referred to as electrolytes, must change their electrical charge to create movement. **Electrolytes** are defined as compounds that are soluble in water and form free ions, which then conduct electricity. The movement of electrolytes during the cardiac cycle causes the heart to beat. The primary electrolyte movement associated with the heart includes the elements of sodium (Na^+), potassium (K^+), and calcium (Ca^{2+}). Electrolytes are regulated by hormones and by filtration through the kidneys, where the excess waste can be flushed from the body. A serious

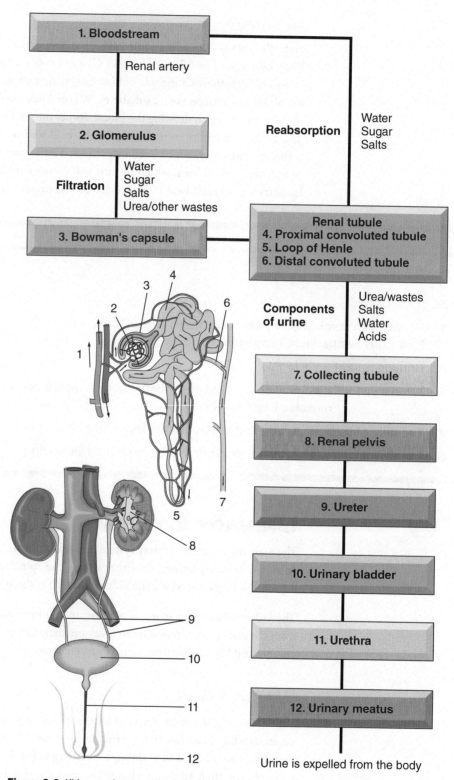

1. Bloodstream

Renal artery

2. Glomerulus

Reabsorption   Water
Sugar
Salts

Filtration   Water
Sugar
Salts
Urea/other wastes

3. Bowman's capsule

Renal tubule
4. Proximal convoluted tubule
5. Loop of Henle
6. Distal convoluted tubule

Components of urine   Urea/wastes
Salts
Water
Acids

7. Collecting tubule

8. Renal pelvis

9. Ureter

10. Urinary bladder

11. Urethra

12. Urinary meatus

Urine is expelled from the body

Figure 2-8 Kidney and surrounding structures

side effect of electrolyte disturbance such as injury, dehydration, or overhydration can cause a cardiac emergency. Electrolyte drinks usually contain sodium and potassium salts to rehydrate the body after dehydration caused by diarrhea, vomiting, diaphoresis, or exercise. More specific information about the electrolyte movement will continue in Chapter 3, on the heart's electrical physiology.

Kidney Filtration

nephrons
Areas in the kidney where urine is produced.

The kidneys eliminate waste, excess electrolytes, and toxins in the form of urine. Urine is expelled from the body after being stored in the bladder through a process called peristalsis. Urine is formed in the kidneys by tiny blood capillary units called **nephrons**. There are several types of nephrons, which perform various filtration functions. Nephrons are responsible for the filtration of waste, reabsorption of blood and other substances, and secretion of urine. **Figure 2-9** magnifies a view of the nephrons and the filtration route of fluids excreted from the body.

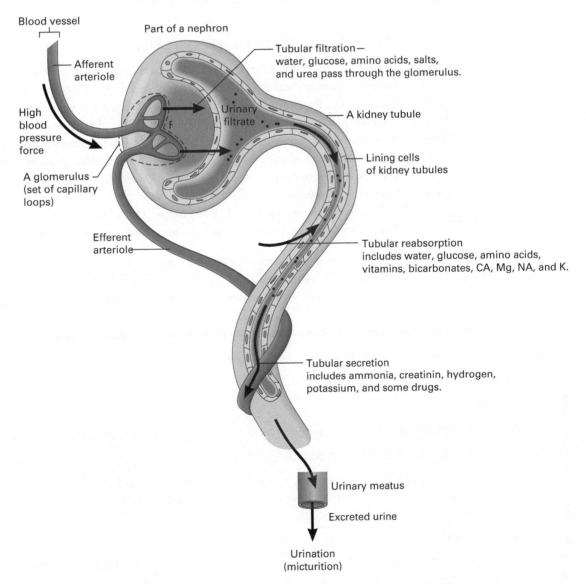

Figure 2-9 A nephron magnified

Although healthy kidneys filter about 47 gallons (approximately 178 liters) of fluid from the bloodstream in one day, only about 40 percent of 1 gallon (approximately 1.5 liters) is expelled as urine. Substances that should be reabsorbed into the bloodstream include amino acids, glucose, electrolytes, vitamins, and water. When a person has hypertensive disease or edema from congestive heart failure, diuretic drugs are often prescribed to increase urine flow, but in doing so, they also inhibit Na ions and water from being reabsorbed. When Na is decreased in the blood, blood pressure can also be reduced. Low sodium reabsorption can impair renal function. The other important ions that need to be reabsorbed in the blood include calcium and potassium. Kidney stones are often a result of the kidney's inability to absorb calcium. Calcium is stored in the bones, and when the kidneys cannot reabsorb calcium adequately, hormones are released from the parathyroid glands to the bones to increase calcium levels in the blood. Potassium is very important to keep the heart beating by circulating blood systemically. This electrolyte allows the heart muscle to move easily and is used by the kidneys to filter blood by removing excess potassium. High blood potassium is called **hyperkalemia** and can cause an irregular heartbeat.

hyperkalemia
High blood potassium.

Blood Pressure Connection

The kidneys' ability to influence blood pressure can cause constriction of the arteries and veins, thereby increasing circulating blood volume. Increased blood volume overstretches the heart muscle, which then causes the heart to generate more pressure with each beat. This is reflected as increased blood pressure. The biggest influence on blood pressure comes in the form of renin secretion. **Renin** produces angiotensin II, which is a powerful arterial and venous constrictor. Excessive production of renin can cause **hypertension** (high blood pressure). Hypertension has a strong link to the body retaining excessive fluids. Uncontrolled hypertension thickens the arterial walls, which can further lead to a stroke, heart attack, or renal disease. This is why hypertension and kidney disease are considered closely related. One of the hallmark symptoms of congestive heart failure is a buildup of excess fluids not only in the heart, but also in the lungs and appendages.

renin
A secretion created in the kidneys that produces angiotensin II which is a powerful arterial and venous constrictor.

hypertension
High blood pressure.

Diabetes is an autoimmune disease and a major noncommunicable disease. Without intervention, it can lead to end-stage renal disease and kidney dysfunction. One early warning sign that a diabetic patient presents with is the development of protein in the urine.

Quick Check 2-7

Fill in the blanks.

1. Excess electrolytes are eliminated by the _____ and regulated within the body by _____.

2. Three free ions necessary for heart conduction include _____, _____, and _____.

3. Substances that should be reabsorbed into the bloodstream and not totally expelled in urine include amino acids, _____, electrolytes, _____, and water.

4. Blood pressure can be reduced when the _____ and water are not reabsorbed during kidney filtration.

5. Uncontrolled blood pressure thickens _____ walls and may lead to a stroke.

ENDOCRINE SYSTEM

The endocrine system is designed to produce hormones that reside in various body glands. These hormones help many of the body's systems, but this book is limited to hormones that directly affect the body systems mentioned in this chapter as they relate to the heart. The major glands to be covered include the adrenal glands, pancreatic islets, parathyroid glands, pituitary gland, and thyroid glands. Hormones use the bloodstream to reach individual cells and organs. **Figure 2-10** identifies major endocrine glands that directly relate to heart health.

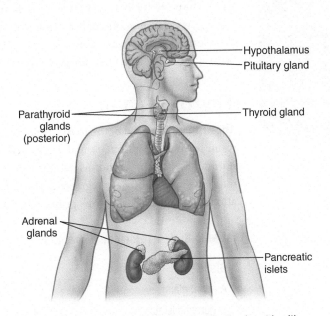

Figure 2-10 Endocrine glands directly affecting heart health

Adrenal Glands

There are two adrenal glands, located on top of each kidney. The primary purpose of the adrenal glands is to control electrolyte levels, regulate metabolism, and interact with the sympathetic nervous system when responding to stress. Chapter 3 will discuss electrolytes in greater detail.

Pancreatic Islets

The pancreatic islets of the endocrine system are very important because they are responsible for secreting glucose, which controls blood sugar levels. The pancreatic islets contain two different types of cells: alpha cells and beta cells. Alpha cells secrete glucagon, which stimulates the liver to increase the glucose level in the body. Beta cells secrete insulin, which also stimulates the liver, but beta cells create energy by converting glucose into glycogen for storage.

Parathyroid Glands

Electrolyte movement in the heart depends heavily on calcium electrolytes. The function of the parathyroid gland is to regulate the calcium levels throughout the body. The body uses calcium that is stored in bones and teeth. The parathyroid needs a hormone called calcitonin, which is released by the thyroid gland in order to function. The parathyroid contains four glands, all of which are located in the posterior portion of the thyroid gland.

Pituitary Gland

Hormones from the pituitary gland control the other glands in the endocrine system. The pituitary gland has two lobes. The anterior lobe has eight hormones stimulated by the pituitary gland. Of these eight, two are significant for heart health. One is the adrenocorticotropic hormone (ACTH), which is important because it stimulates the adrenal cortex and controls cortisol and aldosterone. The second hormone in the anterior lobe is the thyroid-stimulating hormone (TSH), which is significant because it releases the thyroid hormones thyroxine (T4) and triodothyronine (T3). The posterior lobe secretes only two hormones, and one of these, the antidiuretic hormone (ADH), is very important for heart health. Its function is to help regulate blood pressure through the release of urine by the kidneys and to reabsorb water into the bloodstream. This hormone is actually produced in the hypothalamus, but it is stored in the pituitary gland.

Thyroid Gland

The primary function of the thyroid gland is to regulate metabolism. In addition, the thyroid gland secretes calcitonin, which works with the parathyroid to keep the calcium levels at a normal level in the blood. Metabolism is important because through metabolism, all the nutrients in the body are regulated. The five heart hormones are listed in **Table 2-3**, which also identifies each hormone's primary function.

Table 2-3 Heart Hormone Functions

Gland	Primary Function
Adrenal glands	Controls electrolytes
Pancreatic islets	Controls blood sugar
Parathyroid glands	Regulates calcium
Pituitary glands	Regulates blood pressure
Thyroid gland	Regulates metabolism

METABOLIC SYNDROME

The final section in this chapter will discuss a serious health condition that affects more than 20 percent of adult Americans. When covering body systems that relate to heart health, it is important to mention a systematic issue that is increasing in importance, even though it is not one specific disease. Metabolic syndrome is a group of symptoms, mostly related to diabetes mellitus, which, when combined, can be the underlying cause of many cardio-vascular diseases, including heart attack and stroke. The symptoms are grouped into five predominant risk factors, and a person is considered to have metabolic syndrome if he or she has three of the five. These factors include abdominal obesity, high blood pressure, high triglycerides, high fasting blood glucose level, and a low high-density lipoprotein (HDL) cholesterol level.

Abdominal obesity is excess fat around the waist. People with this type of obesity are generally not physically active. People with abdominal obesity usually are also insulin resistant. Insulin is needed by the body to convert starch and sugar into energy, and insulin resistance can lead to diabetes. A woman with a waist of more than 35 inches or a man with a waist of more than 40 inches is considered to have abdominal obesity.

Common Pituitary Hormone Blood Test

A thyroid function test measures how well the thyroid is working by testing TSH, T3, and free T4.

---

metabolic syndrome
A group of symptoms or risk factors including abdominal obesity, high blood pressure, high triglycerides, high fasting blood glucose level, and low HDL cholesterol level, which, when combined, can be the under-lying cause of many cardiovascular diseases, including heart attacks and strokes.

Blood pressure above 130/85 is considered high. People who take blood pressure medication to maintain a healthy level are included in this risk category. Triglycerides are chains of high-energy fatty acids found in the blood that form lipoproteins. Lipoproteins provide energy that is required for tissue functions. Fasting triglycerides should be less than 150 mg/dL without taking medication. High fasting blood glucose is a precursor to diabetes, but blood results must confirm high fasting sugar on at least two occasions to confirm a diabetes diagnosis. A normal range for fasting blood glucose would be 100 mg/dL or less without taking medication. Low HDL cholesterol is a risk factor because HDL cholesterol, when adequate, helps to remove cholesterol from the arteries, thus preventing plaque buildup. People who take medication to maintain a healthy level of HDL cholesterol are included as having a metabolic risk factor. Normal HDL, without taking medication, should be less than 40 mg/dL for women and less than 50 mg/dL for men. **Table 2-4** shows abnormal levels of various conditions that, when combined, can cause a diagnosis of metabolic syndrome.

Table 2-4 Metabolic Syndrome Risk Factors

Risk Factor	Body/Blood Measurements Out of Control (or Being Controlled With Medication)
Abdominal obesity	Women—waist size of more than 35 in. Men—waist size of more than 40 in.
Hypertension	Average blood pressure measurement of more than 130/85
High triglycerides	Fasting lipoprotein analysis blood test showing a triglyceride level at 150 mg/dL or higher
High blood glucose	Fasting blood glucose blood test showing a glucose concentration of more than 100 mg/dL on more than one occasion
Low HDL Cholesterol	Fasting lipoprotein analysis blood test showing an HDL level of less than 40 mg/dL
A person is considered to have metabolic syndrome if he or she has three or more of these risk factors and was tested for these factors on more than one occasion.	

Quick Check 2-8

Fill in the blanks.

1. The endocrine system produces _____, which enter the _____ to reach individual cells.

2. Electrolytes found in the _____ glands and the thyroid glands help to regulate metabolism.

3. The antidiuretic hormone (ADH) is stored in the _____ gland and plays an important role in regulating blood _____ by releasing urine and reabsorbing water into the bloodstream.

4. The function of the parathyroid gland is to regulate _____ levels throughout the body.

5. High blood pressure, high triglycerides, and high _____ are three risk factors found with many people suffering from _____.

SUMMARY

- Five body systems are directly related to heart health, including the respiratory system, nervous system, integumentary system, urinary system, and endocrine system.

- The respiratory system plays an important role in providing oxygen and the exchange of gases necessary for healthy cell growth.

- Two major respiratory conditions that deprive oxygen to the cells are obstructive sleep apnea and chronic obstructive pulmonary disease (COPD).

- The brain is the most complex organ in the body and the primary organ of the nervous system.

- When the heart is under pressure or stress, the ventricles of the heart secrete a hormone called brain natriuretic peptide (BNP). This causes a decrease in blood volume and lowers systemic blood pressure while increasing cardiac output.

- Three types of cerebral vascular accidents (CVAs) include embolic, thrombotic, and hemorrhagic. Another term for a CVA is stroke.

- Strokes occur when blood flow is blocked or greatly reduced to the brain.

- The sympathetic nervous system (SNS) and parasympathetic nervous system (PSNS) are two divisions of the autonomic nervous system (ANS). The SNS and PSNS have opposite effects on the functions they regulate.

- The SNS regulates the rate and force of heart contractions and is often called the heart's "fight-or-flight" response to stimuli.

- The PSNS regulates the conservation of energy in the heart and is often called the "rest-and-digest" response to stimuli or the lack of stimuli.

- Cardiac performance is directly related to the activity of neurotransmitters in the heart that direct the heart on how fast or slow to beat. This is accomplished through the nerve endings in the SNS (called adrenergic) and in the PSNS (called cholinergic).

- The integumentary system includes three primary functions necessary for healthy heart health, including waste removal, control of fluids, and most important, thermoregulation of core body temperature.

- Too high a core temperature or too low a core temperature can become a fatal condition for people who suffer from cardiovascular disease.

- The urinary system also plays an important role in water and waste elimination, but the kidney functions are more closely related to regulation of blood volume than of core temperature.

- Blood volume is directly tied to blood pressure and influence placed on the heart when blood volume is increased, stretching the heart muscle due to constriction of the arteries and veins.

- Uncontrolled high blood pressure can lead to strokes, heart attacks, or renal disease.

- The endocrine system produces hormones that use the bloodstream to reach individual cells and organs. Five endocrine hormones directly affect heart health: the adrenal glands, pancreatic islets, parathyroid glands, pituitary gland, and thyroid gland.

- Metabolic syndrome, when combined with diabetes mellitus, is the underlying cause of many v diseases.

- Obesity and diabetes mellitus play an important role in causing multiple systems to become insulin resistant, which causes cells to become starved for energy.

Critical Thinking Challenges

2-1. Fill in the missing sections in the "Pituitary Hormones" table. In the "Stimulating Hormone" column, be sure to include the name and abbreviation for each hormone. In the "Purpose" column, there are two answers for each hormone; include both. The "Stimulates" column has only one answer each, except for the answer already filled in.

Pituitary Hormones		
Stimulating Hormone	**Stimulates**	**Purpose**
Adrenocorticotropic (ACTH)		
		Releases thyroxine (T4) and triodothyronine (T3)
	Produced in the hypothalamus; Stored in the pituitary gland	

2-2. Fill in the blanks in the following paragraph. Try to complete the paragraph without referring back to the chapter.

Thermoregulation means regulation of the body's _____, which is regulated in the _____ region of the brain. The body has two primary ways of increasing heat. With _____, the body's heat is raised by using a heating pad next to the skin. _____ would be an example of radiation heat gain. _____ is caused when the whole body is overheated, and the skin can consume _____ percent of cardiac output. Cardiac output must increase when the body is overheated to offset a decrease in _____. _____ can occur when the body's temperature is reduced by as little as _____ degrees. When the body is cooled, the blood vessels near the skin _____ to protect the internal organs. An ice pack applied to the skin is an example of _____ heat loss. Another example of heat loss, _____ heat loss, occurs when a person uses cold water to rinse off and cool the skin after getting a mild burn. Heat transfer without physical contact is called _____ heat loss. _____, which is often called sweating, is the only way that the body can physiologically lose heat.

2-3. Design a table on body systems covered in this chapter. Create columns titled "Body System"; "Major Function(s)"; "Major Organs Affecting the Heart"; and "Importance to Heart Health." Then complete your table with the correct answers. Do not create paragraphs for answers, rather, just create lists of the correct information under each column.

Review Activities

2-1. Fill in the blanks under the Sympathetic and Parasympathetic columns identifying the information requested in each numbered row.

Autonomic Nervous System

	Sympathetic	Parasympathetic
1. Origination	_____	_____
2. Neurotransmitter(s)	_____	_____

3. Nerve Endings   _____   _____

4. Heart Rate   _____   _____

5. Blood Vessels   _____   _____

6. Body's Response   _____   _____

7. Function   _____   _____

2-2. Match the thermoregulation with the examples given. Each thermoregulation may be used more than once. Then circle whether the core temperature is increased or decreased with each event.

A. Conduction

B. Convection

C. Evaporation

D. Radiation

Core Temperature Is:

1. _____ Taking a cold shower   increased   decreased

2. _____ Sweating   increased   decreased

3. _____ Using a heating pad   increased   decreased

4. _____ Running a fever   increased   decreased

5. _____ Sunbathing   increased   decreased

6. _____ Using an ice pack   increased   decreased

7. _____ Arterial vasodilatation   increased   decreased

8. _____ Raised hair on the body's surface   increased   decreased

9. _____ Wrapping the body in an electric blanket   increased   decreased

10. _____ Vasoconstriction   increased   decreased

2-3. Using the letters A–E, fill in the blank with the body system that *best* fits the statement.

A. Endocrine system

B. Integumentary system

C. Nervous system

D. Respiratory system

E. Urinary system

1. _____ Brain is primary organ

2. _____ Core body temperature regulation

3. _____ Regulates blood volume

4. _____ Regulates metabolism

5. _____ Fight or flight

6. _____ Obstructive sleep apnea

7. _____ Removes carbon dioxide from the body

8. _____ Controls electrolyte levels

9. _____ Thermoregulation

10. _____ Maintains water balance (pH)

Chapter Two Test

Fill in the blanks.

1. The pituitary stimulating hormone that regulates blood pressure through the release of urine is called _____.

2. When vascular resistance is decreased, _____ must increase.

3. The only way that a body can physiologically lose heat is through _____.

4. The _____ is the body's primary controller.

5. The _____ main purpose is to control breathing.

6. Uncontrolled blood pressure is the primary cause of _____ strokes.

7. _____ strokes are caused by a blood clot that travels to the brain and cuts off the blood supply.

8. The _____ nerve is the primary connector between the brain and the heart.

9. The _____ nervous system stimulates the heart to change its functioning.

10. Acetylcholine influences heart _____ action.

11. A condition or disease of the autonomic nervous system is called _____.

12. A physiological test used to diagnose autonomic dysfunction is called the _____.

13. Another name for excessive sweating is _____.

14. Tiny air sacs where oxygen and carbon dioxide is exchanged are called _____.

15. _____ are water-soluble compounds that can conduct electricity.

Chapter Two Quick Check Answers

Answer order is important except where noted otherwise in parentheses.

When two correct answers are possible, both answers are given, separated by the word "or."

2-1:

1. lungs, capillaries (either order)
2. diaphragm, externally, internal expiration
3. 20
4. lungs, collapsing
5. smoking

2-2:

1. muscle, secretion
2. insulation, metabolic
3. action potential
4. natriuretic peptide
5. oxygen, nutrients (either order)

2-3:

1. vagus
2. sympathetic, parasympathetic (either order)
3. sympathetic, rate, force ("rate" and "force" can be reversed)
4. physical activity, contractile
5. parasympathetic

2-4:

1. Neurons, adrenal
2. epinephrine, adrenalin (either order)
3. fast, slow (either order)
4. diabetes
5. resistance, blood vessels

2-5:

1. waste removal, thermoregulation
2. diaphoresis
3. Homeostasis
4. temperature, glucose, pH
5. water, oxygen (either order)

2-6:

1. blood pressure, heart rate (either order)
2. hypothalmus
3. high, arrector pili
4. evaporation or sweating
5. metabolism

2-7:

1. kidneys, hormones
2. sodium, potassium, calcium (any order)
3. glucose, vitamins
4. sodium ions or sodium electrolytes
5. arterial

2-8:

1. hormones, bloodstream
2. adrenal
3. pituitary, pressure
4. calcium
5. blood glucose, metabolic syndrome

3

HEART ELECTRICAL PHYSIOLOGY

OBJECTIVES

After reading the chapter and completing all Quick Check activities, the student should be able to:

1. Identify the characteristics of specialized myocardial cell functions.
2. Outline polarity-electrolyte movement.
3. Compare the five stages of action potential to electrolyte polarity.
4. Define the terms diastole and systole.
5. Draw the cardiac cycle.
6. Compute cardiac output.
7. Explain electrical conduction.
8. Map the heart's primary pacemakers.
9. List the intrinsic firing ranges.
10. Describe three conduction abnormalities.

KEY TERMS

action potential
afterload
atrial kick
automaticity
bundle branches
bundle of His
cardiac cycle
conductivity
contractility
depolarization
diastole
end diastolic volume
end systolic volume
excitability
extracellular
heart rate
intracellular
internodal pathways
peripheral vascular resistance
polarization
preload
pulse pressure
Purkinje network

refractory period
repolarization

resting state
Starling's Law of the Heart

stroke volume
systole

INTRODUCTION

The average adult human has approximately 5 liters of blood in his or her body. Every minute, a healthy body will pump this amount of blood throughout the circulatory system when the body is at rest. The process begins with a contraction followed by a relaxation of the heart. This chapter begins by describing the cardiac cycle, which identifies the phases of contraction and relaxation of the heart muscle. Then, cardiac cells are revisited from Chapter 1, but in this chapter, their role and ability to conduct and create electrical impulses is explained. Cell conduction will be followed by a discussion of the three major electrolytes that provide polarity and ion movement. This chapter concludes with the identification of the three primary pacemaker sites, their intrinsic firing ranges, and the identification of the electrical path of heart impulses.

SPECIALIZED MYOCARDIAL CELL FUNCTIONS

An understanding of cardiac muscles is essential to understanding what is happening in the heart to create an electrical impulse, which causes the heart to beat. Chapter 1 identified the two types of cardiac muscle cells as either myocardial working cells or specialized pacemaker cells. Recall that their functions are very different. The working cells have a primary function to create a cardiac muscle contraction and then to relax the cardiac muscle, whereas the pacemaker cells have a primary function to generate electrical impulses.

Myocardial cells have a specialized ability to conduct and create electrical impulses through four primary characteristics that make them unique to other cells within the body. These characteristics include three electrical functions named automaticity, excitability, and conductivity, and the fourth is a mechanical function called contractility. Each of the characteristics is different, as is its function. **Automaticity** is the pacemaker cardiac cell's ability to spontaneously generate an electrical impulse without outside stimulation or stimulation by the nervous system. **Excitability** occurs in both pacemaker and working cardiac cells and is the cell's ability to respond to an impulse or electrical stimulus. Excitability is sometimes referred to as irritability of the cardiac cells because the cells are responding to stimuli. **Conductivity** is the unique ability of both pacemaker and working cardiac cells to transmit and receive electrical impulses to and from other myocardial cells. The fourth characteristic of myocardial cells, **contractility**, is a function of the pacemaker cells and occurs in response to the emptying of the ventricles when the cells contract and shorten as they begin to recover after being stretched prior to the contraction. Contractibility is often referred to as the rhythmic cardiac cell function because the myocardial cells produce a heartbeat in response to electrical stimuli created by the pacemaker cardiac cells.

Figure 3-1 summarizes the actions of a cardiac cell as it completes one cycle, which occurs approximately once every 8 seconds. First, the electrical impulse is generated,

automaticity
A unique characteristic of myocardial cells to spontaneously create electricity without outside stimulation or internal stimulation by the nervous system.

excitability
A cardiac cell's unique ability to respond to electrical stimulus; also called irritability.

conductivity
The unique ability of myocardial cells to transmit and receive electrical impulses to and from other myocardial cells.

contractility
The ability of the myocardial cells to shorten and contract before recovering from a ventricular contraction.

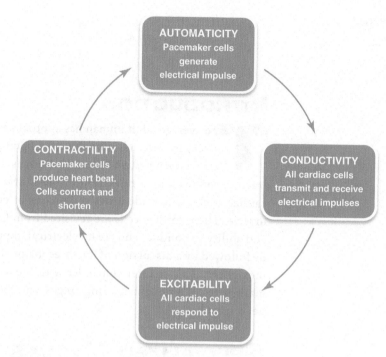

Figure 3-1 Normal cardiac cell cycle

followed by a response of the cells to the impulse. The electrical impulse is then transmitted and received by neighboring cardiac cells, which produce an all-or-nothing response to the stimulus. With a response, a heartbeat is produced when the ventricles contract. After the contraction, the cells return to a normal state and the cycle is repeated approximately 60 to 100 times in 1 minute in a healthy heart.

CELL POLARITY–ELECTROLYTE MOVEMENT

So, how do the myocardial cells actually create electricity? A study of how the cardiac cells move electrolytes through their semipermeable membranes of the cell walls explains this phenomenon. Recall from Chapter 1 that electrolytes are compounds that are soluble in water and form free ions. To further understand electrolytes, the compounds are minerals containing small particles (ions) found in cells that carry a positive or negative electrical charge. In the cardiac cell's resting state, the electrolytes within the cell (**intracellular**) carry a negative charge, but outside the cell (**extracellular**), the electrolyte carries the opposite charge, so at rest the extracellular electrolyte carries a positive charge. Positive ions are called cations and negative ions are called anions. A cardiac cell is considered in a **resting state** (also called resting membrane potential or polarized state) when it is not contracting. When cardiac cells experience automaticity, there is a change in polarity, which then results in an electrical impulse. Through conductivity, the cardiac cell transmits the electrical impulse to other cardiac cells. The cardiac cells then become excitable (i.e., responds to the stimulus), which finally leads to contractility (cardiac muscle contraction). **Figure 3-2** shows the electrolyte charge when the cardiac cell is in a resting state.

intracellular
Located within cell membrane.

extracellular
Located outside a cell membrane.

resting state
A cardiac cell is considered to be in a resting state when it is not contracting; also called resting membrane potential or polarized state.

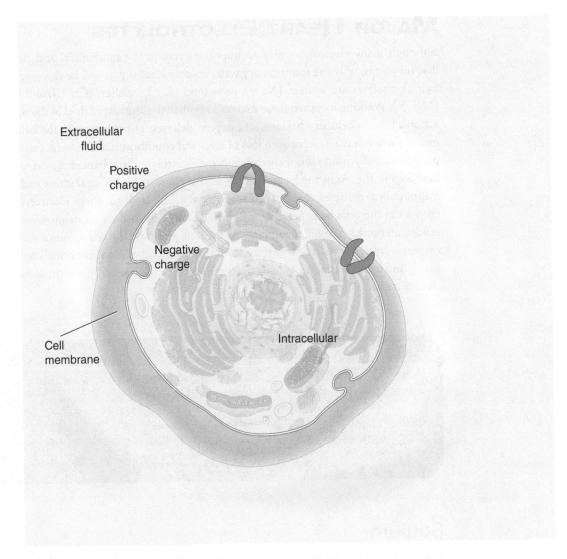

Figure 3-2 Cardiac cell in the resting state

Quick Check 3-1

Fill in the blanks.

1. Cardiac muscle working cells create a(n) _____ before _____ the cardiac muscle.

2. _____ cells have a primary function to _____ electrical impulses.

3. An electrical function that is unique to pacemaker cells is called _____, whereas the unique mechanical function of pacemaker cells is called _____.

4. A normal healthy adult heart will complete the cardiac cycle _____ times in 1 minute, which is approximately once every _____ seconds.

5. In a cardiac cell's resting state, the electrolyte will carry a(n) _____ charge.

MAJOR HEART ELECTROLYTES

Although many electrolytes play an important role in the mechanical and electrical cardiac functions, only the four primary water soluble electrolytes will be discussed here. The four electrolytes are sodium (Na+), potassium (K+), calcium (Ca²+), and magnesium (Mg²+). Working together, these minerals regulate the amount of fluid in the body, muscle actions, blood chemistry balance, and oxygen delivery. Disturbances in the balance of any one of these minerals can cause a loss of electrical equilibrium in the heart that may lead to dangerous arrhythmias if not corrected. Most electrolyte disturbances are caused by severe fluid loss in the body, medications such as diuretics, or health conditions such as kidney malfunctions, diabetes, and heart disease. At the cellular level, these electrolytes produce changes in the cells by generating action potentials, which then create movement of fluids inside and outside the cell membrane. As the ions permeate the cell membrane, an electrical current is created that causes the muscles to contract or relax. A patient urinalysis (electrolyte panel) and blood testing are usually the first diagnostic tools used by practitioners to identify electrolyte imbalance.

The Heart's Primary Water-Soluble Electrolytes

The heart's primary water-soluble electrolytes are sodium (Na+), potassium (K+), calcium (Ca²+), and magnesium (Mg²+). Many cardiac medications (discussed in Chapter 4) address the imbalance of these electrolytes.

Sodium

Sodium is a highly reactive alkali metal. It is classified as a dietary inorganic macromineral that is essential for animal life. Sodium is most abundant in the cell's extracellular fluid and plays a key role in transmitting nerve impulses and maintaining serum concentration and osmolality. It uses regulated voltage by initiating the action potential that triggers a contraction. The body's primary source for sodium is common table salt and processed foods. Most people (Americans) have too much sodium in their diet. The biggest concern of too much sodium is that a person can develop chronic hypertension, a major risk factor for heart failure. Too much sodium is called hypernatremia. Hypernatremia can be caused by excessive sodium intake, inadequate water consumption, or dehydration. It can cause excessive fluid in the blood vessels, which then raises blood pressure and may cause tachycardia heart rhythms. Hyponatremia is too little sodium in the body and can be caused by excessive sweating, water intoxication, kidney disease, diuretics, and illegal drugs. Water follows sodium in the body, so when a person has too much sodium in the body, the brain signals that the body is thirsty and the person wants to drink water, while the antidiuretic hormone (ADH) tells the kidneys to hold onto the water. Likewise, when the body has too little sodium, the release of ADH is inhibited and more water is excreted from the body as urine, thus decreasing plasma osmolality. These are examples of the body's desire to maintain homeostasis, which was described in Chapter 2.

Fast Facts on Sodium (Na+)

Primary source = table salt

Purpose = transmitting nerve impulses, maintaining serum concentration and osmolality

Too much (hypernatremia) causes excessive fluid retention, high blood pressure; too little (hyponatremia) causes reduced plasma osmolality, excessive urination.

Potassium

Potassium is also a highly reactive alkali metal that naturally binds to other minerals and is the most abundant intracellular cation in the body. It is most important to neuromuscular cardiac function (heartbeat) and fluid balance. With high levels of potassium but normal kidney functioning, the hormone aldosterone is released via urine, causing sodium to be retained. Too much potassium in the body is called hyperkalemia, and too little is called hypokalemia. Potassium is required by the body to build protein and muscle. It also is needed to maintain the acid–base balance that the body needs. Potassium is responsible for terminating the action potential and initiating repolarization. It also has voltage-gated channels that open in response to change and slow cardiac impulse conduction. Too much potassium can decrease electrical conduction to the point of disrupting the heart's rhythm. Too little potassium can show up on an electrocardiogram (ECG) as irregular contractions because of premature atrial and ventricular contractions. The source of potassium comes primarily from eating white beans and potatoes and dark leafy vegetables.

The body treats sodium and potassium very differently, even though they are chemically similar. Sodium works opposite of potassium in establishing equilibrium because while they perform many of the same functions, when the muscle is contracting through movement of ions, one electrolyte is causing the contraction while the other electrolyte is causing muscle relaxation.

When sodium has a positive charge, potassium will carry a negative charge and when sodium is pushed out of the cells, blood pressure is increased. Likewise, when potassium enters the cells, blood pressure is decreased. This is why when one of these electrolytes is increased in the body, the other mineral will increase in excretion to try to maintain balance.

Fast Facts on Potassium (K+)

Primary sources = white beans, potatoes, dark leafy vegetables

Purpose = cardiac muscular conduction, fluid balance, builds proteins and muscles

Too much (hyperkalemia) disrupts the heart's rhythm; too little (hypokalemia) causes irregular and premature contractions.

Calcium

Calcium is the most common metal found in animals and is essential in cell physiology. In the heart, calcium plays a role in generating impulses and mediating the heart's pacemaker function. Calcium and sodium work together to cause the heart muscle to contract and work on an opposite charge as potassium and magnesium. Calcium also works to maintain cell wall permeability and muscle contractions. Too much calcium in the body is called hypercalcemia and has several causes, such as an overactive parathyroid gland, kidney disease, or a genetic disorder called familial hypocalciuric hypercalcemia. Too much calcium can cause abnormal heart rhythms (arrhythmia), kidney failure when the blood cannot be cleansed and toxins are not eliminated, and possibly malabsorption of other essential minerals such as magnesium. Too little calcium is called hypocalcemia and can be caused by conditions such as kidney failure or medications such as heparin and can lead to hypotension. Long-term effects of hypocalcemia can include congestive heart failure. The body obtains calcium primarily from ingesting common foods such as dark leafy greens and low-fat cheese, milk, and yogurt.

Fast Facts on Calcium (Ca² +)

Primary sources = dark leafy greens, low-fat cheese, milk, and yogurt

Purpose = mediating heart's pacemaker function

Too much (hypercalcemia) can cause abnormal heart rhythms; too little (hypocalcemia) can cause hypotension and, over time, congestive heart failure.

Magnesium

Magnesium is the second-most-abundant intracellular cation in the body. Magnesium is a metallocoenzyme that activates over 300 other enzymatic reactions and acts as the modulator of the heart's cell functions and in the maintenance of sodium and potassium intra- and extra-cellularly. Of the four minerals named, magnesium is the most likely to be extremely low. Since magnesium regulates the flow of the other electrolytes, it is essential for maintenance of the intracellular potassium concentration. Magnesium also helps muscles relax and has been associated with the regulation of blood pressure and reducing the risk of diabetes. Very low levels of magnesium (known as hypomagnesemia) can cause cardiac muscle irritability to the point of causing an irregular ventricular heart rhythm, particularly in people with recent myocardial infarctions. The body maintaining too much magnesium (known as hypermagnesemia) is rare because the kidneys will usually expel it through urination, but can occur in people with certain diseases such as end-stage renal disease. Hypermagnesemia is often asymptomatic. The body's demand for magnesium increases with exercise because the body utilizes magnesium for muscle contraction. Magnesium is the drug of choice for controlling ventricular tachycardia. Foods such as dark leafy vegetables, nuts and seeds, and beans and lentils are rich in magnesium.

Fast Facts on Magnesium (Mg² +)

Primary sources = dark leafy vegetables, nuts, and seeds

Purpose = essential for maintenance of intracellular potassium and maintaining blood pressure

Too much (hypermagnesemia) is rare; too little (hypomagnesemia) can cause hypertension and irregular ventricular heart rhythms.

Quick Check 3-2

Fill in the blanks.

1. Water follows _____ in the body, and unfortunately, when there is too much of this electrolyte, the brain signals for the person to _____ water.

2. _____ is responsible for terminating the action potential of cardiac muscles, thus when there is too little of this electrolyte, premature _____ can occur.

3. The electrolytes _____ and _____ work together to cause muscle contractions.

4. _____ is the second-most-abundant electrolyte in the body, yet is most likely to be extremely _____ because it is usually expelled.

5. Potassium and magnesium carry a(n) _____ charge when the cardiac cells are at _____.

ELECTROLYTE POLARITY CHANGES

All four electrolytes are positively charged, but in the resting state of cardiac cells, the electrolyte's intracellular charge is negative and the extracellular charge is positive. How can this be? It is because sodium is the most abundant electrolyte in the extracellular fluid, so it carries a stronger charge than the less abundant intracellular electrolyte potassium. Therefore, in the cardiac cell's polarized state, sodium is positively charged outside the cell and potassium becomes negatively charged inside the cell. In this section on polarity changes, three of the minerals—sodium, calcium, and potassium—will be discussed. Magnesium is a coenzyme that works along with potassium; therefore, it is not individually identified. The final part of this section will put everything together in the process of **action potential**, a change in cell polarity.

action potential
A change in polarity of a cardiac cell, from negative charge to positive charge or from positive charge to negative charge.

polarization
A process where, when a cell is at rest, the intracellular membrane is negatively charged.

Polarization

Polarization is the first of three electrical changes that the myocardial cells experience. **Figure 3-3** shows the electrolytes in a cardiac cell and their charges in the polarization state. Remember that polarization is synonymous with resting.

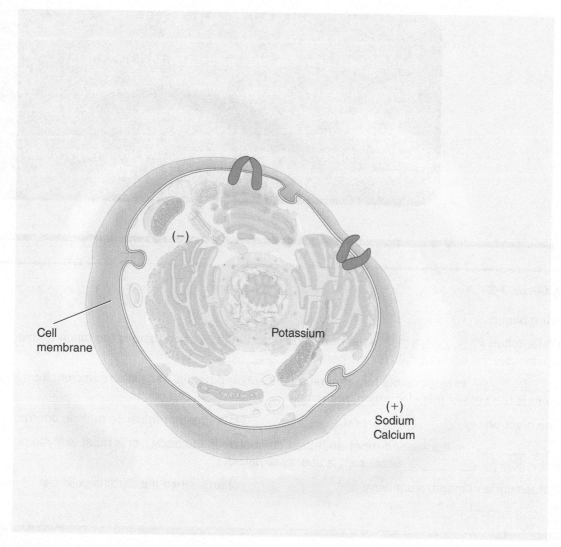

Figure 3-3 Cardiac cell polarization (resting state)

Depolarization

depolarization
Sodium ions cross the cell membrane, causing a reversal of intracellular membrane charges from negative to positive.

The second electrical change of cardiac cells occurs when the cells are stimulated with all-or-none signals, causing a mechanical myocardial contraction. This stage is called **depolarization** because the intracellular charge is changing to positive as the sodium electrolytes rapidly moved into the cell, as shown in **Figure 3-4**. Remember that depolarization is synonymous with action potential.

Repolarization

repolarization
A process where electrolytes cross cell membranes back to the original polarity, thus returning the heart to a resting state and leaving the extracellular charge positive and the intracellular charge negative.

The third electrical change of the myocardial cell, and the longest of the three stages, is a process called **repolarization**. This is a period of cell recovery. In this phase, the heart is returning to a state of negatively charged potassium inside the cell and sodium and calcium positively charged outside the cell. The heart utilizes a mechanism called a sodium–potassium pump to help move the electrolytes to their original polarity, as shown in **Figure 3-5**. Remember that repolarization is synonymous with resting and recovery.

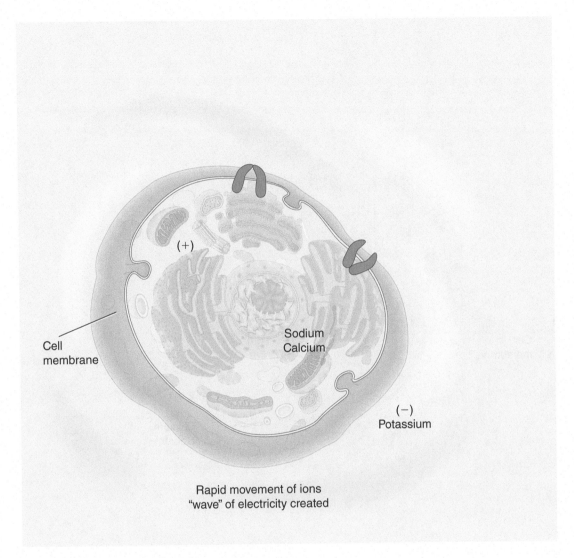

Figure 3-4 Cardiac cell depolarization (action potential)

The cycle of polarization, depolarization, and repolarization is now ready to be repeated for every heartbeat. **Table 3-1** shows the three key electrolyte locations during these processes. Magnesium is not included.

Action Potential

Every cardiac cell goes through the process of producing an electrical current, which then causes a contraction and relaxation of the heart muscles. Look at the action potential of the cell to understand how minerals change polarity during the process of polarization, depolarization, and repolarization. There are actually five phases to review in this process (and remember that this happens typically in 8 seconds). First, the cell is at rest in the polarized state, which is called Phase 4. Then, in Phase 0, the cell becomes excited when sodium rushes into the cell through open channels and changes the cardiac cell's polarity. Phase 0 is called the depolarization state. In Phase 1, the sodium channel closes while calcium begins to enter the cell and potassium begins to move out of the cell. These electrolytes provide a wave of electricity, which causes the heart muscle to contract

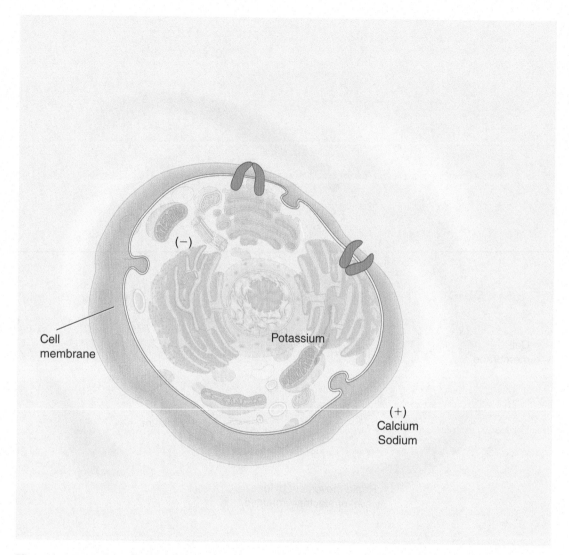

Figure 3-5 Cardiac cell repolarization (recovery)

mechanically. Phase 1 is called early repolarization. In Phase 2, which is called the plateau phase, calcium and potassium continue movement through the cell membrane and the sodium channel reopens. The cells enter a repolarization process where they get ready for the next contraction. Phase 3 is the time where the cells begin to go back to the original polarity, and potassium enters the cell but maintains a negative charge and sodium and calcium returns to the intracellular fluid with a positive charge. During the repolarization phases, the cells cannot receive stimuli as they begin to relax. This period of time is called the **refractory period**.

In the absolute refractory period, the cells cannot accept stimuli, but as the repolarization cycle completes toward the end of Phase 3, which is called late repolarization, a relative refractory period can accept a cardiac cell stimulus prematurely if the stimulus is stronger than normal. **Figure 3-6** shows the action potential and identifies both the stages and the polarization state of the cardiac cell. Notice that the graph shows voltage in comparison to time. In a normal cardiac cell, time is measured from 0 to 300 milliseconds (ms), where the absolute refractory period is shown as being from Phase 0 through the end of Phase 2 and relative

refractory period
A time during the repolarization phase when cardiac cells cannot receive additional electrical impulses.

Table 3-1 Cell Polarity

Location and Charge			
Electrical State	**Electrolyte**	**Intracellular**	**Extracellular**
Polarization	Potassium	(−)	
	Calcium		(+)
	Sodium		(+)
Depolarization	Potassium		(−)
	Calcium	(+)	
	Sodium	(+)	
Repolarization	Potassium	(−)	
	Calcium		(+)
	Sodium		(+)

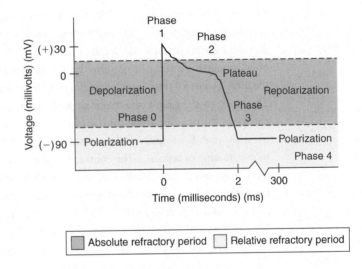

Phases

0   Sodium rushes into cell membrane, calcium channel open, potassium channel closed
1   Sodium channel closes, calcium enters and potassium exits cell membrane quickly
2   Calcium continues to enter, potassium channel continues to move out of cell, sodium channel opens at end of phase 2
3   Calcium channel closed, sodium channel closes, potassium channel closes at end of phase 3
4   Potassium rushes into cell membrane, sodium exits cell membrane, helped by sodium–potassium pump

Figure 3-6 Action potential

refractory is only Phase 3. In addition, notice that Phase 1 is very short (less than 1 ms) and the plateau phase is the longest phase. Voltage begins at −90 membrane potential, measured in millivolts (mV). The plateau phase is at 0 mV and Phase 1 has a positive voltage of 30 mV.

Quick Check 3-3

Fill in the blanks.

1. When cardiac cells are in a polarized state, _____ electrolytes are positively charged outside the cell, while _____ electrolytes are negatively charged inside the cell.

2. Action potential is measured in _____ and _____ to complete one cardiac cycle.

3. A cell can receive a stimulus _____ during the relative refractory period when the stimulus is stronger than normal.

4. The three electrical changes that occur to cardiac cells include _____, _____, and _____.

5. During the _____ refractory period, cells can receive no additional _____.

HEART ACTIONS

heart rate
The number of times the heart beats in 1 minute.

cardiac cycle
The time it takes for the heart to complete one cycle from ventricular contraction to ventricular relaxation.

systole
The contraction phase of a heart muscle.

diastole
The resting phase of a heart muscle, when the chambers fill with blood.

end systolic volume
The volume of blood that remains in the left ventricle after a contraction; typical adult level is 50 mL.

end diastolic volume
The volume of blood in the left ventricle when the ventricle is filled to capacity; typical adult level is 120 mL.

As mentioned previously, a healthy adult's heart typically beats approximately 60–100 times in a minute, but it can go as high as 180 beats per minute (bpm) in an adult with resistance issues. The number of beats in a minute is called the **heart rate**. For each heartbeat, blood is pumped not only through the heart, but also also through the entire cardiovascular system. A **cardiac cycle** is the time it takes for the heart's ventricles to go through one sequence of contraction to relaxation. The heart goes through two major steps to complete each cardiac cycle. These steps include a change in the polarity of the cardiac electrolytes at the cellular level, which then creates an electrical impulse. The impulse follows a predetermined path and causes the heart muscle to respond by contracting or relaxing. The contraction phase in the heartbeat is called **systole**, whereas the relaxation phase is called **diastole**. Systole is often referred to as ventricular systole because when the left ventricle ejects the blood into the aorta, a small amount of blood remains in the ventricle, and the volume is called **end systolic volume**. Normal end systolic volume is approximately 50 milliliters (mL) of blood. During the heart's relaxation phase, when the left ventricle is filled to capacity prior to systole, the blood volume is referred to as **end diastolic volume**. Typically, the left ventricle at capacity can hold approximately 120 mL of blood in an adult. Remember that it is the contraction of the heart that causes the heart valves to open and close.

Heart Sounds

Recall from Chapter 1 that the function of the atria is to receive blood from either the body or the lungs. Because the atria are small and only dump the returning blood into the ventricles, the atria are not under tremendous pressure to move blood like the ventricles are. It is during this filling and expansion of the atria that the heart is considered to be in the relaxed phase called diastole or early ventricular diastole. The actual atrial contraction that forces the blood to move out of the atria into the ventricles is called atrial systole or late ventricular diastole. It makes sense, then, that the thicker-walled ventricles are the source of a heartbeat that can be heard with a stethoscope. When the atrioventricular valves close in early ventricular systole, the first heart sound can be heard. Normally, the mitral valve closes before the tricuspid valve. The second heart sound is heard in late ventricular systole, when the aortic and pulmonary valves close and the ventricles begin to relax. When a person with a normal, healthy heart inhales, one can listen closely and hear the pulmonary valve close after the aortic valve. In healthy adults, one may hear only two heart sounds. Sometimes with children, a third heart sound can be heard during the phase of the ventricles relaxing and filling. It is thought that the tensing of the chordae tendineae causes this sound. Finally, in the elderly, another heart sound sometimes might be heard during atrial contraction, when the ventricular walls vibrate. The purpose of taking deep breaths while a practitioner listens to heart sounds is an important part of a physical exam because abnormal conduction blocks might be heard. **Table 3-2** shows four possible heart sounds.

Table 3-2 Heart Sounds

Normal Adult		
Sound	**Cardiac Phase**	**Cause**
1	Early ventricular systole	Closure of atrioventricular valves
		Mitral valve closes before tricuspid valve
2	Late ventricular systole	Closure of semilunar valves
		Aortic valve closes before pulmonary valve
Additional sounds that might be heard in:		
Children		**Possible Cause**
3	Ventricular diastole	Tensing of the chordae tendineae
Elderly		
4	Atrial systole	Ventricular wall vibration

Cardiac Cycle

The cardiac cycle begins in Phase 1 with atrial systole. This is a short, approximately 1-second period of time after the blood has been received in the atria, when the atrioventricular valves open and blood is dumped into the ventricles. In normally functioning hearts, approximately 70–85 percent of the blood leaving the atria is dumped freely into the ventricles. The atria contraction increases atrial pressure and forces about 10 percent of the remaining blood into the ventricles before the atrioventricular valves close. Atrial blood pressure is greatest just before the atrial contraction. If a person has a high heart rate, as much as 40 percent of the blood from the atria may be forced into the ventricles with an atrial contraction. During the remainder of the cardiac cycle, the atria are in atrial diastole. The first phase of the cardiac cycle is also ventricular preload and ventricular depolarization.

The second phase of the cardiac cycle is called ventricular systole and occurs over a period of approximately 2.8 seconds. No blood enters the ventricles during Phase 2, and all valves are closed so that ventricular pressure can build in preparation of ventricular ejection. As the tension increases in the ventricles, it is important to realize that in a normal heart, when the atria are in a systole phase, the ventricles are in a diastole phase; and likewise, when the atria are in diastole, the ventricles are in systole. In **Figure 3-7**, the overlap between systole and diastole in the atria, and the ventricles is shown in one cardiac cycle. The entire cardiac cycle typically takes only a total of 8 seconds, so Figure 3-7 also identifies the number of seconds to show approximately how much time the heart is contracting in comparison to how much time the heart should be at rest. Notice that ventricular systole is approximately 2.8 seconds per cardiac cycle, while ventricular diastole is about double that time (typically 5.2 seconds per cardiac cycle). Also, atrial systole is very short, at approximately 1 second.

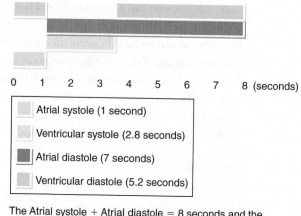

0   1   2   3   4   5   6   7   8 (seconds)

Atrial systole (1 second)

Ventricular systole (2.8 seconds)

Atrial diastole (7 seconds)

Ventricular diastole (5.2 seconds)

The Atrial systole + Atrial diastole = 8 seconds and the Ventricular systole + Ventricular diastole = 8 seconds. However, the diastolic (resting) stage is significantly longer than the systolic (contraction) stage in both heart chambers.

Figure 3-7 One cardiac cycle = approximately 8 seconds

Quick Check 3-4

Fill in the blanks.

1. Blood is ejected from the left ventricle during the contraction phase of the cardiac cycle called _____.

2. During the heart's _____ phase, the term end diastolic volume refers to a time when the _____ventricle is filled to capacity.

3. The actual _____ phase when blood is dumped from the atria into the ventricles is called _____ or late ventricular _____.

4. When a healthy person _____, the health practitioner is listening for the pulmonary valve to close after the aortic valve.

5. No blood enters the ventricles in the _____ stage of the cardiac cycle, which is called _____ systole.

Cardiac Output

atrial kick
An atrial contraction that forces the remaining blood (not previously drained from the atria to the ventricles) to enter the ventricles before the atrioventricular (AV) valves close.

Approximately 70–80 percent of blood flows passively from the atria to the ventricles. The remaining blood is normally forced into the ventricles through a process called **atrial kick** (a contraction). In the process of atrial kick, an atrial contraction causes the remaining blood that did not passively drain to be emptied into the ventricles before the atrioventricular valves close. Both the contraction and relaxation phases of the heart must complete a full cycle properly or blood circulation will be compromised. For example, if the diastolic phase, which allows the heart to rest, is too short, then the atria may not fill completely and the ventricles will not have time to rest between contractions. In addition, the ventricles may not produce a high enough cardiac output, defined as the amount of blood that the heart pumps in 1 minute. Cardiac output varies based on what is happening in the external environment of the body. For example, if a person is at rest or sleeping, the cardiac output is normally as little as 5 liters per minute. Recall from Chapter 2 that when the heart is at rest, the parasympathetic nerve fibers release acetylcholine, which then slows the heart rate. Also, as mentioned previously, the typical heart rate in an adult ranges from 60–100 beats per minute. Heart rate can be measured by taking a person's pulse for 1 minute. The pulse rate measures cardiovascular activity and can be taken by compressing an artery against a bone, such as in the neck (carotid artery) or at the wrist (radial artery). A second way that the heart rate can be measured is through auscultation (listening) to the heart directly through a stethoscope.

If a person is participating in strenuous exercising, cardiac output will increase and can increase normal output up to 35 liters of blood per minute. Increased heart rate occurs when the sympathetic nerve fibers release epinephrine. Not having enough cardiac output can attribute to hypertension, and be a sign of congestive heart failure (CHF), shock, or a myocardial infarction. Tachycardia can also cause low cardiac output.

Stroke Volume

stroke volume
The amount of blood ejected by the ventricles with each contraction.

Cardiac output can be measured by multiplying the heart rate by the **stroke volume**. Stroke volume is defined as the amount of blood ejected by the ventricles with each contraction. The normal adult will have a stroke volume of approximately 70 mL per heartbeat. The stroke volume can be determined by subtracting the normal end systolic volume (which is approximately 50 mL) from the normal end diastolic volume (which is approximately 120 mL). The more blood that can fill the ventricles in one atrial contraction, the greater the stroke volume.

To determine a patient's cardiac output, use the formula

cardiac output = heart rate × stroke volume

Box 3-1 highlights this formula. Each term can be abbreviated as follows: cardiac output = CO; heart rate = HR; and stroke volume = SV.

Box 3-1 Cardiac Output Formula

Cardiac Output = Heart Rate × Stroke Volume

Practice computing cardiac output. Using the formula, determine the cardiac output for a patient who has a heart rate of 66 bpm with a normal stroke volume of 70 mL.

Applying the Formula:

> CO = HR * SV
> CO = 66 * 70
> CO = 4,620 mL per minute

Cardiac output equals 4,620 mL per minute. Recall that 1,000 milliliters = 1 liter (L), so the answer is 4.6 L per minute. The normal range of cardiac output per minute is between 4 and 8 L of blood per minute, so this patient would have a cardiac output within normal limits.

In a second example, the person had just finished strenuous exercising and had a pulse rate of 120 bpm. If the person had a normal stroke volume of 70 mL/beat, would you expect that they would be within normal limits for cardiac output?

Do the math and use the same formula:

$$HR \times SV = CO$$
$$120 \times 70 = CO$$
$$CO = 8{,}400 \text{ mL per minute}$$

Convert milliliters to liters; the answer is 8.4 L per minute, so yes, they are within the upper limits of normal. Notice that when either stroke volume or heart rate increases, cardiac output increases. The reverse is also true.

In the third example, a person has been sleeping for the past 8 hours. He has a resting pulse of 56 bpm and a stroke volume of 60mL/beat. Compute the cardiac output.

Solution:

$$CO = HR * SV$$
$$CO = 56 * 60$$
$$CO = 3{,}360 \text{ mL/minute or } 3.36 \text{ L per minute.}$$

preload
At the end of diastole, the amount of blood in the left ventricle and the pressure used to stretch the muscle fibers.

afterload
A force that interferes with systemic blood flow from the left ventricle, caused primarily by atrial vascular resistance.

This rate is too low. Stroke volume can be affected by cardiac muscle pressure or lack of pressure. To maintain a cardiac output within normal range, the following factors must be as balanced as possible. At the end of diastole, the amount of blood volume in the left ventricle and the pressure used to stretch the muscle fibers determine the next cardiac cycle's **preload**. In other words, preload is directly affected by the amount of blood that returns to the right atrium, which increases or decreases with changes in volume. Next, the amount of resistance that the heart must use to pump the blood through the cardiovascular system, called **afterload**, is important because the more arterial resistance there is, the harder the heart usually has to work. Afterload affects stroke volume and cardiac output, which will be discussed in the next sections.

Quick Check 3-5

Fill in the blanks.

1. External environment affects _____, which is measured by the formula: _____.

2. Exercise causes the sympathetic nerve fibers to release _____, which then _____ the heart rate.

3. The parasympathetic nerve fibers release _____, which then slows the heart rate.

4. Determine the cardiac output when the heart rate is 80 bpm and the stroke volume is 65 mL.

   Answer in milliliters: _____

   Is the answer within normal limits? _____

5. Determine the cardiac output when the heart rate is 88 bpm and the stroke volume is 78 mL.

   Answer in milliliters: _____

   Is the answer within normal limits? _____

Peripheral Vascular Resistance

Resistance can be measured by obtaining a blood pressure reading. The blood pressure measurement records **peripheral vascular resistance**. Vasoconstriction and vasodilatation determine peripheral vascular resistance.

peripheral vascular resistance
Arterial opposition to blood flow; can be measured by a blood pressure reading.

Blood Pressure

Blood pressure can be determined not only by the strength of a contraction or tension placed on the walls of the arteries, but also by the resistance of the arterioles and capillaries, blood volume, and the elasticity of blood vessels. Systolic blood pressure reflects the highest resistance or maximum pressure when the heart contracts. Systolic pressure occurs during the depolarization phase. A second number is called the diastolic blood pressure, which measures the amount of pressure in the arteries between contractions and occurs during the polarization phase. Blood pressure is written like a fraction, with systolic pressure as the numerator (above the line), and the diastolic pressure as the denominator (below the line). Blood pressure can be computed by multiplying cardiac output by peripheral vascular resistance. Box 3-2 highlights the formula. Each term can be abbreviated as follows: blood pressure = BP; cardiac output = CO; and peripheral vascular resistance = PVR. Blood pressure is measured in units of millimeters of mercury (mm Hg) but the units are rarely recorded, just the systolic/diastolic pressure.

> **Box 3-2 Blood Pressure Formula**
>
> Blood Pressure = Cardiac Output × Peripheral Vascular Resistance

Although the above formula will compute blood pressure, use of the blood pressure cuff and a stethoscope are standard tools used to take a persons' blood pressure so the formula above is for reference purposes to help further your understanding of the concept of blood pressure.

Blood pressure will change when there is a change in either cardiac output or in peripheral vascular resistance, or when both CO and PVR change. Normal systolic blood pressure ranges between 110 and 120 mm Hg, and the diastolic blood pressure normal range is 70–80 mm Hg. Systolic pressure has been more strongly correlated with cardiovascular events. Much more information on blood pressure and the different ranges will be presented in several chapters throughout this book. Modest variances in blood pressure can be indications that the heart muscle is not performing at its peak level and the body may not be in homeostasis. Blood pressure provides a snapshot of a person's blood flow at one particular moment in time, so the reading is repeated regularly depending on the previous reading or health indications. Blood pressure is a standard procedure to record whenever a practitioner is treating a person.

Pulse Pressure

Pulse pressure is a good indicator of cardiac output and is a stronger predictor of coronary events than blood pressure alone. Recall that a person's pulse rate can be measured to determine heart rate, but **pulse pressure** is determined by the change in blood pressure when the heart contracts. However, there is not a direct correlation between pulse rate and blood pressure. In other words, increasing your heart rate—say, by exercising—will not increase blood pressure by the same amount of increase in pulse rate. Therefore, ideally blood pressure

pulse pressure
The difference between the diastolic blood pressure and the systolic blood pressure.

should be taken when a person is relaxed because a healthy person who has just finished exercising may have an increased pulse pressure but not have any medical problems.

Pulse pressure is measured like blood pressure in mm Hg. To calculate pulse pressure, subtract the diastolic blood pressure from the systolic blood pressure. For example, if the blood pressure is 120/80, the pulse pressure is 40. (The systolic number is 120, the diastolic number is 80, and 120 − 80 = 40.) Box 3-3 highlights the pulse pressure formula. Usually, no abbreviations are used for the diastolic or systolic part of the formula, but PP can be used to stand for pulse pressure.

Box 3-3 Pulse Pressure Formula

Systolic Blood Pressure
− Diastolic Blood Pressure
Pulse Pressure

Practice computing pulse pressure if the person's blood pressure measures 160/100.

Solution:

$$\begin{array}{r} 160 \\ -\ 100 \\ \hline 60 \end{array}$$

The pulse pressure is 60 mm Hg, which is considered high. A normal, healthy pulse pressure should be in the range of 40 mm Hg but less than 60 mm Hg. Consistent pulse pressure higher than 40 mm Hg may indicate damage to heart vessels (especially the aorta) and may be an indication of atherosclerosis, anemia, aortic dissection, chronic aortic regurgitation, heart block, endocarditis, or many other health issues. This is especially true in older adults who present with pulse pressures at 60 mm Hg or more. Successfully treating a person for hypertension will sometimes keep pulse pressure within normal guidelines if permanent damage has not already occurred.

Low pulse pressure is also dangerous. Pulse pressure is considered abnormally low if the PP number is less than 25 percent of the systolic value. A drop in left ventricular stroke volume or significant blood loss may provide abnormally low pulse pressures. In addition, blood pressure medications may decrease the diastolic blood pressure too much, resulting in reduced pulse pressure.

Pulse pressure is like blood pressure; it needs to be taken over a period of time to establish a person's typical range. Abnormal pulse pressure is an important risk factor for heart disease evaluation.

Contractility

The third factor is contractility. As explained earlier in the chapter, contractility is the ability of the heart's muscle cells to return to normal after being stretched through a contraction. The heart is often viewed as a "demand pump" because the amount of blood that is returned to the right atrium directly influences the amount of blood that can then be ejected from the

Starling's Law of the Heart
The degree of the stretch of the heart muscle; is directly related to the force of the blood being ejected from the ventricles.

left ventricle with the next contraction. **Starling's Law of the Heart** is a theory of muscle contraction stating that the degree of the stretching of the heart muscle directly relates to the force of the blood being ejected from the ventricles.

Blood vessels can increase or decrease the resistance to blood flow. Increases in blood flow are usually attributed to an increase in heart rate; however, when the cardiac muscles are overstretched in diastole, they will contract more forcefully in systole. Cardiovascular diseases, hypertension, and heart failure can all determine peripheral vascular resistance.

Quick Check 3-6

Fill in the blanks.

1. Vasoconstriction and vasodilation determine _____ vascular resistance.

2. Systolic blood pressure reflects the highest _____ or _____ of a heart contraction.

3. Diastolic pressure measures the heart at _____ during the _____ phase.

4. Calculate pulse pressure when blood pressure is 142/88.

   Answer: _____ mm Hg.

   Is this within normal limits? _____

5. A blood pressure is recorded at 92/74, so the pulse pressure is less than 25 percent of the systolic pressure. This may occur with a drop in left ventricular stroke volume or with significant _____.

ELECTRICAL CONDUCTION

This section identifies the normal path that an electrical current takes through the heart. The example that follows is how a normal human heart conducts electricity.

Sinoatrial (SA) Node

The pathway begins in the upper posterior wall of the right atrium, where the sinoatrial (SA) node can be found. Pacemaker cells become excited and polarity begins to change. With the polarity changing, an electrical impulse begins to move from the SA node anteriorly, posteriorly, and centrally through the right and left atria via the internodal pathways. The function of the SA node is to start the electrical impulse, which will cause the heart to contract—first in the atria, then in the ventricles at the end of the electrical path. The SA node is considered the heart's primary pacemaker because of two distinct features. First, the location of the SA node is at the highest point in the heart's electrical pathway. Second, the intrinsic firing rate (generating electrical impulses) is the fastest, at 60–100 bpm in a normal heart.

internodal pathways
Four pathways that provide a route for electrical impulses to travel; three pathways travel from the sinoatrial (SA) node to the atrioventricular (AV) node, and the fourth path carries the impulse from the SA node to the left atrium.

Internodal Pathways

The **internodal pathways** provide four paths for the electrical impulses to follow when leaving the SA node. Three paths flow through the right atrium posteriorly, anteriorly, and medially and lead from the SA node to the atrioventricular (AV) node. The fourth path leaves the SA node and allows the electrical impulse to travel into the left atrium. In addition to providing pathways, the purpose of the internodal pathways is to slow the impulse as the depolarization spreads throughout the atria. Three of the pathways are named for the doctors who first described them. The first and most familiar pathway, which is a subdivision of the anterior nodal pathway and is the electrical impulse that travels to the left atrium, is called Bachmann's bundle. The second pathway is known as Wenchebach's bundle; it leaves the SA node and sends the impulse through the middle of the SA node toward the AV node. The least recognized internodal path is called Thorel's pathway; it leaves the SA node and travels through the right atrial muscle posteriorly toward the AV node.

AV Node

The location of the atrioventricular (AV) node is on the floor of the right atrium near the junction of the atrium and ventricle (AV junction), also near the opening of the coronary sinus, and just above the tricuspid valve. The function of the AV node is to accept and slow the electrical impulse from the SA node so that the atrium can contract and empty blood into the ventricles (atrial systole) before the impulse continues on the path to creating ventricular contractions. The AV node is considered the secondary pacemaker of the heart because if the SA node fails to provide an electrical impulse for any reason, the AV junction pacemaker cells will assume the role of creating an impulse by changing polarity. Two distinct features of the AV node are that it is the second-highest point in the heart's electrical pathway, and the intrinsic firing rate has slowed the depolarization of cells to between 40 and 60 bpm. In addition, it is in the AV junction that the network of muscle fibers that will cause a contraction of the ventricles are located.

Bundle of His

bundle of His
An electrical conduction pathway that connects the upper and lower chambers of the heart.

The electrical pathway continues to the **bundle of His**, which lies at the top of the interventricular septum and eventually splits into a right and left bundle branch before continuing into the ventricles. Just like the internodal pathways, the bundle of His is named after a person: Dr. Wilhelm His, because he first described this conduction pathway. The purpose of the bundle of His is to act as a passageway between the upper and lower chambers of the heart. The bundle of His does not actually contain pacemaker cells, but the junctional muscle tissue surrounding the bundle of His does, so there is an intrinsic firing rate of 40–60 bpm in this area.

Bundle Branches

bundle branches
Two electrical conduction pathways that send impulses to the ventricles by connecting the bundle of His to the Purkinje network.

As mentioned in the previous section, the **bundle branches** split into two main branches with the purpose of transferring the electrical impulse down to the Purkinje network, where the ventricles can then contract. The location of the bundle branches is lateral and posterior, and then through the respective right and left ventricles. The left bundle branch divides to send impulses to the anterior and posterior walls of the left ventricle. As the depolarized impulses move toward the apex of the heart, both bundle branches end in the Purkinje network.

Purkinje Network

Purkinje network
A group of network fibers that serve as the third pacemaker of the heart, generates electrical impulses at a rate of 20–40 bpm.

The **Purkinje network** is made of a conduction network of fibers called Purkinje fibers. The fibers carry the electrical impulses directly to the ventricular muscle walls. Through these fibers, the ventricles are capable of serving as a backup pacemaker for the heart, but the intrinsic firing rate is slowest of all heart pacemaker cells (at 20–40 bpm). Depolarized cells cause the ventricles to contract simultaneously. **Figure 3-8** shows the location of the heart electrical conduction system.

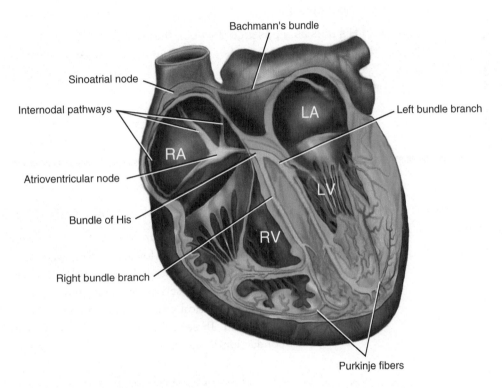

Figure 3-8 Heart electrical conduction system

Analysis of Electrical Conduction

Recall that the intrinsic firing rate is always fastest closer to the base of the heart and continues to slow down as the impulse moves closer to the apex of the heart. Normal intrinsic firing ranges are summarized in **Table 3-3**. When the heart does not conduct electricity normally, the pacemaker cells will try three times, in different positions along the conduction path, to create an impulse.

Table 3-3 Pacemaker Firing Ranges

Firing Order	Location	Speed
First	Sinoatrial (SA) node	60–100 bpm
Second	Atrioventricular (AV) node	40–60 bpm
Third	Purkinje fibers	20–40 bpm

bpm = beats per minute

Quick Check 3-7

Fill in the blanks.

1. The sinoatrial node is considered the heart's primary pacemaker because it is the _____ in the heart's electrical pathway and has an intrinsic firing rate of 60–100 bpm.

2. The _____ node is located near the opening of the coronary sinus, just above the tricuspid valve, and has an intrinsic firing rate of _____ bpm.

3. The bundle of His acts as a passage between the upper and lower chambers of the heart. Even though it does not actually contain pacemaker cells, it creates an intrinsic firing range of _____ bpm.

4. Through the _____, the heart has a final pacemaker that fires at a rate of _____ bpm directly through the ventricular walls.

5. Intrinsic firing rates are fastest when closest to the _____ of the heart and slowest near the _____ of the heart.

ABNORMAL CONDUCTION ISSUES

Cardiac conduction problems can be of a structural or functional nature. Structural issues include problems with impulse formation, propagation, synchronization, or blockage. The functional malfunctions may occur during depolarization, repolarization, or polarization. It is the conduction system that sets the proper heart rate based on the body's demand for oxygen. In addition, if the electrical system is not working correctly, the heart is unable to maintain the correct rhythm. Three of the more common ways that the heart responds to abnormal cardiac conduction are by abnormal automaticity, ectopic beats, and impulse reentry cycles.

Abnormal Automaticity

Recall that automaticity is the spontaneous creation of electricity by specific myocardial cells. All cardiac cells can create an electrical impulse, but only some of them are specifically designed to create the impulse. Those cells are located in the SA node, AV node, bundle of His, and Purkinje fibers. If cells in other areas of the heart create electrical impulses, one effect is premature heartbeats, which can then cause instability of the myocardial cell membrane. Another effect can be a conduction delay or conduction blocks. Conduction delays and blocks can cause the heart to beat slower the farther the block is from the SA node. The most significant blocks occur in the ventricles because the block prevents blood flow, which then puts additional stress on the heart. Increased automaticity may also be caused by sympathetic nervous system conditions or hypoxia (low oxygen levels).

Ectopic Beats

Ectopic events occur because an electrical impulse is being created in a region of the heart other than at the SA node, thereby affecting cardiac rhythm. Ventricular escape beats and junctional escape beats are the most common types of ectopic beats. The ectopic beat can occur occasionally, occur consistently, occur more often than the SA intrinsic firing, or even be absent altogether. Occasionally occurring ectopic fluctuations are common in adults and are not of major clinical significance. They tend to occur more frequently as a person ages.

If the ectopic focus fires more often than the SA node, the rhythm can produce sustained poorly coordinated contractions and can become a pathogenic situation. Ectopic beats may be caused by electrolyte imbalance or by a decreased blood supply to the heart and can be agitated by stress, alcohol consumption, smoking, or use of illicit drugs. Premature heart beats are classified as either premature atrial contractions or premature ventricular contractions. Rhythm variations are most often classified as dysrhythmias (abnormal rhythms), arrhythmias (irregular or lost rhythms in time or force), or extrasystole (premature rhythms).

Impulse Reentry Cycles

In normal conduction, an action potential impulse will travel through the atrium into the ventricles and into the Purkinje fibers very quickly to create one contraction. Impulses can travel on two parallel paths, each of which has beginning and ending connection pathways and different refractory periods, which allow an electrical circuit to be completed when the impulses reach the ending connection point. However, sometimes the refractory period becomes delayed, slowing conduction, and a new impulse will attempt to enter one of the pathways before the depolarization process is complete in that path. This causes timing errors because the additional impulse cannot be conducted, so the impulse can be reexcited and will "cycle," or create a loop through the unblocked or depolarized path. Depending on the location of the timing error, the abnormal circuit rhythm can lead to atrial flutter, fibrillation, and supraventricular or ventricular tachycardia. A different problem, called triggered beats or triggered activity, can occur when ion channels in individual cardiac cells abnormally propagate, creating an abnormal rhythm due to repetitive ectopic firings that lead to spontaneous or secondary depolarization. Triggered events can be an undesirable side effect of antiarrhythmic drugs, hypokalemia, or hypercalcemia.

Heart conduction problems may cause a cerebral vascular accident, congenital heart failure, coronary artery disease, endocarditis, a myocardial infarction, or sudden death syndrome. Abnormal conduction issues are introduced in Chapter 3 to bring a connection to the topics of myocardial cell functions, electrolyte polarity changes, and electrical conduction and are topics covered further in the advanced study of cardiac arrhythmias.

Quick Check 3-8

Fill in the blanks.

1. Cardiac conduction problems are classified as either _____ or _____ in nature.

2. It is the conduction system that sets the proper heart _____ based upon the body's demand for _____.

3. Three issues of concern that can occur when heart cells outside the normal conduction paths create electrical impulses include premature heartbeats, conduction _____, or conduction _____.

4. Cardiac rhythm disturbances, known as _____, occur when the electrical impulse does not begin in the SA node.

5. Timing errors caused by multiple electrical impulses creating triggered events can cause an abnormal _____ which may further lead to spontaneous or secondary _____.

SUMMARY

- Four specialized characteristics of myocardial cells are automaticity, excitability, conductivity, and contractility.

- Contractility is a mechanical function, whereas the other three myocardial characteristics create an electrical impulse.

- Electrolytes move between the intracellular and extracellular fluids and permeate the cell membrane, causing action potential.

- A myocardial cell in resting state has a negative polarity intracellularly and a positive polarity extracellularly.

- The major heart electrolytes include sodium, potassium, calcium, and magnesium.

- Sodium, potassium, and calcium ions cause the cells to go through the process of action potential with every contraction.

- Every myocyte experiences three electrical changes called polarization, depolarization, and repolarization in order to cause the contraction and relaxation of heart muscles.

- Polarization is synonymous with the myocyte at rest.

- Depolarization occurs with action potential.

- Repolarization is synonymous with the resting and recovery period of the heart muscle.

- There are five phases in the process of a single contraction and relaxation of the cardiac cell. The process begins in Phase 4, when the cell is at rest.

- Phase 0 is the depolarization state where sodium quickly rushes into the cell, causing action potential.

- In Phase 1, called early repolarization, the sodium channels close and calcium begins to enter the cell while potassium moves out of the cell.

- Phase 2, called the plateau phase, is a continuation of the depolarization state, a period of time when the calcium and potassium ions continue moving in and out of the cell membrane until, toward the middle of the phase, sodium channels reopen.

- In Phase 3, potassium rushes back into the cell, sodium and calcium return to the outside of the cell, and the cell begins to go back into original polarity and back into Phase 4 (resting).

- During the repolarization phases, the cells go through a refractory period where they cannot respond to any additional stimuli.

- The entire process of a contraction, relaxation, and resting occurs in approximately 8 seconds and is called one cardiac cycle.

- The cardiac cycle corresponds with one heartbeat in a process called diastole and systole. Diastole is where blood is filling the atria and the heart is in a relaxed state.

- Systole is the contraction phase, which results in blood systemically nourishing the body's cells with nutrients and oxygen.

- Cardiac output measures how much blood the heart is pumping in a minute and is measured by taking a person's pulse to determine heart rate multiplied by stroke volume, which is the amount of blood ejected by the ventricles in one contraction.

- Blood pressure measures the highest systolic resistance during the repolarization phase with the diastolic or resting vascular resistance.

- The electrical conduction path begins with an impulse in the sinoatrial (SA) node continuing through the internodal pathways to the atrioventricular (AV) node, continuing through the bundle of His and bundle branches, and the Purkinje network of fibers before concluding with a ventricular contraction.

- The heart responds to abnormal cardiac conduction through abnormal automaticity, ectopic beats, and impulse reentry cycles.

Critical Thinking Challenges

3-1. Draw a picture showing three cells, one representing each stage of the cardiac cell's cycle. For each cell, label the stage, the cell membrane, the intercellular ions and their charges, and the extracellular ions and their charges.

3-2. Heart Conduction Directions:

Part 1: On the heart, draw a line to each conduction location (you should have at least six locations identified).

Part 2: Name each conduction location—do not use abbreviations.

Part 3: Using six different colored pencils, completely color each conduction area.

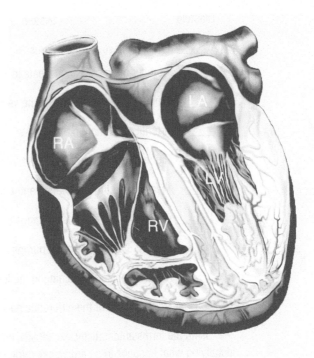

Figure 3-9

3-3. Fill in the blanks in the following paragraph. Try to complete the paragraph without referring back to the chapter.

A change in the electrical polarity of a cardiac cell is called _____. Ions move through the _____ when they become excited. When cardiac cells are resting they are in a(n) _____ state. The cells become excited when _____ rushes _____.

This action is called _____ and lasts less than a second. _____ moves into the cell while _____ moves out, and this action provides a wave of electricity, which causes the heart muscle to _____ contract. Toward the middle of the _____ phase, _____ channels reopen and the cell begins to return to original polarity. It is during the _____ phases that the cell cannot receive any additional stimuli. This period is called the _____ period.

Review Activities

3-1. Match the correct term with the definitions given. Use each term once; not all terms will be used.

A. Automaticity

B. Blood pressure

C. Cardiac cycle

D. Cardiac output

E. Conductivity

F. Depolarization

G. Diastole

H. End diastolic volume

I. End systolic volume

J. Heart rate

K. Peripheral vascular resistance

L. Pulse pressure

M. Stroke volume

N. Systole

1. _____ Resting phase of a heart muscle

2. _____ Number of times a heart beats in 1 minute

3. _____ Amount of blood ejected by the ventricles with each contraction

4. _____ Arterial opposition to blood flow

5. _____ Highest resistance or maximum pressure of blood vessels when heart contracts

6. _____ Measured in time between ventricular contraction to ventricular relaxation

7. _____ Changes when there is a change in cardiac output or peripheral vascular resistance

8. _____ Amount of blood the heart pumps in 1 minute systemically

9. _____ Amount of blood remaining in the left ventricle after a contraction

10. _____ Measurement of the difference between diastolic and systolic blood pressure

3-2. Using the terms automaticity, excitability, conductivity, and contractility, create a chart identifying what happens to a cardiac cell during one cardiac cycle. Be sure to include whether the function of the cell is an electrical or mechanical function.

3-3. Fill in the chart with the letters A–E by choosing the best response to this question: In what direction and speed are the electrolytes moving through the cardiac cell's membrane during action potential?

Hint: Answer each action potential independently. You will repeat choices A–E.

A. Rushing In

B. Movement In

C. Channel Closed

D. Rushing Out

E. Movement Out

F. Channel Open

Action Potential	Minerals		
Phase	Calcium	Potassium	Sodium
0	_____	_____	_____
1	_____	_____	_____
2	_____	_____	_____
3	_____	_____	_____
4	_____	_____	_____

Chapter Three Test

Match the term with its description. Each letter will be used only one time.

1. _____ Starling's Law of the Heart

2. _____ SA node

3. _____ Repolarization

4. _____ Diastole

5. _____ Resting membrane potential

6. _____ Stroke volume

7. _____ Cardiac output

8. _____ Depolarization state

9. _____ Atrial kick

10. _____ Automaticity

11. _____ Contractility

12. _____ Afterload

A. Small particles that carry a positive or negative electrical charge

B. Heart is at rest

C. Creation of spontaneous electrical impulses

D. Resistance needed to pump blood throughout cardiovascular system

E. Intrinsic firing rate of 60–100 bpm

F. Amount of blood that heart pumps in 1 minute through cardiovascular system

G. Atrial contraction that contributes 20–30 percent of cardiac output

H. Amount of blood that leaves ventricles with each contraction

I. Uses a sodium–potassium pump to help myocytes return to resting state

J. Mechanical function of myocardial cell

K. Number of times the heart beats in 1 minute

L. Extracellular carries positive charge; intracellular carries negative charge

13. _____ Heart rate

14. _____ Systole

15. _____ Electrolytes

M. Potassium rapidly moves outside of myocyte and carries a positive charge, while sodium and calcium move into the cell

N. Contractions of the heart that causes the heart valves to open and close

O. The degree of stretch of the heart muscle directly relates to the force of the blood being ejected from the ventricles

Chapter Three Quick Check Answers

Answer order is important except where noted otherwise in parentheses.

When two correct answers are possible, both answers are given separated by the word "or."

3-1:

1. muscle contraction, relaxing
2. Pacemaker, generate
3. automaticity, contractility
4. 60–100, 8
5. negative

3-2:

1. sodium, drink
2. potassium, contractions
3. calcium, sodium (either order)
4. magnesium, low
5. negative, rest

3-3:

1. sodium, potassium
2. voltage, time (either order)
3. prematurely
4. polarization, depolarization, repolarization (any order)
5. absolute, stimuli

3-4:

1. systole
2. relaxation, left
3. contraction, atrial systole, diastole
4. inhales
5. second, ventricular

3-5:

1. cardiac output, CO = HR × SV or cardiac output = heart rate × stroke volume
2. epinephrine, increases
3. acetylcholine

4. CO is 80 × 65 = 5,200 mL = 5. 2 L per minute; yes, normal limit is 4–8 L per minute

5. CO is 88 × 78 = 6,864 mL = 6.8 or can be rounded to 6.9 L per minute; yes

3-6:

1. peripheral

2. resistance, maximum pressure

3. rest, polarization

4. PP is 142 − 88 = 54 mm Hg; yes normal average limits is 40 mm Hg

5. blood loss

3-7:

1. highest point

2. atrioventricular or AV, 40–60

3. 40–60

4. Purkinje fibers, 20–40

5. base, apex

3-8:

1. structural, functional (either order)

2. rate, oxygen

3. delay, blocks

4. ectopic events

5. rhythm, depolarization

CARDIOVASCULAR MEDICATIONS

4

OBJECTIVES

After reading the chapter and completing all Quick Check activities, the student should be able to:

1. Explain the difference between primary and secondary prevention drugs.
2. List five categories of cardiac medications.
3. Explain the function of the angiotensin hormone.
4. List three major classifications of arrhythmia.
5. Identify the long-term goals for beta blocker drugs.
6. Identify the purpose of antihyperlipidemic drug therapy.
7. Explain the difference between antiplatelet and anticoagulant agents.
8. List three types of potential drug interactions with prescribed medications.
9. Identify three ways that patients can take ownership of their heart health.

KEY TERMS

angina

angiotensin

antianginal

antiarrhythmic

antihyperlipidemic

antihypertensive

arrhythmia

antithrombotic

bioavailability

cardiomegaly

dysrhythmia

fibrillation

fibrin

heart disease

heart failure

hypertrophy

pharmacodynamics

pharmacokinetics

pharmacogenetics

platelets

premature atrial complex (PAC)

premature ventricular complex (PVC)

primary prevention drug

rhabdomyolysis

secondary prevention drug

sinus bradycardia

sinus tachycardia

supraventricular

syncope

thrombosis

thrombus

vasodilators

INTRODUCTION

On the list of the top 200 selling drugs for 2014, approximately 25 percent were medications prescribed for people experiencing some type of cardiovascular issue. This chapter introduces medications that would be typically prescribed to cardiovascular patients. Throughout this chapter, the generic brand is always listed first, with brand names following in parentheses. Also in this chapter, many broad categories of cardiovascular medications will be explained. Drug actions and interactions will be introduced. The specific cardiac drugs most commonly prescribed according to the American Heart Association will be identified, with the generic name, brand name, classification, dosage information, and potential adverse cardiac effects given in a table format. The chapter will conclude with cardiac drug interaction information.

MAJOR PURPOSES OF CARDIAC MEDICATIONS

primary prevention drug
A drug prescribed before a cardiovascular event, such as before a stroke or myocardial infarction (MI).

Drug therapy can help patients in two major ways. **Primary prevention drugs** are prescribed before a cardiovascular event, such as a stroke or myocardial infarction, happens. The health care provider will determine if a person is at risk for heart issues based on blood testing, blood pressure, lifestyle, and other factors and will determine whether to prescribe medications, encourage lifestyle and diet changes, encourage a moderate exercise routine, or a combination of actions. Through patient education and early medicinal therapy, some people are able to improve their quality of life and ward off a major cardiovascular event. Other people do not seek medical intervention until after symptoms of heart disease, pain, or a cardiovascular event has occurred. People under this category will be prescribed **secondary prevention drug** therapy. The purpose of drugs in the secondary prevention group is to limit the disease from further damage or progress or to reduce symptoms.

secondary prevention drug
A drug prescribed to limit heart disease from further damaging the heart or to reduce the symptoms.

There are five broad categories of cardiovascular medications that can be identified further by the purpose of the drugs within the categories. Many cardiac medications do not fit into only one category and may be prescribed for different purposes. The first major category of drugs includes those that will change blood pressure. The second broad category of cardiac medications includes drugs prescribed to address blood clotting issues. A third major effect of cardiac medications changes the rate or rhythm of the heart. A fourth major category is utilized to reduce chest pain, and the fifth major category addresses medications used to lower blood cholesterol.

CARDIAC MEDICATIONS PRESCRIBED TO CHANGE BLOOD PRESSURE

Recall that the purpose of the blood is to carry oxygen, nutrients, and waste products throughout the body. The effectiveness of how the blood accomplishes these tasks is directly related to the heart because the heart is the "pump" that moves the blood. How well the blood is being pumped throughout the body can be measured in several ways, the least invasive being by a blood pressure measurement. Patients with blood pressure problems usually have high blood pressure, known as hypertension. These patients are usually prescribed drugs called **antihypertensive** agents, or drugs used to lower blood pressure. Every patient should have his or her blood pressure recorded during every visit. Cardiac medications used to modify the blood pressure can be classed into any of five categories: angiotensin converting enzyme (ACE) inhibitors, angiotensin II receptor blockers (ARBs), beta blockers, calcium channel blocker (CCBs), and diuretics.

antihypertensive
A category of drugs used to lower blood pressure.

Cardiac Medications That Modify Blood Pressure

- Angiotensin converting enzyme (ACE) inhibitors
- Angiotensin II receptor blockers (ARB)
- Beta blockers
- Calcium channel blocker (CCB)
- Diuretics

Angiotensin Hormone

angiotensin
A hormone created in the liver as a protein responsible for regulating sodium and water balance in the body.

ACE inhibitors and ARBs are directly affected by a hormone called **angiotensin**, which is responsible for regulating sodium and water balance in the body. This hormone begins in the liver as a protein called angiotensinogen, which then moves through the bloodstream and is broken up in the kidneys by an enzyme called renin, forming angiotensin I. As the hormone continues the loop through the body, further metabolism in the lungs produces angiotensin II, which binds to receptors in the blood vessels, causing the blood vessels to constrict. The constricted blood vessels also cause platelets to aggregate, thus raising blood pressure and causing the heart to work harder to move the blood. Angiotensin II also affects other body systems. For example, too much of this hormone affects the kidneys by causing sodium retention and increases water reabsorption, resulting in increased blood volume, which also can cause an increase in blood pressure. Angiotensin II stimulates the adrenal glands to produce aldosterone, which causes the body to retain sodium but lose potassium during urination. The angiotensin II protein also encourages the release of noradrenaline from the sympathetic nerves. Too little of the angiotensin hormone can cause problems such as low blood pressure and retention of potassium or loss of too much sodium through increased urination.

Angiotensin Converting Enzyme (ACE) Inhibitors

ACE inhibitors are intended to work by expanding the blood vessels and preventing angiotensin II to form on the blood vessels. The relaxed blood vessels should reduce blood pressure by allowing the blood to flow from the heart with reduced resistance. The reduced resistance allows the heart to work more efficiently. ACE inhibitor drug therapy can also reduce **hypertrophy**, thickening of the heart, thus reducing a person's risk of death through heart disease. Besides improving blood pressure, symptoms in diseases including coronary artery disease, heart failure and myocardial infarctions, diabetes, and even migraine headaches can be reduced. Commonly prescribed angiotensin converting enzyme medications are shown in Box 4-1.

hypertrophy
Abnormal thickening of the walls and structures of the heart.

Notice that all generic angiotensin converting enzyme drug names mentioned in Box 4-1 end with the letters pril.

Box 4-1 Angiotensin Converting Enzyme Medications

Generic Name	Brand Name
lisinopril	Prinivil
enalapril maleate	Vasotec
rampril	Altace
benazepril hydrochloride	Lotensin
quinapril hydrochloride	Accupril

Angiotensin II Receptor Blocker (ARB)

ARB drugs work by causing the blood vessels to dilate because angiotensin II is blocked from binding to the blood vessels. The main difference between ACE inhibitors and ARBs is that ARB drugs work to prevent the blood pressure from rising to begin with. ARB drugs are also a first choice for people that cannot tolerate the side effects of ACE inhibitors. ARBs will often be combined with a diuretic to reduce fluid retention and increase urine output. The diuretic most commonly added is called hydrochlorothiazide (HCTZ). Like ACE inhibitors, ARB medication can do more than just treat hypertension. ARB medication is commonly prescribed to treat or improve chronic kidney disease and kidney failure manifested from diabetes. Commonly prescribed ARB medications are included in Box 4-2.

Notice that all angiotensin II receptor blocker generic drug names mentioned in Box 4-2 end with the letters sartan.

Box 4-2 Angiotensin II Receptor Blocker Medications

Generic Name	Brand Name
valsartan	Diovan
losartan potassium	Cozaar
irbesartan	Avapro
telmisartan	Micardis

Quick Check 4-1

Fill in the blanks.

1. Angiotensin is a(n) _____ that regulates _____ and water balance in the body.

2. Angiotensin I is broken up in the _____ by an enzyme called _____.

3. Angiotensin II is metabolized in the _____ and binds to blood vessel receptors, causing the blood vessels to _____.

4. _____ medication can reduce blood pressure by allowing reduced resistance as blood leaves the ventricles, thus improving heart efficiency.

5. Angiotensin II receptor blocker (ARB) medication is often combined with a _____ to reduce fluid retention and _____ urine output.

Beta Blockers

Beta blockers are also called beta-adrenergic blocking agents. Beta blockers obstruct the hormone epinephrine (adrenaline) and norepinephrine in the body's beta receptors found in the autonomic nervous system. This action releases noadrenalin, which blocks electrical impulses from the sympathetic nervous system from stimulating the heart so that it doesn't need as much blood and oxygen. Beta blockers, therefore, can reduce the heart's workload by reducing cardiac output, can slow the heartbeat, and can also be used to control irregular rhythms by reducing heart rate and blood pressure. Beta blockers are often prescribed after a person suffers a myocardial infarction because the medication relieves stress on the heart muscle by reducing the force of a heartbeat, therefore improving survival rates. Beta blockers may also be prescribed to reduce **angina**, caused by a lack of oxygen to the heart muscle. Long-term use of beta blockers has shown to help manage chronic heart failure and to reduce mortality and additional myocardial infarctions. Beta blockers are usually not prescribed until other categories of medications, such as ACE inhibitors or diuretics, were tried and found to be ineffective. As in the previous categories of drugs, beta blockers may also be prescribed for other medical conditions including migraine headaches, anxiety, glaucoma, or thyroid problems. Commonly prescribed beta blocker medications are included in Box 4-3.

angina
Heart pain caused by inadequate oxygen to the heart caused by blocked or constricted arteries and veins.

Notice that all beta blocker generic drug names included in Box 4-3 end with the letters lol.

Box 4-3 Beta Blocker Medications

Generic Name	Brand Name
atenolol	Tenorim
metoprolol tartrate	Lopressor
carvedilol	Coreg
propranolol hydrochloride	Inderal
bisoprolol fumarate	Zebeta

Calcium Channel Blocker (CCB)

Recall from Chapter 2 that calcium plays an important role in the health of a cardiac cell. Calcium must enter the cells to create cardiac cell contractions. However, too much calcium entering the cells is not good for the heart because too much calcium causes the heart muscle cells to work too hard, which increases systemic vascular resistance, arterial blood pressure, and heart rate, as well as causing large vessel stiffness. CCBs work by restricting some calcium from entering the cells of the blood vessels, thus preventing the blood vessels from becoming too constricted, and can slow the heart rate, which may relieve angina and control an irregular heartbeat. CCBs are also prescribed for hypertension. There are different types of CCBs, which differ by how they are metabolized and the duration of time that they work. CCB medications come in extended-release and short-acting forms. The short-acting CCBs do not change heart rate or contractions and are preferred for use with a slow heart rate. The longer-lasting CCBs work to reduce heart rate by reducing the strength and rate of heart contractions. Commonly prescribed CCB medications are included in Box 4-4.

Notice that the short-acting forms of the generic CCB drug names shown in Box 4-4 end with the letters pine.

Box 4-4 Calcium Channel Blocker Medications

Generic Name	Brand Name
amlodipine	Norvasc
verapamil	Calan, Isoptin
diltiazem hydrochloride	Cardizem
nifedipine	Procardia, Adalat

Diuretics

Diuretics stimulate the kidneys to release more urine. Diuretics come under three different categories. Cardiac patients might be prescribed any one or a combination of two different types of diuretics. The health care provider might also prescribe a diuretic in combination with a drug from another category already mentioned, such as an ACE inhibitor. Diuretics remove excess fluid from the body, which builds up because the heart is not pumping blood efficiently, thus causing peripheral edema, pulmonary edema, or both.

The first category of diuretics is called thiazide diuretics. These diuretics are designed to increase the excretion of water and salt through urination, and are good for long-term use because they are not as potent as the next category of diuretics, which are called loop diuretics. Thiazide diuretics are also used to reduce blood pressure because unlike the other two types of diuretics, thiazide diuretics can cause a dilation of the blood vessels.

Loop diuretics are often used in emergencies when a person has evidence of fluid overload. Fluid overload may present with congested symptoms such as orthopnea, edema, or shortness of breath. Loop diuretics are used to restore normal fluid volume, especially in patients diagnosed with heart failure. They are usually short acting and may be prescribed in large doses over several days, twice or three times a day. When loop diuretics are ineffective, thiazide diuretics may be added, but patients will need additional monitoring of their electrolytes for abnormalities and of blood pressure for hypotension, as well as kidney function tests.

The third type of diuretics is called potassium-sparing diuretics. These diuretics can also be combined with other diuretics. Potassium-sparing diuretics also reduce the fluid in the body, but unlike other diuretics, they do not cause the body to lose potassium. Since diuretics are designed to increase urination, they are often prescribed to be administered in the morning so that they can work within the body all day and not disrupt sleep. Commonly prescribed diuretic medications include medications listed in Box 4-5.

Box 4-5 Diuretic Medications

Generic Name	Brand Name(s)
hydrochlorothiazide	Microzide, Esidrix, Hydrodiuril
furosemide	Lasix
triamterene	Dyrenium
spironolactone	Aldactone

Quick Check 4-2

Fill in the blanks.

1. _____ medication is designed to reduce the force of a heartbeat, therefore relieving stress on the heart muscle.

2. Calcium channel blocker medication works by _____ calcium from entering the cells of blood vessels, which then prevents blood vessel _____, and it also may slow the heart rate and control irregular heartbeats.

3. _____ diuretic medication can reduce blood pressure by causing a(n) _____ of blood vessels.

4. _____ diuretic medications are used to restore a normal fluid _____ in patients diagnosed with heart failure.

5. Potassium-sparing diuretic medication _____ fluid in the body but does not cause the body to _____ potassium.

MEDICATIONS PRESCRIBED FOR ANTITHROMBOTIC THERAPY

antithrombotic
A category of drugs used to prevent or treat blood clots.

Cardiac medications can also be prescribed to affect blood clotting. These medications are called **antithrombotic** agents and come under two categories: anticoagulants and antiplatelet agents.

Antithrombotic Agents

- anticoagulants
- antiplatelet agents

thrombus
A blood clot that is attached to the vessel wall where it formed.

Fibrin blood cells mainly form in veins.

Platelet blood cells mainly form in arteries.

thrombosis
A condition in which a blood clot has become dislodged from the vessel wall and is now circulating within the bloodstream.

fibrin
A protein that forms a mesh to keep platelets together.

platelets
A type of blood cell that can create a mass of thrombin.

A **thrombus** is a blood clot. It can be very beneficial to a person who is bleeding due to an external injury to the body, such as in a car accident, because a thrombus will stop the bleeding by forming a clot in the injured area. However, if the injury is internal, the thrombus attaches to an artery or vein because the cardiovascular system is a closed loop; so a thrombus can become potentially life threatening if the clot begins to block the flow of blood. When this happens, the term **thrombosis** is used. The main difference between the terms thrombus and thrombosis is that in a thrombus, the clot is still attached to the vessel wall where it formed, whereas in a thrombosis, the clot has become dislodged from the vessel wall and is now circulating within the bloodstream. The main components of a blood clot are fibrin and platelets. **Fibrin** is a fibrous protein that forms a mesh to keep platelets together, sort of like a sticky glue or spiderweb in the blood. Fibrin mainly forms in the veins. **Platelets** are a type of blood cell that assists in blood clotting by aggregating cells into a mass; they mainly form in the arteries.

There are two main types of antithrombotic drugs. They are called antiplatelet and anticoagulant drugs. People often believe that antithrombotic drugs "thin" the blood. Actually, this is not true—in fact, these drugs help keep the blood flowing but do not thin the blood. The characteristics of each type of medication will be discussed next. Both types of antithrombotic drugs are designed to work as primary or secondary prevention drugs to cerebrovascular or cardiovascular events.

Antiplatelet Agents

Antiplatelet drugs are designed to keep the blood moving by preventing protein in the platelets from being able to clump up and bind together to form blood clots. Interestingly, platelets are always present in the blood, but they normally just move with the blood unless there is injury, inflammation, or disease within the body. When there is injury, inflammation, or disease, blood coagulation causes the platelets to come into action, moving to the affected area and beginning to bind into blood clots. Many arterial blood clots in the body are platelet based. When the blood clot reduces blood flow in the brain, it is called a transit ischemic attack (TIA), or if it stops the flow of blood in the brain the result is called a stroke or cerebral vascular accident (CVA). When the arteries of the heart have a reduced blood flow from blood clots, a person may experience angina. More serious blockage in the heart may induce a myocardial infarction.

Antiplatelet medication inhibits the production of thromboxane; therefore, the platelets have a decreased responsiveness to aggregate and form clots. Aspirin was the first recognized antiplatelet drug. Although considered a weak antiplatelet, aspirin is the preferred nonsteroidal anti-inflammatory drug (NSAID). Commonly prescribed antiplatelet medications are included in Box 4-6.

Box 4-6 Antiplatelet Medications

Generic Name	Brand Name
ticlopidine hydrochloride	Ticlid
dipyridamole	Persantine
clopidogrel bisulfate	Plavix

Anticoagulant Agents

Anticoagulant agents target clotting factors and are usually the first antithrombotic medication prescribed. Vitamin K is used by the liver to create clotting factors. Anticoagulants work on chemical reactions of liver proteins to lengthen the time it takes for blood clots to form in the blood vessels. If a blood clot already exists, anticoagulant drug therapy can keep the blood clot from enlarging, but these agents cannot dissolve clots that have already formed. Anticoagulants cause interference with the formation of the fibrin web. For more than 60 years, the only oral anticoagulant was warfarin. People taking warfarin had to also be prescribed Vitamin K. People with coagulation problems had to be hospitalized for about five days and administered heparin to block the activities of thrombin and to monitor the effectiveness of the warfarin. Heparin was for short-term use and had to be administered either intravenously or by injection. A breakthrough came in the 1980s, when low-molecular-weight heparin (LMWH) was developed. LMWH was advantageous because it could be injected subcutaneously in a fixed-dose syringe, so patients could omit the hospital stay and medicate at home. Patients also did not need to have blood tests to monitor the effectiveness of the medication. Anticoagulants are considered more aggressive antithrombotic therapy than antiplatelet agents and are much more expensive. Anticoagulant agents are primarily used for stroke patients, in patients when the clot originates in the heart, and for atrial fibrillation patients. Commonly prescribed anticoagulant medications are included in Box 4-7.

> Notice that generic anticoagulant drug names listed in Box 4-7 end with the letters arin, except for warfarin sodium.

Box 4-7 Anticoagulant Medications

Generic Name	Brand Name
warfarin sodium	Coumadin
enoxaparin	Lovenox
dalteparin	Fragmin

Quick Check 4-3

Fill in the blanks.

1. A thrombus is a blood clot that is still _____ to the vessel wall where it _____.

2. A(n) _____ is a blood clot that has become dislodged from a vessel wall and is now _____ within the bloodstream.

3. Antithrombotic drug therapy is designed to work as a prevention drug to _____ and cardiovascular events.

4. Many _____ blood clots are platelet based. A transit ischemic attack (TIA) is a blood clot that has reduced blood flow to the _____. When blood flow to the _____ has stopped, a cerebral vascular accident (CVA) occurs.

5. Vitamin _____ is used by the _____ to create blood clotting factors.

CARDIAC MEDICATIONS THAT CHANGE HEART RATE OR RHYTHM

The heart's electrical system can cause the heart to malfunction in four different ways: the heart can stop beating, beat irregularly, beat too fast, or beat too slow. Cardiac medications that change the heart rate or rhythm usually fall into one of these four categories. The malfunctions can be the result of internal issues within the body such as abnormal electrolyte levels or abnormal hormone levels, or the malfunctions may be due to external causes such as drinking too much caffeine, ingesting illegal drugs, or the body being in a state of hypothermia. Keep in mind that many cardiac medications can be used for more than one symptom. For example, blood thinners are used for some types of arrhythmias but are covered under antithrombotic therapy, and rate control medications are covered under beta blockers and calcium channel blockers.

dysrhythmia
Regularly occurring abnormal, faulty, or disordered rhythms.

This section will begin by discussing **dysrhythmias**, which are *any* regularly occurring abnormal, faulty, or disordered rhythms. An example of a common disordered or disorganized rhythm is called atrial fibrillation (also known as A-Fib). **Fibrillation** is caused by electrical signals that produce a quiver, not a contraction, in the heart muscles of the atria or ventricles.

fibrillation
Electrical signals that produce a quiver (not a contraction) in the heart muscles of the atria or ventricles.

The second section will discuss **arrhythmias**, which are heartbeat rhythms caused by alterations in time, quality, force, or sequence of the heartbeat. In severe cases, arrhythmia irregularity not only can cause a loss of rhythm, but also can become fatal if immediate intervention is not provided. However, in most cases, arrhythmias can be successfully treated if treatment is needed at all. An arrhythmia can feel like your heart just "skipped a beat."

arrhythmia
Heartbeat rhythms caused by alterations in time, quality, force, or sequence.

Often the terms dysrhythmia and arrhythmia are used interchangeably because they both can be defined as abnormal rhythms or abnormal heartbeats.

Dysrhythmias

When the heart maintains a regular rhythm—whether too fast, too slow, or irregularly regular—one of the first assessment tools will be the electrocardiogram. The clinician will want to determine if the dysrhythmia is originating above the atrioventricular (AV) node, which is called a **supraventricular** arrhythmia, or from the ventricles (below the AV node). In addition to where the malfunction occurs, dysrhythmias are classified by how the malfunction affects the heartbeat. For example, a rhythm that is too slow can be just as fatal as a rhythm that is too fast.

supraventricular
Originating above the atrioventricular (AV) node.

premature atrial complex (PAC)
A heart rhythm disturbance, an extra beat originating in the atrium; also called premature atrial contraction.

When the heart beats too early or provides an extra beat, if the cause is located within the atria, the condition is known as **premature atrial complex (PAC)**. When the cause is from a ventricular malfunction, the condition is known as **premature ventricular complex (PVC)**.

premature ventricular complex (PVC)
A heart rhythm disturbance, an extra beat originating in the ventricles; also called premature ventricular contraction.

If the heartbeat is normal, meaning that the electrical impulse originates from the sinoatrial (SA) node, but is beating too fast, the rhythm is called **sinus tachycardia**. Sinus tachycardia can be a temporary condition caused by exercise, stress, dehydration, or trauma. Sinus tachycardia causes the heart to pump more blood to meet the body's demand for more oxygen, and is a common rhythm issue. Ventricular tachycardia can become fatal if not addressed quickly.

sinus tachycardia
A heartbeat with a normal rhythm but beating too fast (at more than 100 beats per minute).

sinus bradycardia
A heartbeat with a normal rhythm but beating too slowly (at less than 60 beats per minute).

Sinus bradycardia is the opposite of sinus tachycardia. The heart is beating with a normal rhythm but beating too slowly, meaning the heartbeat is less than 60 beats per minute. In athletes, this may be their normal rhythm. Drugs such as beta blockers and calcium channel blockers may also slow the heartbeat. The vagus nerve can play an important role in a slow heartbeat by releasing acetylcholine when the parasympathetic nervous system has been engaged, such as in situations of severe pain. In addition, a person may become lightheaded or even faint, a condition called **syncope**, when the heart is beating too slowly.

syncope
A condition when a person becomes lightheaded or faints.

If a person is otherwise in good health, having sinus bradycardia or sinus tachycardia may not require any medical intervention or drug therapy. Clinicians may only need to monitor the abnormal rhythm over a period of time.

Quick Check 4-4

Fill in the blanks.

1. Examples of internal issues with the body which can cause irregular heartbeats include abnormal _____ levels and abnormal _____ levels.

2. External environmental issues that may cause heart _____ include drinking too much coffee, ingesting _____ drugs, and hypothermia.

3. Heart _____ is produced by faulty electrical signals, which causes the heart to _____ instead of contract.

4. A(n) _____ can determine if abnormal rhythms originate above the _____ node or from the ventricles.

5. A normal, but fast, heartbeat rhythm is called sinus _____. A normal, but slow heartbeat rhythm is called sinus _____.

Arrhythmias

Like a dysrhythmia, an arrhythmia includes any disturbance in the rhythm of a heartbeat. There are three major common classifications of arrhythmias, which are identified as supraventricular, ventricular, and bradyarrhythmias. Supraventricular arrhythmias and ventricular arrhythmias indicate where the dysrhythmia originates—either in the upper or lower heart chambers. Bradyarrhythmias occur somewhere within the heart's conduction system, such as the SA or AV node. Heart blocks usually have a pathology of the AV node; hence, they are often referred to as AV blocks.

Major Common Classifications of Arrhythmias

- Supraventricular arrhythmias
- Ventricular arrhythmias
- Bradyarrhythmias

The study of the major classifications of arrhythmias are further subdivided into specific areas of disturbance, which in many cases can be detected from a good tracing of the electrocardiogram. The subdivided arrhythmias are classified by heart rate and mechanism. Heart rate classifications include normal sinus rhythm, bradycardia, and tachycardia. Mechanism classifications include automaticity, reentry, junctional, or fibrillation. **Table 4-1** identifies the three major classifications and some of the common subcategories.

Table 4-1 Arrhythmia Classifications

Major Classification	Subclassifications
Supraventricular	Premature atrial contractions
	Multifocal atrial tachycardia
	Atrial flutter
	Atrial fibrillation
	Paroxysmal supraventricular tachycardia
	Accessory pathway tachycardia
	AV nodal reentrant tachycardia
Ventricular	Premature ventricular contractions
	Ventricular tachycardia
	Ventricular fibrillation
	Long QT syndrome
Bradyarrhythmias	Sinus node dysfunction
	Heart blocks

antiarrhythmic
An agent (drug) used to control or prevent arrhythmias.

When medications are necessary, **antiarrhythmic** drugs can be administered to control irregular heartbeat, premature beating or extra beats, and supraventricular or ventricular irregular beating. Antiarrhythmic drugs work to change the rhythm by trying to correct or compensate for the irregular rhythm because the heart may not be pumping enough blood to the body due to the disorganized rhythm. The two main categories of antiarrhythmic drugs include sodium channel blockers and potassium channel blockers. A third category combines both sodium and potassium channel blockers. Box 4-8 identifies the most common antiarrhythmic medications.

Box 4-8 Antiarrhythmic Medications by Common Categories

Category	Generic Name	Brand Name
Sodium channel blockers	disopyramide phosphate	Norpace
	flecainide acetate	Tambocor
	propafenone hydrochloride	Rythmol
Potassium channel blockers	doletilide	
	sotalol hydrochloride	Betapace
Sodium and potassium combination	amiodarone	Cordarone, Pacerone

Sodium Channel Blockers

Recall from Chapter 3 that sodium channels allow electrical heart conduction to occur. Therefore, sodium channel blockers decrease the speed of the electrical conduction in the heart, stabilizing the cardiac membrane by inhibiting automaticity.

Potassium Channel Blockers

Potassium channels allow the heart to receive nerve impulses. Therefore, potassium channel blockers would slow nerve impulses within the heart, which in turn decreases heart rate and oxygen requirements.

Sodium and Potassium Combination

The most effective antiarrhythmic drug combines both sodium and potassium channel blockers. By using a combination of sodium and potassium channel blockers, the duration of the action potential is extended, which in turn decreases peripheral vascular resistance. The biggest concern with antiarrhythmic drugs is that there are many possible side effects, including damage to other organs such as the lungs, liver, and thyroid gland. Antiarrhythmic channel blockers may be counterindicated for people diagnosed with coronary disease or heart failure. Potassium channel blockers may have adverse effects on the kidneys, and dofetilide must be first administered in the hospital to make sure that the patient can tolerate the medicine and not have adverse complications such as a ventricular arrhythmia.

A list of all drug preparations for the cardiac medications that change the heart rate or rhythm would be extensive; entire textbooks are dedicated to each of the three main categories, and not all subcategories are described in this text. For example, atrial fibrillation is one of the most common arrhythmias. There are three different categories of medications used in treating atrial fibrillation, including antithrombotic drugs, rate control drugs, and antiarrhythmic drugs. Within the three categories, there are many different blood-thinning medications, which are covered in the section entitled "Medications Prescribed for Antithrombotic Therapy," earlier in this chapter. One category of medications that has not been previously mentioned but that belongs in the category of irregular heartbeat medications (especially for the treatment of atrial fibrillation or atrial flutter), and is used to slow irregular heartbeat arrhythmias while increasing the force of the contraction, are digitalis preparations. The primary digitalis preparation is the cardiac glycoside called digoxin, which can be prescribed under the brand name Lanoxin. This classification of medications can also be used when patients fail to respond to ACE inhibitors or diuretics, or have symptoms of congestive heart failure. Other categories used for long-term antiarrhythmic medications include beta blockers and calcium channel blockers.

More information about these classifications of arrhythmias is covered in advanced courses on interpreting electrocardiograms. Therefore, this topic will not be covered in further detail in this book.

Quick Check 4-5

Fill in the blanks.

1. Arrhythmias are subdivided by heart _____ and _____.

2. _____ medication works to correct an irregular rhythm when the heart is not pumping enough blood due to a(n) _____ rhythm.

3. Sodium channel blocker medication _____ the speed of electrical conduction, inhibiting _____.

4. Potassium channel blocker medication slows _____ impulses within the heart, which _____ heart rate and oxygen requirements.

5. Using a combination of sodium and potassium channel blocker medication extends the cell's _____, which then decreases peripheral vascular resistance.

CARDIAC MEDICATIONS PRESCRIBED TO REDUCE CHEST PAIN

antianginal
A category of drugs used to reduce angina.

vasodilators
Medications that reduces the heart's workload by relaxing and dilating the blood vessels, which allows them to hold more blood, therefore increasing the flow of oxygen-rich blood to the heart; also called nitrates.

The drug category of cardiac medications used to reduce angina are called antianginal drugs. Vasodilators are prescribed to treat angina, or chest pain, caused by blocked or constricted arteries and veins in the heart. The way that vasodilators work is by reducing the heart's workload by relaxing and dilating the blood vessels, which allows the blood vessel to hold more blood, therefore increasing oxygen-rich blood to the heart.

Vasodilators

Vasodilators are also called nitrates. Vasodilators can be prescribed for people who do not have hypotension but do have acute heart failure, and for people who cannot tolerate ACE inhibitors. Organic nitrates are also prescribed for coronary artery disease patients for management of ischemic syndrome. Nitrates can be combined with hydralazine blood pressure medication to treat congestive heart failure.

Nitrates come in three compounds: nitroglycerin, isosorbide dinitrate, and isosorbide mononitrate. These compounds are available in rapid preparations, short-acting preparations and long-lasting preparations. Different forms of nitrate drug administration include buccal and sublingual pills or spray, oral pills, chewable pills, topical ointment, or as a transdermal patch.

Commonly prescribed vasodilator medications are included in Box 4-9.

Box 4-9 Vasodilator Medications

Generic Name	Brand Names
isosorbide dinitrate	Isordil
nesiritide	Natrecor
hydralazine hydrochloride	Apresoline
nitroglycerin	Nitrostat

MEDICATIONS PRESCRIBED TO LOWER BLOOD CHOLESTEROL

antihyperlipidemic
A category of drugs used to lower cholesterol.

heart failure
A condition when the heart can no longer function normally and the pumping action of the heart muscle is greatly reduced, causing insufficient systemic blood flow.

cardiomegaly
An enlarged heart.

heart disease
A structural or functional abnormality of the heart or cardiovascular system.

Drugs used to lower blood cholesterol come under a class of medications called **antihyperlipidemics**. Although many studies have been completed suggesting that statin drug therapy may help individuals with heart disease, there has not been a general consensus that lowering cholesterol levels will help all coronary patients. There is a difference between heart failure and heart disease that seems to divide researchers' opinions.

Heart failure occurs when the heart can no longer function normally and the pumping action of the heart muscle is greatly reduced, causing insufficient systemic blood flow. This usually results in fluid accumulation in the lower extremities and the lungs, causing fatigue and shortness of breath. With heart failure, the heart will become enlarged, a condition known as **cardiomegaly**.

There are two types of heart failure: systolic heart failure and diastolic heart failure. Systolic heart failure occurs in the lower heart chambers, so it affects the force of the blood flowing from the heart. Diastolic heart failure occurs during the resting phase, when the heart is filling with blood and the heart cannot relax long enough to allow the chambers to fill with blood between heartbeats. This causes the heart muscle to become stiff. **Heart disease** occurs when there is a structural or functional abnormality of the heart or cardiovascular system. An example of heart disease is coronary artery disease (CAD), a condition that is created when the arteries become constricted, usually with cholesterol, and this prevents the blood from circulating within the body correctly. Heart disease is responsible for about 40 percent of deaths in the United States each year. The blood test for low-density lipoprotein (LDL) measures plaque in the arteries. In people with heart disease, LDL is usually too high and can result in sudden blood clots, causing myocardial infarctions, cerebral vascular accidents, and often death.

Statins

The class of medications referred to as statins are shown in Box 4-10. Statin drugs work by blocking the liver enzyme that produces cholesterol. Some of the side effects of statin drug therapy include fatigue, muscle weakness and soreness, and depletion of coenzyme Q10, which is a fat-soluble antioxidant needed by the body to remove free radicals from the blood.

Box 4-10 Medications Prescribed to Lower Blood Cholesterol

Generic Name	Brand Name
rosuvastatin	Crestor
atorvastatin calcium	Lipitor
fluvastatin sodium	Lescol
lovastatin	Mevacor
pravastatin	Pravachol
simvastatin	Zorcor
pitavastatin	Livalo

Quick Check 4-6

Fill in the blanks.

1. Vasodilator medication, also called _____, works by reducing the heart's workload, which allows the blood vessels to hold more blood and increase _____ rich blood to the heart.

2. _____ medication is used to lower blood cholesterol.

3. Insufficient systemic blood flow is caused by _____, a condition which also _____ the heart.

4. _____ heart failure occurs in the lower heart chambers, whereas _____ heart failure occurs during the resting phase of the heart.

5. Structural or functional abnormalities of the heart or cardiovascular system is the definition of _____.

REVIEW OF CARDIOVASCULAR DRUGS BY CATEGORIES

This next section will identify and condense, through the use of tables, the function of each category of medication, how each medication is supplied, the typical dose, and possible side effects. The tables provide a faster review and easier comparison of the different cardiovascular drug categories. The medications described here are provided in nonemergency dosages. Emergency cardiac medications are discussed in Chapter 8.

Drug Functions by Category

Table 4-2 identifies the major classifications of cardiovascular drugs and how the drugs within the category function overall.

Table 4-2 Cardiovascular Drug Functions

Drug Category	Function
Angiotensin converting enzyme inhibitors	Expand blood vessels, prevent angiotensin II from forming
Angiotensin II receptor blockers	Dilate blood vessels, prevent blood pressure from increasing
Beta blockers	Reduce the heart's workload by slowing heartbeat
Calcium channel blockers	Prevent blood vessels from becoming too constricted by restricting calcium from entering the cells
Diuretics	Remove excess fluids from the body by stimulating the kidneys to release more urine
Antiplatelet agents	Keep the blood moving by preventing protein in the platelets from binding and forming clots
Anticoagulant agents	Create chemical reactions in liver proteins to lengthen the time it takes for blood to clot
Sodium channel blockers	Decrease the speed of the electrical conduction, which then stabilizes the cardiac membrane by inhibiting automaticity
Potassium channel blockers	Slow nerve impulses within the heart, which in turn decrease heart rate and oxygen requirements
Sodium and potassium combinations	Cause the duration of the action potential to be extended, which in turn decrease peripheral vascular resistance
Vasodilators	Used for management of ischemic syndrome and to treat congestive heart failure
Statins	Block the liver enzyme that produces cholesterol, therefore reducing LDL (i.e., bad) cholesterol

Cardiovascular Medications

Table 4-3 is divided into five columns. Column one contains the generic name for a cardiac medication listed in this chapter. Column two identifies at least one brand name for the generic drug. (Although many drugs have numerous brand names, only a partial list of U.S. brand name drugs has been included on the chart.) Column three identifies the drug classification. Many drugs come under more than one classification, as noted in this column. Column four provides dosage information. The drugs listed may have additional injectable versions, but they are not included in this list. Drugs will be identified by the route of administration, the type of drug available (such as a tablet, capsule, ointment, etc.), and the daily therapeutic range. In the same column, the frequency that the drug is taken is identified. Column five lists some potential adverse reactions the drugs have been identified with. Although many of these drugs come in extended-release form or injectable form, only standard dosage information is found in the table.

As the health provider collects the patient's history, information about the various drugs prescribed will enhance information that the health provider needs to know, and also will identify areas where a patient may need more guidance in order to comply with the way the drug should be taken to maximize its potential.

Table 4-3 Cardiovascular Medications

Generic Name	Brand Name	Classification	Dosage Information	Possible Adverse Cardiac Effects
lisinopril	Prinivil	antihypertensive, angiotensin converting enzyme (ACE) inhibitor	Tab, 2.5–40 mg, QD	hypotension, A-Fib, TIAs, PVCs
enalapril maleate	Vasotec	angiotensin converting enzyme (ACE) inhibitor, antihypertensive	Tab, 2.5–20 mg QD or bid	A-Fib, tachycardia, bradycardia, angina, syncope, dysrhythmias
rampril	Altace	angiotensin converting enzyme (ACE) inhibitor, antihypertensive	Caps, 1.25–10 mg QD or bid	hypotension, angina, palpitations, syncope, dysrhythmias
benazepril hydrochloride	Lotensin	antihypertensive, angiotensin converting enzyme (ACE) inhibitor	Tab, 20–40 mg QD or bid	symptomatic hypotension, syncope, palpitations
quinapril hydrochloride	Accupril	angiotensin converting enzyme (ACE) inhibitor	Tab, 20–40 mg, QD	vasodilation, tachycardia, heart failure
valsartan	Diovan	antihypertensive, angiotensin II receptor antagonist	Caps, 80–320 mg, QD	palpitations
losartan potassium	Cozaar	antihypertensive, angiotensin II receptor antagonist	Tab, 25–100 mg, QD	angina, CVA, MI, ventricular tachycardia or ventricular fibrillation
irbesartan	Avapro	antihypertensive, angiotension II receptor antagonist	Tab, 75–300 mg, QD	tachycardia, hypertension, MI, hypertensive crisis
telmisartan	Micardis	antihypertensive, angiotensin II receptor antagonist	Tab, 20–80 mg, QD	angina, hypertension, peripheral edema
atenolol	Tenorim	beta-adrenergic blocking agent	Tab, 25–100 mg, bid	low BP, chronic HF, bradycardia
metoprolol tartrate	Lopressor	beta-adrenergic blocking agent	Tab, 50–100 mg, QD	edema
carvedilol	Coreg	alpha/beta adrenergic blocking agent	Tab, 3.125–25 mg, bid	bradycardia, postural hypotension, AV block
propranolol	Inderal	beta-adrenergic blocking agent, antiarrhythmic	Caps, 10–80 mg, bid	contraindicated bronchial asthma, COPD
bisoprolol fumarate	Zebeta	beta-adrenergic blocking agent	Tab, 5–10 mg, QD	
amlodipine	Norvasc	antihypertensive, calcium channel blocking (CCB) agent	Tab, 2.5–10 mg, QD	peripheral edema, palpitations, hypotension, syncope, bradycardia

(Continued)

Table 4-3 Continued

Generic Name	Brand Name	Classification	Dosage Information	Possible Adverse Cardiac Effects
verapamil	Calan, Isoptin	calcium channel blocking (CCB) agent	Tab, 40–120 mg, tid	CHF, bradycardia, AV block, peripheral edema
diltiazem hydrochloride	Cardizem, Tiazac	calcium channel blocking (CCB) agent, antihypertensive, Group IV	Tab, 30–120 mg, qid	AV block, bradycardia, CHF, hypotension, syncope, palpitations
nifedipine	Procardia, Adalat	calcium channel blocking (CCB) agent, Antihypertensive	Caps, 10–20 mg, tid	peripheral and pulmonary edema, MI, hypotension, palpitations, syncope, CHF
hydro-chlorothiazide	Microzide, Esidrix, Hydrodiuril	diuretic, thiazide type	Tab 25–50 mg, Caps 12.5 mg, QD	allergic myocarditis, hypotension
furosemide	Lasix	loop diuretic	Tab, 20–80 mg, QD	orthostatic hypotension, chronic aortitis, thrombophlebitis contraindication: never use with ethacrynic acid
triamterene	Dyrenium	diuretic, potassium sparing	Caps, 50–100 mg, bid	electrolyte hyperkalemia, anaphylaxis
spironolactone	Aldactone	diuretic, potassium sparing	Tab 25–100 mg, bid or qid	electrolyte hyperkalemia, hyponatremia
ticlopidine hydrochloride	Ticlid	platelet aggregation inhibitor	Tab, 250 mg, bid	bleeding times may be prolonged
dipyridamole	Persantine	platelet adhesion inhibitor	Tab, 25–75 mg, qid	peripheral vasodilation, flushing
clopidogrel bisulfate	Plavix	antiplatelet	Tab, 75 mg, QD	edema, hypertension
warfarin sodium	Coumadin	anticoagulant	Tab, 1-10 mg, QD	hemmorrhage
disopyramide phosphate	Norpace	antiarrhythmic Class 1A	Caps, 100–150 mg, qid	hypotension, CHF, worsening of arrhythmias, edema, weight gain, syncope, angina, AV block
flecainide acetate	Tambocor	antiarrhythmic Class 1C	Tab, 50–150 mg, q 12 hr	new or worsened ventricular arrhythmia and CHF
propafenone hydrochloride	Rythmol	antiarrhythmic Class 1C	Tab, 150–300 mg, tid or qid	new or worsened arrhythmias, angina, CHF, atrial fibrillation
sotalol hydrochloride	Betapace	beta-adrenergic blocking agent	Tab, 80–240 mg, bid	new or worsened ventricular arrhythmias
amiodarone	Cordarone, Pacerone	antiarrithythmic	Tab, 400-600 mg, QD	bradycardia

(Continued)

Table 4-3 Continued

Generic Name	Brand Name	Classification	Dosage Information	Possible Adverse Cardiac Effects
isosorbide dinitrate	Isordil	vasodilator, antianginal	Chewable Tab, 5–10 mg, q 2–3 hr, Sublingual Tab, 2.5–10 mg, q 2–3 hr, Tab, 5–40 mg, q 6 hr	vascular headaches
hydralazine hydrochloride	Apresoline	antihypertensive	Tab, 10–100 mg, qid	orthostatic hypotension, hypotension, MI, angina
nitroglycerin	Nitrostat	antianginal vasodilator	Sublingual Tab, 0.3–0.6 mg prn before stressful activity no more than 3 tab in 15 min.	
rosuvastatin	Crestor	antihyperlipidemic	Tab, 5-20 mg, QD	angina
atorvastatin	Lipitor	antihyperlipidemic	Tab, 10–40 mg, QD	
fluvastatin sodium	Lescol	antihyperlipidemic	Caps, 20–40 mg, QD-hs	fatigue
lovastatin	Mevacor	antihyperlipidemic	Tab, 10–40 mg, QD	angina
pravastatin	Pravachol	antihyperlipidemic	Tab, 20-80 mg, QD	angina
simvastatin	Zorcor	antihyperlipidemic	Tab, 5–80 mg, QD	vasculitis
digoxin	Lanoxin	inotropic antidysrhythmic, cardiac glycoside	Caps, 0.05–0.2 mg, bid, Elixir, 0.05 mg/mL, q 6–8 hr	ventricular fibrillation, ventricular tachycardia

Note: Tab = tablet, QD = once daily, bid = twice a day, tid = three times a day, caps = capsules, qid = four times a day

DRUG INTERACTIONS

pharmacodynamics
The study of how drugs act in living organisms.

pharmacokinetics
The study of how the body metabolizes a drug and how the body distributes or excretes drugs.

pharmacogenetics
The study of how drugs interrelate based on genetics.

When a person ingests any type of drug, whether prescribed or taken illegally, there is always a possibility of undesired reciprocal actions within the body caused by anything else the person also ingested at the time. There are two broad categories of interactions. The first is called **pharmacodynamics**, which is the study of how drugs react to living organisms. A pharmacodynamic interaction occurs when a drug counteracts with another drug, herb, vitamin, or food that has a similar effect on the body. The second group of interactions is classed as pharmacokinetics. **Pharmacokinetics** is the study of how the body metabolizes a drug and how the body distributes or excretes drugs. When the pathway in absorption is the same (such as being metabolized in the liver), health providers can better predict treatment success by combining different drugs. The study of how drugs interrelate based on genetics is called **pharmacogenetics**.

Patient education about the warning signs and when to seek help with a drug interaction cannot be stressed enough. Patient education should also include directions on usage to prevent or lower the risk of drug interactions. It is important that the patient understands how and when to take particular medications, such as before meals, after meals, on an empty stomach, before bed, etc. The patient should also be made aware that a drug interaction could take place with foods they eat, alcoholic and nonalcoholic drinks, herbs, vitamins, dietary supplements, or even other prescribed or illegal drugs. When a patient history is taken, if the patient suggests that he or she may have had an adverse reaction to prescribed medication, always inquire how the prescribed medication was taken, how the patient responded if a suspected interaction occurred (many patients will continue taking the medicine), whether the patient had also changed the diet or took over-the-counter (OTC) supplements such as herbs or vitamins, and how much and when the patient drinks fluids, including water. Something as simple as not drinking enough water on a daily basis may cause some drugs to have undesired effects on the body, especially in elderly people. Always document what the patient or patient representative states about the medication, even if the information seems irrelevant to you at the time.

bioavailability
The rate a drug is absorbed or the degree at which a drug is absorbed into the body.

Bioavailability is the rate a drug is absorbed or the degree at which a drug is absorbed into the body. The absorption rate can be altered through a delay or decreased absorption, or it could be enhanced by the drug's potency. Consumers need to be aware that interactions can occur. This section will look at the three main categories of interactions with bioavailability that may occur when taking cardiovascular drugs.

Drug and Food or Beverage Interactions

To prevent medication side effects, the beverage that should be avoided with most medications is alcohol, because alcohol will usually either increase or decrease the effect of the prescription drugs. The other beverage that is still being studied as to the effects on antihypertensive medications is grapefruit juice. Studies have shown that grapefruit juice can cause medication toxicity in some antihypertensive classes of medication because it strengthens the dosage, which in turn can be the cause of side effects. The food that poses the most known danger for some cardiovascular medications is natural licorice, which can cause toxicity with some medications used to treat congestive heart failure. Licorice may also increase edema or induce electrolyte imbalance. Cardiovascular drugs, including antihypertensives and diuretics, have shown negative effects in reaction to licorice consumption because licorice may reduce the effect of these medications. Known licorice interactions have been recorded with digoxin (Lanoxin), hydrochlorothiazide (Hydrodiuril), and spironolactone (Aldactone). Vitamin K is found in high concentrations in many foods, such as dark leafy vegetables, egg yolks, and dairy products. Vitamin K is used by the liver to create blood-clotting proteins. When a person is taking an anticoagulant drug such as warfarin (Coumadin), a drug–food interaction can occur because the warfarin works by inactivating Vitamin K, therefore increasing the time for blood clots to form. This is an example of how information on diet is important to the health care professional because the amount of medication may need to be adjusted so that a person on anticoagulants can continue to eat healthy foods.

Always ask a patient about alcohol consumption when taking cardiac medication. Be sure to document patient responses in the patient chart.

Drug and Dietary Supplement Interactions

Many people consume herbs, not only in oral forms such as tablets or capsules, but also as part of their dietary intake in salads, dressings, sauces, and meat flavoring. When discussing a person's intake of herbs, be sure to ask about the foods they eat in general because often people will say that they do not take supplements or herbs, yet they will forget that the food they eat may be seasoned with herbs. Herb extract is much more potent than standardized extracts, small amounts of tincture, fresh foods, or by drinking a cup of tea. Some known herb interactions occur with common garlic, ginger, ginkgo, ginseng, goldenseal, and feverfew. Garlic, ginger, ginkgo, and feverfew may increase bleeding in patients who are on antithrombotic therapy drugs. Ginseng may increase hypertension and heart rate, and decrease the effectiveness of antithrombotic agents. Goldenseal may cause an increase in edema and may increase hypertension. The antiplatelet drug warfarin (Coumadin) has been named in several studies as having a strong potential for herb–drug interactions, especially with the herbs ginseng and ginger and Vitamin E. Ginkgo has also been reported to interact with aspirin and other antiplatelet drugs such as clopidogrel (Plavix) and ticlodipine (Ticlid) by increasing the toxicity of these drugs. When toxicity is expected, a simple blood test called a prothrombine test (PT) can be confirmed to check if modifications in drugs or diet are called for.

> Cup of tea, anyone? Patients do not realize the potency of many of the teas purchased in grocery stores today. Many hot teas are made with a single-serve tea bag that includes ingredients such as gingko and ginseng.

Drug-to-Drug Interactions

Often, people do not consider OTC drugs (including cough syrups and cold remedies, antipyretics, and creams and ointments used transdermally) as drugs that can interact with prescription medications. Many people often do not recognize drug interactions as what they are—often, they place the blame on other conditions instead. Many drug-to-drug interactions can be avoided by patients if they understand what to take and when to take it. Health care providers cannot always predict how an individual patient will respond to a drug because of individual variables, including environmental and stress issues, morbidity and eating habits, smoking, comedications, age, and gender.

A drug's therapeutic effect can be obtained when the target concentration is found in the bloodstream. The target concentration is a combination of the dose administered and how the body metabolizes a drug. When the drug does not reach a target concentration, it may be ineffective. Likewise, when the drug reaches higher concentrations than the planned therapeutic effect, adverse reactions tend to occur.

Studies have shown that pharmacogenetics plays an important role for health providers in deciding which drugs to administer and in what concentrations. Early identification of risk and drug dosage adjustments can limit adverse reactions. When health care providers individualize drug therapy based on a person's genetic makeup, drug interactions can be minimalized while still achieving the treatment goals. For example, in diuretic drugs, drug absorption takes place in numerous locations within the body, which then creates variances according to a person's gene makeup of how the drug is absorbed.

A few examples of drug-to-drug interactions include the use of OTC antihistamines with hypertensive medications. When combined, OTC drugs may increase blood pressure and tachycardia. Another example involves amiodarone (Cordarone), an antiarrhythmic, and the use of simvastatin (Zocor), an antihyperlipidemic, at the same time. The Food and Drug Administration (FDA) warned that taking these drugs together increases the risk for a patient to develop **rhabdomyolysis**, a rare muscle injury that can lead to kidney failure or death. Amiodarone (Cordarone) was also found to inhibit the effect of the blood thinner warfarin (Coumadin). Finally, some drugs have a narrow therapeutic range, which can cause drug-to-drug interactions. An example would be digoxin (Lanoxin). When the therapeutic level of digoxin increases due to a drug-to-drug interaction, the result can be irregular heart rhythms.

rhabdomyolysis
A rare muscle injury that can lead to kidney failure or death.

Avoiding Interactions

Patient education can help people take ownership of their health. The most important person on a health care team is the patient, but patients often do not actively participate in their own care for many reasons, including that they feel intimidated, they feel they are at the mercy of a doctor's decisions, they have little or no insurance, or they believe that they cannot afford options that could change their overall health. Culture, employment, family, and patient attitudes also play important roles in patients' overall health. Box 4-11 identifies tips that the medical office can offer to patients to improve compliance to taking medications, preparing for medical office visits, and taking ownership of their own health care.

Box 4-11 Tips to Encourage Patient Ownership of Their Health Care

Before a Visit

- List all drugs, herbs and dietary supplements, and any over-the-counter medications on a paper to give to the provider.
- List common foods and beverages, including alcohol, coffee, tea, or energy drinks consumed regularly.
- Prepare a list of questions about your treatment plan.
- Mention possible drug interactions, including what happens, the frequency and length of each event, what you ate and drank prior, and what you did to stop the event.

During the Visit

- Ask questions!
- Answer questions truly and as completely as possible.
- Ask for information about your condition.
- Listen to (and maybe write down) suggestions and instructions provided by the health care team.
- Bring a caring friend or family member to document your visit.

(Continued)

> **Box 4-11 Continued**
>
> *After the Visit*
> - Use one pharmacy to fill all your prescriptions.
> - Clarify with the pharmacist any questions about the medications you might have, such as what medications can be taken together, the time of day to take the drugs, whether to take before or after meals or at the time of sleep, if refrigeration is necessary, refills, and warnings on the drugs.
> - Read the drug labels carefully.
> - Keep drugs in the original containers.

Chapter 5 will discuss patient assessment and further identify patient questioning techniques so that the health care team can best address a successful patient health plan, which includes correctly identifying drug interaction issues.

Quick Check 4-7

Fill in the blanks.

1. Pharmacodynamic interaction occurs when a drug _____ the effects of another drug, herb, vitamin or food that provides a similar effect to the body.
2. How the body _____ a drug and how the body _____ or _____ a drug is defined by pharmacokinetics.
3. Adverse reactions to licorice include medication toxicity, increased _____, and induced _____ imbalance.
4. Herbal toxicity can be found by consuming tablets or capsules or in dietary supplements, especially in potent _____.
5. Drug-to-drug interactions can be best avoided when the patient understands _____ drug to take and _____ to take the varieties of medications prescribed.

SUMMARY

- Cardiovascular medications are classified as primary prevention drugs, which are prescribed before an event happens, or secondary prevention drugs, which are prescribed to reduce symptoms or limit further damage after events occur.
- Cardiac drugs fall within five major categories, including drugs that will change blood pressure, drugs that address blood clotting issues, drugs that can change heart rate or rhythm, drugs that address chest pain, and drugs used to lower blood cholesterol.

- Angiotensin is a very important hormone used by several body systems, including the heart, and regulates sodium and water balance within the body.

- Arrhythmias are grouped into three categories: supraventricular, ventricular, or bradyarrhythmia.

- Beta blocker medication relieves stress on the heart muscle by reducing the force of the heartbeat.

- Antihyperlipidemics are medications used to control blood cholesterol levels and can help all coronary patients.

- Two types of antithrombotic medication affects blood clotting. Antiplatelet medication is designed to keep the blood moving, and anticoagulant medication causes interference with the formation of the fibrin web.

- Statin drug therapy is used to control hyperlipidemia.

- Drug interactions include food and beverage interactions, drug and dietary supplement interactions, and drug-to-drug interactions.

- Patients need to take ownership of their health by better preparing before a health visit, participating during the health visit, and following suggested protocols after their visit.

Critical Thinking Challenges

4-1. Using Table 4-3, match the possible adverse cardiac effect with each generic drug listed.

1. _____ irbesartin	a) Hemorrhage
2. _____ lisinopril	b) Weight gain
3. _____ losartan potassium	c) Heart failure
4. _____ propranolol	d) Hypertensive crisis
5. _____ warfarin sodium	e) Vasculitis
6. _____ simvastatin	f) Transit ischemic attack
7. _____ isosorbide dinitrate	g) Ventricular fibrillation
8. _____ disopyramide phosphate	h) Symptomatic hypotension
9. _____ benazepril hydrochloride	i) Chronic obstructive pulmonary disease (COPD)
10. _____ quinapril hydrochloride	j) Vascular headaches

4-2. Match the drug category with its function.

1. _____ Potassium channel blockers	a) prevents blood pressure from increasing
2. _____ Anticoagulant agents	b) decreases heart rate and oxygen requirements by slowing nerve impulses
3. _____ Angiotensin II receptor blockers	c) prevents angiotensin II from forming
4. _____ Statins	d) inhibits automaticity
5. _____ Beta blockers	e) lengthens the time it takes for a blood to clot

6. _____ Diuretics

f) decreases peripheral vascular resistance by extending duration of action potential

7. _____ Sodium and potassium combinations

g) treats congestive heart failure

8. _____ angiotensin converting enzyme inhibitors

h) reduces low–density lipoproteins

9. _____ Vasodilators

i) stimulates the kidneys to increase urine output

10. _____ Sodium channel blockers

j) decreases heartbeats

4-3. Five categories of drugs are used to control blood pressure and are usually given as a first-line treatment for hypertension. Some of the drugs are designed to manipulate the three electrolytes discussed in Chapter 3 at the cellular level by blocking calcium channels (CCBs), or blocking or sparing potassium channels (potassium-sparing diuretics).

Identify a drug from each of the five categories of cardiac medications used to modify blood pressure. Then describe how the drug is designed to work.

Review Activities

4-1. Many medications sound the same but have totally different actions. It is very important to recognize the correct spelling of cardiovascular medications so that errors are reduced by health care providers. Below are 10 terms commonly misspelled. Circle the correct spelling.

1. flurosemide   furosemide   furosimede

2. nesiritide   neseritide   nesirytide

3. bisoprolol   bysoprolol   bysoprelol

4. metraprolol   meteprolol   metoprolol

5. nefedipine   nifedipine   nifadipine

6. ramepril   ramaparil   rampril

7. telemisartan   telmisartan   telmesartan

8. clopidogrel   copidogrel   copidegril

9. warferin   warefarin   warfarin

10. rosevastatin   rosuvastatin   rosavastatin

4-2. Match the brand name with the generic drug name.

1. _____ Persantine

a) triamterene

2. _____ Dyrenium

b) irbesartan

3. _____ Cardizem

c) simvastatin

4. _____ Norvasc

d) diltazem hydrochloride

5. _____ Tenorim   e) benazepril hydrochloride

6. _____ Avapro   f) lisinopril

7. _____ Lotensin   g) dipyridamole

8. _____ Betapace   h) atenolol

9. _____ Prinivil   i) sotalol hydrochloride

10. _____ Zocor   j) amlodipine

4-3. Match the brand name drugs with their actions. Note that some drugs may have more than one action.

1. _____ Zocor   a) antihypertensive

2. _____ Lopressor   b) angiotensin converting enzyme inhibitor

3. _____ Isoptin   c) beta-adrenergic blocking agent

4. _____ Aldactone   d) calcium channel blocker

5. _____ Lanoxin   e) loop diuretic

6. _____ Coumadin   f) potassium-sparing diuretic

7. _____ Vasotec   g) anticoagulant

8. _____ Prinivil   h) antianginal

9. _____ Nitrostat   i) antihyperlipidemic

10. _____ Lasix   j) cardiac glycoside

Chapter Four Test

Fill in the blanks.

1. The main components of a blood clot are _____ and _____.

2. _____ are a category of cardiovascular drugs whose function is to reduce electrical conduction.

3. Mixing over-the-counter antihistamines with _____ medications can induce drug-to-drug interactions.

4. Sinus _____ is the opposite of sinus tachycardia.

5. An extra beat originating from the atria is called a(n) _____.

6. Sodium and water balance are regulated by a hormone named _____.

7. Bioavailability can best be described as a process when drug _____ is enhanced.

8. Atrial fibrillation is an example of a(n) _____ arrhythmia.

9. The drug category that reduces pain is called _____.

10. A heartbeat of 117 bpm is called _____.

Chapter Four Quick Check Answers

Answer order is important except where noted otherwise (in parentheses).

When two correct answers are possible, both answers are given separated by the word "or."

4-1:

1. hormone, sodium
2. kidneys, renin
3. lungs, constrict
4. ACE inhibitor
5. diuretic, increase

4-2:

1. Beta blocker
2. restricting, constriction
3. Thiazide, dilation
4. Loop, volume
5. reduces, lose

4-3:

1. attached, formed
2. thrombosis, circulating
3. cerebrovascular
4. arterial, brain, brain
5. K, liver

4-4:

1. electrolyte, hormone (either order)
2. arrhythmias, illegal
3. fibrillation, quiver
4. electrocardiogram, atrioventricular
5. tachycardia, bradycardia

4-5:

1. rate, mechanism
2. Antiarrhythmic, disorganized
3. decreases, automaticity
4. nerve, decreases
5. action potential

4-6:

1. nitrates, oxygen
2. Antihyperlipidemic
3. heart failure, enlarges
4. Systemic, diastolic
5. heart disease

4-7:

1. counteracts
2. metabolizes, distributes, excretes
3. edema, electrolyte
4. herb extracts
5. what, when

5

PATIENT ASSESSMENT

OBJECTIVES

After reading the chapter and completing all Quick Check activities, the student should be able to:

1. Interpret HIPAA privacy laws.
2. List six primary vital sign measurements.
3. Explain the purpose of a pulse oximeter.
4. Describe heart rate variability.
5. Describe the purpose of measuring jugular venous pressure (JVP).
6. Calculate an ankle brachial index (ABI) systemic blood pressure.
7. Contrast the major classifications of diabetes.
8. List routine cardiac blood tests.
9. Define SAMPLE assessment.
10. Define OPQRST assessment.

KEY TERMS

ankle brachial index (ABI)

electrocardiogram (ECG)

glycation

Health Information Portability and Accountability Act (HIPAA)

heart rate variability (HRV)

insulin resistance

jugular venous pressure (JVP)

noninvasive

open-ended questioning

OPQRST

primary hypertension

pulse oximeter

SAMPLE

secondary hypertension

SOAP

sphygmomanometer

within normal limits (WNL)

INTRODUCTION

While serving in the U.S. Navy, I was taught a saying that has been with me all my adult life. We were taught "Loose lips sink ships," meaning that sharing confidential information can have adverse effects. Translated to the medical field, privacy and confidentiality, along with personal ethics, are always of upmost importance and should be a part of your everyday routine and practiced daily. For this reason, the federal laws surrounding health care will be introduced in this chapter because health care begins with patient assessment.

This chapter provides insight into common initial assessment testing that is completed in a nonemergency situation. The chapter also discusses two major diseases that can be attributed to cardiac emergencies when left undiagnosed or untreated. Both of these diseases are considered "silent killers" because many people may not have identified any previous issues before complaining of chest pains or other heart conditions. Also included in this chapter is an explanation of how to perform the ankle brachial test, an advanced test that is becoming more routinely used as an assessment tool.

The text continues with tables of common laboratory blood tests used in assessment and concludes with an overview of two assessment tools: the SAMPLE system (commonly used to complete a patient history) and the OPQRST system (to determine pain issues). Completing and documenting a good patient assessment is vital in being able to optimize not only the patient's condition, but also in creating a productive work flow in the ambulatory clinic by documenting assessments in the electronic medical record at the time of service.

Patient assessment includes obtaining previous medical lab reports and diagnostic tests prior to patient arrival, as well as completing a patient history and vital signs when a patient is about to be seen by the clinician. Patient assessment is necessary before a diagnosis or treatment plan can begin. With a move in the United States toward total patient care, almost every patient that will be seen by medical professionals will need a minimum of current vital signs and blood pressure taken and recorded at each visit. Each vital sign procedure will provide a quick snapshot of a patient's condition at that moment in time. Collecting a complete patient history can improve patient outcome.

Health Information Portability and Accountability Act (HIPAA) (1996) A federal law that established national standards in several health care areas, including the quality, efficiency, effectiveness, and cost of health care; and in protecting patient rights, safety, security, access, confidentiality, and disclosure of identifiable health information by all types of media; and established notification standards, penalties, and enforcement activities for noncompliance by every member of all areas in the health care industry.

HEALTH INSURANCE PORTABILITY AND ACCOUNTABILITY ACT (HIPAA)

Before discussing assessment techniques, it is necessary to provide important features of the federal guidelines for health professionals that all levels of caregivers must adhere to in order to be in compliance with the federal law called the **Health Information Portability and Accountability Act (HIPAA)**. Failure to understand or to practice the guidelines not only can put your career in jeopardy, but there are also substantial monetary penalties attached for failure to adhere to the federal guidelines. HIPAA guidelines are constantly being improved, with new provisions being added on a timely basis. The law provides protection in three distinct areas of health care that everyone involved with health care needs to know, understand, and comply with. These areas include patient privacy, security protection of patient information, and privacy in electronic transactions of medical records. There are additional standards in the HIPAA guidelines relating to patient insurance that are not covered in this text.

HIPAA was originally established in 1996, with different provisions being implemented at established timelines over several years. These national standards covered a number of health care areas, including the quality, efficiency, effectiveness and cost of health care; protecting patient rights, safety, security, access, confidentiality, and disclosure of identifiable health information by all media means; and establishing notification standards, penalties, and enforcement activities in response to noncompliance by individuals and every member of all areas in the health care industry for sharing information without patient consent. Outlined next are several important features of HIPAA that you need to comply with.

HIPAA Standard: Privacy

The first area involves privacy standards, with a rule requiring health professionals to protect personal health information. Personal health information not only includes the patient's history, diagnosis, and treatment, but also all demographic information (name, address, phone number, etc.). Furthermore, the patient is entitled to have appointments, hospitalizations, and testing information kept private from family, friends, coworkers, and clinical staff. Trust in the health care provider by patients can be accomplished only when they consider that the information they provide will remain securely entrusted except when disclosure is required by law (such as in cases of births, deaths, communicable diseases, and certain crimes). Clinical staff who do not need the information in order to provide medical care are not entitled to privileged information simply because they work at the facility. Confidentiality in the health care setting is of upmost importance. Simply stated: *never* gossip or look up information not necessary to perform your ECG technician duties.

HIPAA Guideline: Privacy

Private personal health information includes anything about the patient's existence in the health care setting.

HIPAA Standard: Security

The second area of patient protection includes security standards. Within the security category, administrative, technical, and physical standards must be implemented. Under the administrative area, clinical administrators are required to provide written standards for privacy and confidentiality. Patients must be provided written guidelines concerning their right to privacy and disclosures, and is often located in a document called the "Patient's Bill of Rights." Staff must be provided training and time to review, understand, and implement HIPAA guidelines. When new protocols are being implemented, all staff should be trained or retrained. Training may include areas such as new or improved computerized medical record documentation requirements, providing or updating staff access coding to patient records, and assigning specific levels of access to computerized patient data.

Physical and technical standards refer to the method of maintaining confidentiality while using various media methods. Since federal law provides patients the right to access or to obtain a copy of their medical records, knowing the office protocol is important for the ECG technician. For example, the ECG technician needs to know the protocol for giving a copy of the

electrocardiogram (ECG)
A noninvasive diagnostic test performed on a patient in which electrodes are placed on the body to measure the electrical activity of the heart.

ECG to a patient on the same day as the test is performed, before the doctor sees the patient, or when the interpretation is provided on the computerized **electrocardiogram ECG**. A patient owns the information in a medical record; however, a practitioner may determine to what extent, and when, the information may be given to the patient. Often, a computerized analysis of a patient ECG is incorrect or incomplete, so the protocol may include release of the ECG, but it may be in the patient's best interest not to release ECG interpretation. Finally, the law gives patients the right to know who else has viewed or obtained a copy of their personal information. Patients must give written consent for release of personally identifiable information.

HIPAA Guideline: Security

Health professionals have a legal responsibility to keep patient information private and secured.

HIPAA Standard: Electronic Information Transfer

Patient information must remain confidential whether the information is being transferred to pharmacies, insurance companies, other doctor offices or clinics, hospitals, etc. Technical guidelines involve the transfer of information electronically at all levels of patient care, including via email, fax, mobile media, and all other forms of media. A confidentiality disclaimer is attached to many of the transfer protocols that specifies that the information is confidential, and if received in error, the receiver should inform the sender. Inappropriate use or transfer of personally identifiable patient information without the patient's written approval is not acceptable. Get the patient's written approval before transferring any information. Knowing the office protocols are a requirement to provide patients with optimal, timely service.

HIPAA Guideline: Electronic Information Transfer

Confidentiality must be maintained by everyone who deals with identifiable patient information.

Ethics

Ethics defines a person's inner self—who we are. What this means is that ethics are formed by individual beliefs, which are often based on upbringing, religious beliefs, and education. Knowing the difference beyond what is right or wrong and how situations are handled in our personal life forms our ethical point of view. Laws are often created by civilized societies that define many of the rules of ethics to specific populations. Other times, organizations such as the World Health Organization (WHO) develop common goals or guidelines that may define the health or welfare of world populations. In the health care field, most professionals agree to follow a Code of Ethics or a Code of Conduct that defines how to handle situations based on common professional beliefs and training. Ethics plays a role in the ECG technician's daily routine and with patient interactions, such as collecting a patient history or asking a patient personal information. ECG technicians should document information as provided by the patient but should not add their personal point of view, personal biases, attitudes, or preconceptions about what the patient has disclosed, either while interacting with the patient or while documenting the patient's medical record. Observations can be included, but each one should be clearly noted in the patient's medical record as "I observed …". Health care professionals should maintain high ethics by knowing and following established office protocols.

Quick Check 5-1

Fill in the blanks.

1. Privacy under HIPAA guidelines includes _____ concerning the patient.

2. HIPAA training is a responsibility of the health care _____, but understanding and implementing HIPAA standards are the responsibility of the health care _____.

3. Patients have a right to _____ their personal information; however, the ECG technician must adhere to _____ in providing that information.

4. A(n) _____ is attached to many transfer protocols, which informs the receiver that private patient information has been sent, and if received in error, the receiver should notify the sender.

5. Ethics plays a role in the technician/patient _____ when collecting a patient history or when asking for and documenting _____ patient information.

IMPORTANCE OF VITAL SIGN MEASUREMENTS

noninvasive
Patient tests or procedures that do not penetrate the skin and body orifices are not entered.

within normal limits (WNL)
A range of numbers given to medical tests or procedures that show the results to be within a medically selected normal healthy range for a specific population of people (i.e., children, adults, geriatric, etc.).

Vital signs are considered **noninvasive**, standard protocol assessment testing because these tests can give a snapshot into a patient's immediate health situation. Six patient vital statistics, typically called "vital signs," are completed with patients prior to having an ECG. These measurements include temperature, pulse, respirations, pulse oxygen level, weight, and blood pressure. Normal vital signs in adults are not just one specific number; rather, each vital has a range of numbers that a person's statistics can fall within while still being considered **within normal limits (WNL)**. According to the National Institutes of Health (NIH), the normal range for each vital statistic (except weight) has been listed in **Table 5-1**. Note that the values given are for an average healthy adult while the adult is in a resting state.

Table 5-1 Healthy Adult Vital Sign Ranges

Vital Sign	Normal Range
Temperature	97.8°–99.1°F (36.5°–37.2°C)
Pulse	60–100 beats per minute
Respirations	12–18 breaths per minute
Pulse Oxygen Saturation Level	95–100% (SpO$_2$)
Blood Pressure	90/60–120/80 millimeters of mercury (mm Hg)

Pulse Oximeter

Taking a patient's pulse oxygen level as standard protocol is relatively new in clinics and doctor offices. Prior to 2010, emergency rooms, critical care units, and surgical units were the predominant users of the **pulse oximeter**. A pulse oximeter found in a clinic is typically a portable, battery-operated device that is put on a patient's finger and used to measure arterial oxygen saturation and heart rate. This nonevasive test is used as a screening tool in diabetic patients and patients with pulmonary diseases, or it can be used to detect whether a patient is in need of oxygen (perhaps due to heart blockage or poor systemic circulation). Normal blood saturation levels are considered to be in the 95 percent–100 percent range. Pulse oxygen saturation levels taken with a pulse oximeter are documented with the abbreviation SpO_2. **Figure 5-1** shows a pulse oximeter that can give a printout of the oxygen level. Smaller portable units only include a finger probe with a digital analysis. Hospital units typically are connected to a monitor that gives continuous feedback on all the vital signs. The pulse oxygen reading cannot detect circulatory sufficiency or ventilation issues, and the pulse oximeter is not as effective as the invasive arterial puncture for determining oxygen saturation, but for most patients, as part of the initial vital signs, the pulse oxygen reading is sufficient.

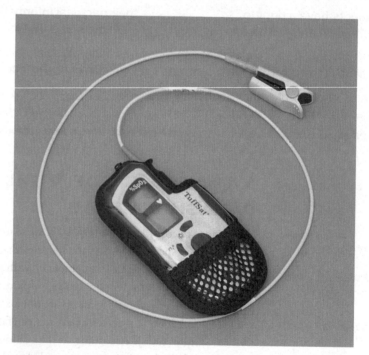

Figure 5-1 Pulse oximeter

Additional Vital Sign Measurements

Cardiac patients may have additional procedures or tests performed during a typical visit with a specialist that are included with the vital signs. One of these tests is called a **heart rate variability (HRV)** analysis, which is documented from the standard ECG and measures the load on the resting heart mediated by respiratory gating. With HRV, specific variations to the beat-to-beat intervals of a patient's heartbeat are recognized and documented. Performing an ECG procedure that displays HRV can often be used as an assessment tool to moderately predict the likelihood of a particular cardiac event occurring in the future. These variations have also been linked to certain medical conditions being found before any other symptoms have appeared or have been documented. HRV is considered an assessment tool for the autonomic regulation of the heart and in the future may be recognized as a newly required additional vital sign. HRV will be further explained in Chapter 7, which discusses ECG measurements.

Several additional tests may be routinely completed at a cardiologist's office along with the standard noninvasive vital signs already mentioned. For example, if peripheral artery disease is suspected, a carotid ultrasound, abdominal ultrasound, or ankle brachial index may be obtained. The ankle brachial test will be described in further detail under the blood pressure section in this chapter. Ultrasound testing is not covered in this book.

It is very important to always take the patient's vital signs during each visit. Ethically, health care personnel should never substitute the vitals taken on a previous visit in lieu of completing all vitals completely and correctly just before the patient is seen by the practitioner. Accuracy taking the vital signs and documenting each vital sign with the date, time, results, and health care personnel's identification is usually in the patient's electronic medical record.

Quick Check 5-2

Fill in the blanks.

1. Vital signs are _____ procedures that provide a(n) _____ of a patient's current health.
2. A pulse oximeter measures _____ oxygen saturation and _____.
3. The pulse oxygen reading does *not* measure circulatory _____ or _____ issues.
4. Heart rate variability measures the _____ on a resting heart mediated by respiratory gating.
5. When peripheral _____ is suspected, a carotid or abdominal ultrasound may be ordered.

ROLE OF BLOOD PRESSURE

sphygmomanometer
A device used to measure arterial blood pressure in a noninvasive manner.

Recall that blood pressure measures heart rate. There are two ways to take blood pressure measurements—directly and indirectly. The direct method is an invasive procedure that requires a sterile needle or catheter that is inserted into the lumen of an artery or within a chamber of the heart. In patient assessment, the indirect measurement of blood pressure is always used. The indirect method is noninvasive and requires the use of a **sphygmomanometer**. Taking a blood pressure reading on a patient gives caregivers an immediate snapshot of the patient's overall condition. Many factors can change a patient's blood pressure from minute to minute; therefore, understanding the importance of blood pressure to the heart's immediate condition is important. Not all heart conditions will create a variance from a normal reading. In fact, some heart conditions will continuously show a current normal reading even if heart damage occurred in the past. Though introduced in this chapter, the importance and role of blood pressure readings will be referred to throughout the remainder of this book.

Previous chapters have covered the flow of blood, systemic circulation, pulmonary circulation, and the cardiac cycle. This chapter puts these terms into perspective by showing their relationships in a simple blood pressure reading. To understand blood pressure, recall that in one cardiac cycle, the heart is at rest or the heart is contracting. Both processes need to be able to complete their part of the cycle for the heart to be healthy. Next, recall from Chapter 3 that in one cardiac cycle, the resting stage of the cycle is called diastole and the contraction stage is called systole. When recording the patient's blood pressure, always record the numbers side by side, separated by a slash. The systolic number is always written first because the systolic pressure records the heart's highest pressure, which occurs during a ventricular contraction. Blood pressure is measured in units of millimeters of mercury (mmHg). Blood pressure readings have a range of measurements, such as "normal" being any measurement between 90/60 mmHg to 120/80 mmHg.

Blood Pressure

$$\text{Blood Pressure} = \frac{\text{Systolic Pressure (heart contraction)}}{\text{Diastolic Pressure (heart relaxation)}}$$

Blood pressure readings in a clinical setting use a sphygmomanometer. Two types of sphygmomanometers are used: digital and analog (manual). Both types use a blood pressure cuff, but the analog method also requires the use of a stethoscope by health care personnel to detect heart sounds. With the digital method, once the blood pressure cuff has been placed, typically the health care professional only needs to push a button, and the machine does the measuring. In some cardiology offices, only analog (manual) blood pressure readings are taken and recorded because some cardiologists believe that the calibration of manual sphygmomanometers is superior to that of electronic devices. Proper calibration of either device is an important but often overlooked task in many clinics. It is important to always use the proper size of blood pressure cuff on a patient in order to obtain an accurate reading. **Figure 5-2** shows various sizes of blood pressure cuffs available.

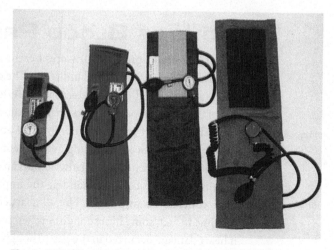

Figure 5-2 Different sizes of blood pressure cuffs

Blood Pressure Measurement in Relation to the Heart

Chapter 2 describes the circulatory system as the human body's transportation system for nutrients, gases, and waste products. Blood is either flowing through the arteries, veins, or capillaries. Taking this information to a new dimension, consider the force at which the blood is moved through the body and what causes this force to change. The change in force is called blood pressure variance. Changes in variance can be created from internal changes (from within the body) or by external change (such as a sudden injury). This section will concentrate on internal changes not caused by physical activity. Internal changes in blood pressure are primarily caused by constriction or dilation of the arteries or veins, which prevents or hinders the completion of the cardiac cycle. The variance is noted in blood pressure readings and on an ECG. When the blood pressure is too high, the patient can be at increased risk for a stroke, cardiovascular illness, or kidney disease. **Table 5-2** shows the normal range for blood pressure readings, as well as the range for prehypertension (high normal) and the four progressive stages of hypertension. Again, every patient should have their blood pressure checked at every medical visit. Keep in mind that pulse pressure (as discussed in Chapter 3) is also an important variable. Notice the slight overlap in numbers. A person's blood pressure can fall within two different ranges—for example, a blood pressure of 130/70 would fall within the high normal systolic range, but also within the normal diastolic range.

Table 5-2 Blood Pressure Ranges

Condition	Systolic Pressure Range (mmHg)		Diastolic Pressure Range (mmHg)
Hypotension	90–50	/	60–35
Normal	120–90	/	80–60
High Normal	140–120	/	90–80
Hypertension—Stage 1	160–140	/	100–90
Hypertension—Stage 2	180–160	/	110–100
Hypertension—Stage 3	210–180	/	120–110
Hypertension—Stage 4	240–210	/	130–120

Note: Keep pulse pressure in mind (normal pulse pressure range is 30–40 mmHg).

When the arteries are not open and cannot move nutrients, gases, or waste products through them, pressure builds up and the blood circulation slows down. Over a period of time, the arteries can become clogged or blocked with waste products, and this can eventually cause heart blockage. The body tries to compensate for the smaller blood passage by increasing arterial pressure, which causes an increase in blood pressure. This increase in blood pressure, which usually occurs over time, is called hypertension, which is abbreviated in medical records as HTN.

Hypertension and Heart Disease

Long-term, uncontrolled hypertension can cause many cardiac problems. Therefore, it is important to take and record blood pressure readings carefully. Medical diagnosis of hypertension must be identified over a period of time, usually confirmed by a higher-than-normal blood pressure on at least three different office visits during a period of weeks or months. A complete physical exam, blood work, and an ECG will confirm the diagnosis. Once a diagnosis of hypertension has been made, the person is then classified by the type of hypertension. The two types of hypertension classifications are **primary hypertension** (also referred to as essential hypertension or idiopathic hypertension) and **secondary hypertension. Table 5-3** compares the differences between primary and secondary hypertension. Primary hypertension has no known cause but may be linked to one or more of four distinct factors: genetics, lack of exercise, obesity, and poor diet. Primary hypertension usually develops over a period of many years. Primary hypertension is not curable, but it can be managed and controlled. Because there is not yet a cure, primary hypertension is often referred to as hypertension disease. Secondary hypertension is caused by a medical condition that might be curable or treatable. Secondary hypertension might be alleviated if the underlying medical condition that caused the sudden spike in blood pressure is addressed. Some known causes of secondary hypertension include complications with diabetes such as diabetic nephropathy, sleep apnea, and high alcohol intake. Diabetes is a leading cause of secondary hypertension.

Table 5-3 Primary/Secondary Hypertension Comparison

Primary Hypertension
CAUSE: Unknown, but believed to be linked to:
• Genetics
• Lack of exercise
• Obesity
• Poor diet
ONSET: Occurs over a period of time, perhaps years
OUTLOOK: Cannot be cured but can be controlled and managed.
Secondary Hypertension
CAUSE: Underlying medical conditions
May be linked to:
• Complications of diabetes
• Sleep apnea
• High alcohol intake
ONSET: Acute
OUTLOOK: May be curable or treatable if the underlying condition that caused the sudden spike in blood pressure is placed under control.

Unfortunately, many people with hypertension do not know that they have hypertension, or that they are at an increased risk for cardiac events. There may be no symptoms until after complications occur. Once a patient has been diagnosed with hypertension, the medical goal becomes to monitor and maintain a healthy blood pressure. Hypertension disease can usually be managed through drug therapy, lifestyle changes, and exercise. Patient education is very important because hypertension management protocol cannot be accomplished by medical personnel alone. Patients should be taught how to self-monitor their blood pressure between office visits, understand the need for complete compliance of drug therapy, and remember to document events that occur when they note blood pressure increases. Patient education can greatly improve the patient's long-term success in maintaining the targeted rate and may improve quality of life through lifestyle changes and exercise.

Hypertension

Primary hypertension = hypertension disease; no cure, only control

Secondary hypertension = usually sudden onset; medical condition, possibly curable

---

Quick Check 5-3

Fill in the blanks.

1. One _____ process consists of the heart at rest, followed by the heart contracting.

2. The resting stage of the heart is called _____ and the contracting stage is called _____.

3. The change of _____ at which blood moves through the body is called blood pressure _____.

4. Smaller blood passages caused by blockage cause arterial pressure to _____ and blood pressure to _____.

5. _____ hypertension has no cure and no known cause, but _____ hypertension is usually caused by a medical condition and may be cured if the medical condition is resolved.

Specialized Cardiac Blood Pressure Testing

Two additional tests may be performed in medical offices on a routine basis. They are called the ankle brachial pressure test and the jugular venous pressure test, and are described next.

Ankle Brachial Pressure Index (ABPI) Test

ankle brachial index (ABI)
A noninvasive test performed to obtain a ratio of the systolic blood pressure in the lower legs in comparison to the systolic blood pressure in the arms; also called ankle brachial pressure index (ABPI).

Many practitioners request that an ankle brachial pressure index (ABPI) test, more commonly referred to as an **ankle brachial index (ABI)**, be performed as part of the vital signs. The purpose of the test is to compare blood flow in the extremities by obtaining a ratio of the systolic blood pressure in the lower legs compared to the systolic blood pressure in the arms.

ABI Advantages

The ABI test can be used to screen, diagnose, and monitor systemic blood pressure in a noninvasive manner. The results can be used as part of a preliminary assessment of peripheral arterial disease (PAD) or for determining treatment options for patients already diagnosed with PAD. The ABI test is also used for leg ulcer assessment and to determine the use and nonuse of high compression bandaging for ulcers. Because a person may present with symptoms or may be asymptomatic, once a person has been diagnosed with PAD, the ABI test is repeated annually to assist in the assessment of how medications are working and whether the disease has progressed.

ABI Limitations

One of the current concerns in using the ABI as a routine test is that there is a lack of standardization with the blood pressure recordings based on variables such as cuff placement and size, speed of inflation and deflation, and the length of time the patient needs to rest prior to testing. Other concerns include improper administration of the test by repeatedly inflating and deflating the blood pressure cuff, or that the patient may have an irregular pulse that might cause improper reading of the systolic pressure. The test results for the ABI test may be unreliable if patients suffer from arterial calcification, as is commonly found in diabetic patients and the elderly; if patients are heavy smokers; or if patients are suffering from renal disease.

Performing the ABI Test

To perform the ABI test, the health care technician needs a Doppler wand or probe, ultrasound gel, and correctly fitting blood pressure (BP) cuffs for the arm and ankle. The blood pressure cuff is considered the correct size if the bladder section's length in proportion to the upper arm is approximately 80 percent; and the width of the cuff is approximately 140 percent of the circumference of the upper arm. The patient should remove his or her shoes and socks, and if he or she is wearing a long-sleeved shirt, the sleeve needs to be rolled up or the shirt removed if it obstructs the blood flow in the arm. The patient should be in the supine position for approximately 10 minutes before the test is performed. After the procedure is explained to the patient, gel is applied to the brachial artery. To find the ABI value in the arm, position the cuff as normal, then locate and listen to the loudest sound in the brachial artery using the Doppler. Continue listening to the brachial artery as the cuff is inflated to about 20 mmHg above the patient's usual systolic pressure, which should cause the Doppler sound to cease. Slowly deflate the cuff and listen for the Doppler sound to reappear. When the sound of the Doppler brachial pulse is heard with cuff deflation, record the measurement to determine the brachial systolic pressure. Only the systolic pressure is used to obtain the ABI, in order to make a determination of the maximum arterial pressure at the time of the contraction of the left ventricle. The process is repeated in the same manner for the other arm, remembering to record only the systolic pressure. It may be easiest to use the initials BA_L and BA_R to mark the left and right brachial artery. **Figure 5-3** shows the cuff placement and location of the brachial artery for Doppler placement.

To find the ABI value in the leg, place the cuff just above the ankles and locate, with the Doppler, the dorsalis pedus artery and posterior tibial artery in the foot. Be sure to find the strongest sound. Measure the systolic pressure for each artery, inflating the cuff only until the sound of the artery is diminished. After slowly deflating the cuff, record the systolic pressure when the Doppler sound reappears. After recording the systolic pressure for each artery, use only the higher pressure of the two arteries to calculate the ABI for that leg. Repeat the process for the other leg. **Figure 5-4** shows an example of cuff placement, as well as the artery locations for leg ABI.

Although most patients will have similar arm systolic pressures, using the highest pressure increases the accuracy of the central systolic pressure. The formula to use to find the ABI for each leg is to divide the highest pressure in one foot by the highest pressure in either arm. Box 5-1 highlights this formula. Be sure to record each foot separately, and round the answer to two decimal places. For quality control purposes (because blood pressures may change), the recommended order of obtaining the ABI is to obtain the right arm first, followed by the right leg, then the left leg, and finally the left arm.

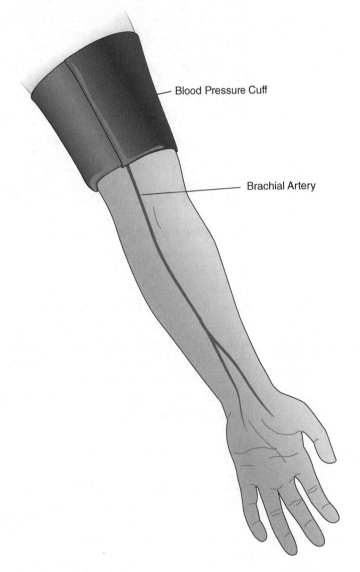

Blood Pressure Cuff

Brachial Artery

Figure 5-3 Arm ABI

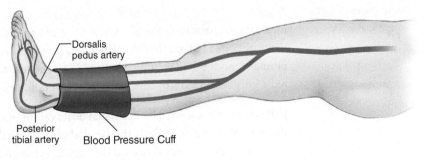

Dorsalis
pedus artery

Posterior
tibial artery

Blood Pressure Cuff

Figure 5-4 Leg ABI

Box 5-1 ABI Formula

Each leg is calculated separately.

Right Leg

$$ABI_R = \frac{\text{Highest Ankle Systolic Pressure in Right Leg}}{\text{Highest Brachial Systolic Pressure of the Two Arms}}$$

Left Leg

$$ABI_L = \frac{\text{Highest Ankle Systolic Pressure in Left Leg}}{\text{Highest Brachial Systolic Pressure of the Two Arms}}$$

Interpreting the Results of the ABI Test

There has not been enough evidence-based literature to overwhelmingly interpret the results of the ABI test, but generally accepted methodology has used a range of numbers to identify a normal range, acceptable range, and variances above and below the normal and acceptable ranges. Researchers are concerned about two factors—the person's age and blood pressure, which are not addressed in the interpretation. **Table 5-4** shows the generally accepted ABI values. Previous studies have also shown that auscultation with a stethoscope to find the brachial systolic blood pressure has resulted in comparable Doppler readings, so the preferred method to obtain the arm blood pressures is really up to the clinician. Whichever method is chosen, it is imperative that the technician pays meticulous attention to detail to obtain valid measurements.

Table 5-4 Ankle Brachial Index Test Interpretation

ABI Value	Interpretation
Above 1.4	Abnormal, possible calcification or vessel hardening from peripheral vascular disease (PVD)
1.0–1.4	Normal
0.8–1.0	Acceptable; may be insignificant arterial disease
0.5–0.8	Moderate arterial disease
Less than 0.5	Severe arterial disease

Jugular Venous Pressure (JVP)

jugular venous pressure (JVP) The observation and measurement of the jugular vein in the neck to determine venous blood pressure and volume.

Jugular venous pressure (JVP) is another example of an assessment tool used by some medical clinicians to aid in the assessment of cardiac and pulmonary dysfunctions. A correctly obtained JVP can indicate whether a person has a normal venous blood pressure and a normal venous blood volume. Elevated JVP typically reflects congestive heart failure, tricuspid regurgitation, constrictive pericarditis, or pulmonary hypertension.

JVP is normally assessed by the visual observation of the right side of a patient's neck while the patient is reclining with the head slightly turned to the left and the chin extended. Adequate light is directed toward the jugular veins on the neck to observe the jugular pulse while the patient inhales and exhales. In a normal JVP, the practitioner should notice a rise in the JVP when a person exhales and the pressure falling during inspiration. It is most difficult to notice the JVP on obese people and people with short necks. If no venous movements are noticed, gentle pressure applied to the upper right abdominal cavity for about 10 seconds may produce a transient rise in JVP, which is normal. It is considered an abnormal response if the JVP remains elevated the entire time that the abdomen is compressed, and this could be an indication of impaired right heart function. Finally, it is difficult to measure venous pressure when the pulse rate is greater than 100 beats per minute.

It is important to note some differences between the carotid artery and the jugular vein. Some observations to note include:

- The jugular vein does not have a palpable pulsation, but the carotid artery does.
- The level of the pulse wave should decrease on inspiration and increase on expiration in the jugular vein, whereas the respiration has no effect on the carotid artery, but an outward pulse is usually the carotid artery.

Quick Check 5-4

Fill in the blanks.

1. A concern in using the ankle brachial index test is based on the lack of _____ with blood pressure recordings.

2. Improper administration of the ABI test can be caused when the patient has a(n) _____ pulse, which can cause an inaccurate reading of the _____ pressure.

3. The equipment needed to perform the ABI test includes a(n) _____ wand, ultrasound gel, and a correctly fitting blood _____.

4. To calculate the ABI for each leg, divide the _____ pressure in one _____ by the highest pressure in either arm.

5. In a normal jugular venous pressure, the JVP should _____ when a person exhales and _____ during inspiration.

DIABETES AND HEART DISEASE

As mentioned in Chapter 2, the circulation system of the body is a closed loop, meaning that the blood flows from the heart systemically and returns to the heart to repeat the process. In a normal nondiabetic body, glucose is metabolized as insulin in the pancreas from foods that were ingested and enters the bloodstream to provide for cell growth and energy. The circulatory system is the main means of transportation of the insulin to the cells. During systemic circulation, the blood picks up waste products in the capillary beds and uses the kidneys as a major route to dispose of the waste. A person who has diabetes is not able to metabolize glucose; therefore, the insulin that should have been produced in the pancreas does not permeate the cells, and the cells are starved of fuel and energy. The diabetic person excretes glucose, unmetabolized, in the urine. High blood glucose levels raise the risk of people for developing diabetes, and a major complication of diabetes is heart disease. Although not typically performed as part of the cardiac assessment, while collecting a patient history, the patient's fasting blood sugar should be documented. If a patient does not know his or her blood sugar level, the clinician will most likely order routine blood work to be completed prior to the next visit.

Adult diabetics are considered high-risk patients for cardiovascular disease. There are three primary types of diabetes—Type 1, Type 2, and gestational diabetes. Type 1 diabetes is considered an autoimmune disease because the body's own immune system attacks and then destroys the insulin-producing cells in the pancreas. Type 1 diabetics must take insulin daily to survive because the pancreas does not produce insulin. The cause of Type 1 diabetes is not known, but it is thought that genetics, environmental factors, or viruses may contribute to this autoimmune disease. Type 2 diabetes, which includes the majority of people that present with cardiac problems related to long-term diabetes, do produce insulin in the pancreas, but the body does not use the insulin effectively. This ineffective use of insulin is called **insulin resistance**. Causes for Type 2 diabetes include being an adult, often over the age of 40, overweight or obese, and having a sedentary lifestyle. Unfortunately, more children today are being diagnosed with Type 2 diabetes. It is thought that the high usage of processed foods in children's diets and lack of exercise may be contributing factors, but current studies are inconclusive as to the exact cause. If symptoms are present for Type 1 or Type 2 diabetes, they may include one or several of the following: increased thirst, increased urination, constant hunger, weight loss, blurred vision, or extreme fatigue. Gestational diabetes occurs primarily in the third trimester of pregnancy and is thought to be caused by hormones or a shortage of insulin. Gestational diabetes usually disappears after childbirth, but women who have had gestational diabetes are usually about 50 percent more likely than those without gestational diabetes to develop Type 2 diabetes within 10 years. A fourth type of diabetes, named latent autoimmune diabetes in adults (LADA), usually appears in people over 30. Much research is currently under way, but LADA seems to show a combination of Type 1 and Type 2 symptoms. Early in this disease, the patient is usually still creating insulin (Type 2 diabetes), so glucose is still being managed with a combination of lifestyle changes, exercise, and medication. As the disease progresses, the patient must go on insulin to stay alive (Type 1 diabetes) because the body stops producing insulin.

insulin resistance
The human body's inability to utilize insulin produced in the pancreas, which then causes too much glucose to build up in the blood.

An important part of the patient assessment for diabetic patients is to document blood pressure, weight, eating habits, physical activity, family history, smoking history (the strongest controllable risk factor for heart disease), and a complete record of all medications, including the name of the drug, dosage, frequency of dosage, and patient compliance to dosage. Many patients will also know their cholesterol levels [both low-density lipoprotein (LDL) and high-density lipoprotein (HDL)] and HbA1C. Clinicians will normally order labs to confirm these numbers.

ROUTINE CARDIAC BLOOD TESTS

An important part of clinician assessment is a review of current patient blood results. Blood tests have the advantage of being quick, assessable, and relatively inexpensive, and yet blood tests can enhance other diagnostic assessment tools. The cardiac patient is usually monitored for one or more of the following blood tests. Although clinicians may add more blood tests, the common types of blood tests, their importance, and normal values are mentioned. It is vital when confirming appointments with patients that they are asked if they recently had blood work completed so that any current lab tests can be made available to the clinician at the time when patients are being seen. Levels outside the normal range typically increase a patient's risk of a cardiovascular event.

Cholesterol

Cholesterol blood tests are often collectively called a lipid panel because cholesterol levels are primarily the measurement of fats (lipids) in the blood. These lipids can be affected by lifestyle [except for Lp(a)] and eating habits. There are several numbers that are commonly looked at. Cholesterol, triglycerides, and apolipoproteins are found in the liver and create lipoproteins.

The first measure commonly looked at is total cholesterol. Total cholesterol is the sum of all the blood's cholesterol. Next are a category of cholesterol tests called the lipoproteins, which are a combination of cholesterol, protein, and triglycerides. Low-density lipoprotein (LDL) cholesterol measures plaque in the arteries; hence, LDL is usually called the "bad" cholesterol. Another type of LDL lipoprotein is called lipoprotein(a), or Lp(a). This type of LDL protein is determined by genes, not lifestyle. Another major type of LDL is classified as very low-density lipoprotein (VLDL). VLDL is usually measured as a percentage of the triglyceride value. High levels of VLDL may indicate an increased risk for coronary artery disease. Finally, there is high-density lipoprotein (HDL) cholesterol, which is often called "good" cholesterol because this number indicates how open the arteries are, which can further indicate how freely the blood is flowing. The final cholesterol category is called triglycerides, which are a type of fat. Triglycerides are very important to heart health because this measurement indicates the calories burned in relationship to the amount of food ingested. High triglycerides indicate that the patient is consuming more calories than he or she is burning. **Table 5-5** shows the ranges of cholesterol values for each cholesterol blood test mentioned. The values shown are measured in milligrams per deciliter (mg/dL).

Table 5-5 Cholesterol Values

	Value (Range)	Category
Total Cholesterol	200 mg/dL or less	Optimal
	200–239 mg/dL	Borderline high
	240 mg/dL or higher	High
LDL Cholesterol	129 mg/dL or less	Optimal, however, recommended level for at-risk heart disease patients is 70 mg/dL or less
	130–159 mg/dL	Borderline high
	160–189 mg/dL	High
	190 mg/dL or higher	Very high
HDL Cholesterol	60 mg/dL or higher	Optimal
	50–59 mg/dL (women)	Borderline low
	40–59 mg/dL (men)	Borderline low
	50 mg/dL or less (women)	Low; major risk factor of heart disease
	40 mg/dL or less (men)	Low; major risk factor of heart disease
Triglycerides	150 mg/dL or less	Optimal
	150–199 mg/dL	Borderline high
	200–499 mg/dL	High
	500 mg/dL or higher	Very high

Glycated Hemoglobin (HbA1C)

The glycated hemoglobin blood test measures a weighted average plasma glucose concentration over prolonged periods of time. The glycated hemoglobin blood test is referred to as the HbA1C or the hemoglobin A1c. HbA1C test results are reported as a percentage. Some physicians prefer to show the HbA1C results in terms of eAG, which means "average glucose." Results given in eAG are shown as milligrams per deciliter, the measurement shown on most home glucose monitors. The main difference between a glucose monitor and the eAG measurement is that the monitor records the glucose at a specific moment in time, whereas the eAG measures the glucose over a 24-hour period.

Recall that diabetes is often one of the main root causes of cardiovascular events. Long-term elevated glucose increases the risk of coronary disease and heart failure, stroke, or myocardial infarction (MI).

glycation
Having too much glucose in the blood, which causes the glucose to bind to hemoglobin.

The purpose of the HbA1C blood test is to diagnose diabetes and to provide an analysis of a patient's glucose control over the previous 120 days. Hemoglobin is an oxygenated protein found in the red blood cells. The purpose of hemoglobin is to carry oxygen from the lungs to all the cells in the body. Too much glucose in the blood causes the glucose to bind to the hemoglobin, which is called **glycation**. Glycation causes microvascular damage in nerves throughout the body and in the nephrons of the kidneys. The HbA1C test measures average blood glucose as a percentage of glycated hemoglobin in the blood. Identifying the average blood sugar will determine if diabetic medication prescribed is working (if the patient is compliant) or whether a new treatment plan needs to be implemented. A person is considered to be diabetic if, on two different occasions, the HbA1C is ≥ 6.5 percent or the person has an impaired fasting glucose, impaired glucose tolerance test, or a random plasma glucose measurement of more than 200 mg/dL, along with symptoms of hyperglycemia. In 2013, changes in the standardized American Diabetes Association (ADA) tables were recognized to meet new patient-centered needs and values, instead of just placing every patient on one predetermined scale. This means that the individualized goal for HbA1C still recognizes a general goal of < 7.0, but a goal of < 8.0 may be acceptable, as well as a goal of < 6.5, as shown in Box 5-2.

Box 5-2 Individualized Diabetic Goals

HbA1C < 6.5	May be an appropriate goal if the patient has no coronary vascular disease, has had diabetes for a short period of time, and tolerates treatment well
HbA1C < 7.0	General goal
HbA1C < 8.0	May be an appropriate goal for patients with long-standing diabetes with limited life expectancy, extensive comorbid conditions, severe uncontrollable hyperglycemia, or severe hypoglycemia

---

The HbA1C test can give abnormal results because hemoglobin can be depleted if a person has chronic or heavy bleeding, anemia, low iron, or other conditions causing low hemoglobin. In addition, supplements such as Vitamins C and E, high cholesterol levels, and conditions such as kidney or liver disease can cause abnormal results. Therefore, this test should be

Table 5-6 2013 American Diabetes Association® HbA1C and eAG Comparison Values

	Glycated Hemoglobin HbA1C	Mean Plasma Glucose eAG
Measured in:	Percentage	Milligrams per deciliter
	6	126
	6.5	140
	7	154
	7.5	169
	8	183
	8.5	198
	9	212
	9.5	227
	10	240
	10.5	255
	11	269
	11.5	284
	12	298

Source: American Diabetes Association®, 2013

Note: HbA1C is measured by percentage (%). eAG is measured by milligrams per deciliter (mg/dL).

used along with other assessments. **Table 5-6** compares the 2013 ADA HbA1C values by percentage to the estimated blood sugar (measured in milligrams per deciliter) for the same period of time.

B-Type Natriuretic Peptides (BNP)

B-type natriuretic peptides (BNP) is a brain protein hormone that acts on blood vessels and is also found in the kidneys. BNP is released when ventricular pressure changes due to worsening symptoms of heart failure. BNP is designed to protect the heart from stress and compensate the body for congestive heart failure by promoting the excretion of sodium and water in urine and by lowering blood pressure by relaxing blood vessels. When a patient presents with chest pain along with hypertension, shortness of breath, or fluid retention, clinicians can use this quick and inexpensive fasting blood test to diagnose, monitor, and aggressively treat current heart conditions. When the heart is under stress or has been damaged, the body secretes high levels of BNP into the bloodstream as a natural defense. The net effect of the release of BNP is a decrease in blood volume, which increases cardiac output.

BNP increases with age, and females tend to have greater levels of BNP than males have. **Table 5-7** shows the BNP level in relationship to indications of heart failure. A high level of BNP in the blood indicates that there is increased fluid or pressure within the heart, unstable angina, the person recently had a myocardial infarction, or the person may have an acute pulmonary embolism. The BNP blood test is not used to diagnose heart failure by itself; it is one of the newer assessment tools used, and the results are combined with results from other testing to design treatment plans.

Table 5-7 BNP Levels Compared to Risk of Heart Failure

Level	Analysis
0–99 pg/mL	Normal
100–299 pg/mL	Potential heart failure
300–599 pg/mL	Mild heart failure
600–899 pg/mL	Moderate heart failure
Above 900 pg/mL	Severe heart failure

Note: BNP is measured in picograms per milliliter (pg/mL).

High-Sensitivity C-Reactive Protein (hsCRP)

C-reactive protein (CRP) is produced in the liver. The high-sensitivity C-reactive protein (hsCRP) blood test is used to detect inflammation within the body. The inflammation may be due to many physical conditions such as burns, trauma, or infections, as well as many inflammatory disease processes such as rheumatoid arthritis, lupus, and vasculitis. The Centers for Disease Control (CDC) recommends two CRP tests be administered, two weeks apart, to determine if infection or inflammation have influenced the readings. The average of the two numbers is then used to determine cardiovascular risk (see **Table 5-8**). An elevation of hsCRP has been linked to atherosclerosis, blood clot formation, and heart disease. Although the hsCRP blood test is not monitored as an independent risk factor, in atherosclerosis, it is the formation of the plaques that were caused by the inflammation restricting blood flow that is thought to be the cause for heart attacks or strokes. Current research suggests that the hsCRP blood test is best utilized to assess asymptomatic adults for statin therapy or for low to intermediate risk of myocardial infarction patients, but the hsCRP is not recommended for risk assessment in high-risk cardiac patients, nor is the CRP level alone typically used as the assessment tool to determine cardiovascular disease. CRP testing is most often used to treat the risk factors that are believed to be causing the increase in CRP, such as hypertension, diabetes mellitus, and obesity. As with most of the blood tests mentioned in this section, when results are considered overall as a group of indicators, cardiovascular disease can be more accurately diagnosed and treated.

Table 5-8 hsCRP Levels and Cardiac Risk Assessment

CRP Level	Risk for Future Cardiovascular Disease
0–1.0 mg/dL	Low risk
1.0–3.0 mg/dL	Intermediate risk
3.0–10 mg/dL	High risk

There are many additional blood tests available, especially for cardiac emergencies. Students should research these tests further if they are involved with emergency medicine.

Quick Check 5-5

Fill in the blanks.

1. Type _____ diabetics use insulin ineffectively. This condition is referred to as insulin _____.

2. Lipoprotein cholesterol tests for cholesterol, protein, and _____, which is a type of _____, are all important blood tests used to assess heart health.

3. Glycated hemoglobin blood tests measure weighted average plasma _____ concentration over _____ periods of time.

4. BNP is a brain hormone that is designed to protect the heart from _____ by _____ blood vessels.

5. An elevation of C-reactive protein (CRP) has been linked to atherosclerosis, blood clot formation, and _____.

ASSESSMENT TECHNIQUES

There are many different types of assessment tools used to obtain vital information from a patient. Patient interviewing, whenever possible, is the dominant acceptable method across the different techniques. If a patient is unable to speak or is unconscious, be sure to get the name, phone number, and relationship to the patient of the person who is providing the details for the assessment questions.

open-ended questioning
An interview technique used to obtain information that allows and encourages more response from an individual than a simple yes or no answer.

The key to remember, regardless of which assessment tool is used, is that the information obtained should be recorded as accurately and completely as possible. Only state facts provided by the patient or person being interviewed; do not add your personal opinion or bias. Questioning techniques should include **open-ended questioning**, which means that the interviewer should not ask a patient a question that can be answered with a yes or no answer. Instead, ask a question that will allow the patient to add additional comments. For example, instead of asking a patient "Do you drink alcohol?" ask "How much alcohol would you say you drink in a typical week?" Remember that any personal information a patient shares should be documented for the clinician, but the technician should take care to keep the information private and not discuss it with others who do not need this knowledge.

HIPAA Review

HIPAA requires health personnel to protect patients' personal information and to safeguard the electronic exchange of personal information.

In the following sections, three of the more common types of assessment tools—SOAP, and the SAMPLE and OPQRST interviewing techniques—are explained. SOAP, SAMPLE, and OPQRST are mnemonic acronyms that will be explained individually. SAMPLE and OPQRST are often used in emergency medicine. Box 5-6 at the end of this section combines important data from both SAMPLE and OPQRST methods to create a more comprehensive patient assessment questionnaire. Even though most facilities use a fill-in style form, understanding how to obtain the most complete answer and establishing a time frame around the event should always be your goal.

SOAP Assessment System

SOAP, meaning Subjective, Objective, Assessment, and Plan, is the most common mnemonic acronym assessment ever taught, but the SOAP method is not complete enough to obtain vital cardiac patient information, so other, more detailed assessments are often used. Box 5-3 shows the SOAP mnemonic acronym. It is important to recall SOAP, though, because the part of SAMPLE and OPQRST assessment being introduced next falls under the subjective category in SOAP.

Box 5-3	SOAP Assessment Mnemonic	
S	Subjective	What the patient states
O	Objective	What medical personnel observe
A	Assessment	What labs or testing shows, initial determination of diagnosis made by clinician
P	Plan	Care or plan of action taken by clinician

Subjective

Recall that subjective information is information that is provided from the patient's point of view, the family members' point of view, or the point of view of another person being interviewed because the patient cannot speak. Subjective information may not always be accurate or realistic, but it is vital in creating a history for the patient. Always record the subjective information as closely as stated by the respondent. The other sections of SOAP are not covered in this section, but a short recap of their definitions is included.

Objective

The objective section is what is observed by the medical personnel. An example of objective information includes documenting slurred speech or excessive sweating (hyperhidrosis).

Assessment

Assessment includes the review of results from lab work, x-rays, subjective history, and objective history to create a diagnosis. Unless the medical personnel are out in the field, such as emergency medical technicians (EMTs), the assessment part of SOAP is always completed by a clinician, not the technician.

Plan

The final section of SOAP is the plan of action to be taken after all other vital information—subjective, objective, and assessment—has been reviewed. Again, the clinician is the person in a clinical setting who documents and creates the plan.

Quick Check 5-6

Fill in the blanks.

1. Patient interviews should allow the patient to offer input other than just answering yes or no to the questions asked. This technique is called _____ questioning.

2. Subjective information provided by the patient is not always _____ or _____, but should always be recorded as closely as stated by the respondent.

3. _____ information is provided by observing the patient while trying to get the most _____ answers to your questions.

4. In a nonemergency clinical setting, the ECG technician only records the _____ and _____ information in a medical record.

5. The actual ECG test would be used as one tool in the _____ of a patient's condition, from which the clinician can then design a(n) _____ for treatment.

SAMPLE Assessment System

SAMPLE
A mnemonic acronym meaning Signs and symptoms, Allergies, Medications, Past medical history or injuries or illnesses, Last oral intake, and Events that led up to the current illness or injury.

SAMPLE is a mnemonic acronym meaning Signs and Symptoms; Allergies; Medications; Past medical history, injuries, or illnesses; Last oral intake; and Events that led up to the current illness or injury. There is more to the SAMPLE method than just asking these six questions to compile a patient's history. SAMPLE assessment is often used in an emergency room, urgent care center, or at the scene of an accident. The SAMPLE method encourages the patient to actively provide answers and to provide additional information that may be relevant. Rarely is the SAMPLE method assessment completed in the exact order necessary for documentation because one question may spark new pertinent information that needs to be recorded when the information is offered by the patient. Good SAMPLE assessment techniques can be time consuming. Box 5-4 shows the SAMPLE mnemonic acronym.

Box 5-4	SAMPLE Assessment Mnemonic	
S	Signs and symptoms	Subjective and objective assessment, including vital signs.
A	Allergies	Include food, medicine, herbs, and environmental allergies.
M	Medications	Include prescribed, over-the-counter (OTC), herbs, vitamins, minerals or other supplements, and recreational drugs.
P	Past medical history	Include previous injuries, illnesses, prior hospitalizations, diseases (including when they were diagnosed), and oral health. Also ask about last oral intake (food and drink), and about social history and family history.
L	Last oral intake	Record eating or diet habits, daily routines, social circle, and life stressors.
E	Events of today	Record anything out of the ordinary that happened within the last 24 hours.

Signs and Symptoms

The signs and symptoms section of SAMPLE assessment is usually a combination of subjective and objective information used in the SOAP method. The subjective part is what the patient is experiencing if conscious, whereas the objective part is what the vital signs are showing and what the medical personnel observe, such as bleeding or contusions. Subjective questioning can be thought of as asking the patient: "What happened, when, and why do you think it happened—what were you doing just before the event happened?"

Allergies

Three main types of allergies should be recorded as subjective information given by the patient. They include allergies to food, allergies to medications or herbs, and allergies from the environment, such as seasonal allergies from pollen. Medication allergies should include not only prescription drugs, but also over-the-counter (OTC) medications and recreational drugs. Always ask what the reaction was that made the patient think he or she was allergic to the food, medication, or environment. Also, ask what symptoms the patient experienced, how many times the allergy occurred, and what methods the patient uses to control or inhibit the allergy from returning, keep the allergy under control, or deal with the allergy. Environmental allergies are often overlooked by medical personnel. Environmental allergies include anything the patient could come in contact with, such as insect bites or stings; pollution caused by factories, cars, or trees, plants, and flowers; or everyday products such as latex.

Medications

Medication assessment should include prescription medications, over-the-counter medications, recreational drugs used, and herbs or supplements such as vitamins and minerals used on a regular basis. Important assessment information to record each time includes the amount of medication taken; the method or form used to take the medication, such as inhalation, injection, oral, or sublingually; the frequency that the medication is taken, including the typical time of day when multiple doses are taken; and dosage usually taken each time. Be sure to ask patients when the last time they took each medication.

Often, patients may not know the names of individual prescription medications, but they can tell you how many types of medications they take, how often they take the medication, and what conditions they take the medication for. For example, a patient might state that she takes two medications for high blood pressure, a cholesterol medication, and three diabetes medications. Record only what the patient can tell you. A final question to ask about prescription medications is about patient compliance. Often, patients will know what they should be doing, but they may be skipping doses, not refilling prescriptions, or avoiding the medication due to undesirable side effects, so always ask patients to clarify typical usage.

Past Medical History

Past medical history is easier to obtain if you have an accurate picture of the patient's view of his or her allergies and medications. Ask about any medical history the patient remembers, even if the patient does not feel it is necessary or relevant information for this event. Types of information being collected should include prior hospital stays, how many, and for what condition. Ask about prior illnesses or diseases such as diabetes, hypertension, and cancer. Ask when they were first diagnosed and if they consider the condition to be under control. Include questions about oral health, such as when they last saw a dentist, if they have dentures or partials, or if they have implants or their own teeth. Ask if they have had any major dental work, such as crowns, done recently. Ask if this current event has happened in the past, and if so, how it was taken care of previously. Ask patients how they consider their overall health status to be and if there are any concerns mentioned by their regular doctor. Ask patients what tests they have had recently, and where they were done. Finally, ask patients if they are aware of any risks to their health, such as asthma, difficulty breathing, or memory loss. Record what the patients say, and do not document what questions were asked but yielded no pertinent information unless you are using a fill-in type questionnaire.

Last Oral Intake

Last oral intake is a very important part of the assessment process because the skilled interviewer will uncover a wealth of information about the patient's everyday life, such as eating or diet habits, daily routines, social circle, and life stressors. The information obtained from this assessment can even be used in assessing risk factors for cardiovascular disease. The interviewer should ask about the last medications taken, last liquids taken, and last foods eaten. Ask when, where, and how much was consumed in each category. Ask about the approximate time of consumption. For example, if a patient stated that he takes recreational drugs, ask if he had any today, and where he was when he took the drugs. Continue by asking if he eats or drinks when he takes the drugs, or if he had anything to eat or drink before or after the drugs. If the patient states that he only had alcohol in a public place, ask if the establishment also serves food. If he did not eat and drink, ask why not.

To find out how much food a person might have eaten, ask her if the establishment serves good food or if she would recommend the establishment as a good place to dine. Ask the patient how often she visits this establishment. Ask about tobacco use. If the patient was at a party outside of his home, ask if others became ill after consuming the same food, alcohol, or drugs. The information taken from a patient in the last oral intake section is vital if the patient is going to have surgery, have additional drug therapy, or to be correctly assessed for additional lab work, screenings, or procedures.

Events of Today

The events of today section questions the patient on what happened immediately preceding the current event. The interviewer is trying to document anything out of the ordinary that may have occurred in the daily routine that aggravated the current event. By completing a good last oral intake section, variances of the daily routine can be more readily determined. For example, chest pain occurring after a day of extreme physical activity at a family reunion is much different from symptoms of chest pain that came from sitting quietly at a bar or in front of a television at home. However, the interviewer can assess if levels of aggravation or stress occurred due to a patient watching his favorite team lose on television. The purpose of the event section is to try to document what occurred and the time frame before the event that may play a role in the patient's current condition. It is also important to establish if other conditions may have aggravated the condition the patient is presenting for. Examples of some other conditions that the patient may not recognize as important but that the interviewer should ask about include fatigue, nausea, syncope, confusion, or exertional dyspnea.

One of the main objections to using only the SAMPLE assessment technique is that not enough information is usually asked about family and social history. This is often missed because of the emergency nature of the event occurring or because the patient was unconscious, mentally impaired, or unable to answer the questions being asked. Often, families simply do not know the answers, especially if the adult children of the patient are the informants. Sometimes the patient or even the family will hide drug or alcohol abuse, or they may not see diet as a source of the problem.

Quick Check 5-7

Fill in the blanks.

1. SAMPLE assessment is often used in a(n) _____ situation.

2. The _____ and _____ section of the SAMPLE assessment condenses the subjective and objective areas in SOAP assessment into one category.

3. Important drug information to obtain from the patient includes the _____ of medication taken, _____ of medication taken, method of medication taken, and _____ of medication taken.

4. The last oral intake section in the SAMPLE assessment should include questions relating to the last _____, _____, and _____ ingested.

5. In the events of today section of SAMPLE assessment, what happened immediately _____ the current event is documented.

OPQRST Assessment System

OPQRST

A mnemonic acronym meaning Onset, Provocation, Quality, Radiation, Severity, and Time. The OPQRST assessment is used primarily for cardiac events.

OPQRST is a mnemonic acronym for pain as assessed by the patient. The acronym stands for: Onset, Provocation, Quality, Radiation, Severity, and Time of pain associated with a current event. The OPQRST assessment is used primarily for cardiac events and is used mostly in emergency situations. The OPQRST assessment system is often used along with the SAMPLE system to collect a more complete picture of subjective patient information about pain. As with the SAMPLE assessment, the questions are asked to the patient if possible, to family members if they are present and the patient cannot respond, or to other parties who were with the patient at the time of the event. The main difference between the SAMPLE and OPQRST assessment plans is that the OPQRST usually follows the SAMPLE assessment when cardiac assessment is needed, as well as assessment of other types of severe pain. OPQRST is considered a focused assessment for the evaluation of pain that brought the patient in for this particular event. Box 5-5 identifies the components of the OPQRST assessment.

Box 5-5 OPQRST Assessment Mnemonic		
O	Onset	Patient identifies what he or she was doing at the time of the first signs and symptoms of pain.
P	Provocation	Patient identifies what makes the pain worse. Ask about movement, pressure, and external factors.
Q	Quality	Patient describes the nature of the pain and its duration.
R	Radiation	Patient describes how pain exists (moves) in the body.
S	Severity	Patient identifies the level of pain.
T	Time	Patient compares pain now with the onset pain and previous pain; length of time that the patient has suffered the pain.

Onset

Onset questions relate to what the patient was doing when the signs and symptoms first started to occur. The interviewer should document by questioning if the pain started when the patient was active or inactive, or under a lot of stress. Additional questioning should describe if the onset of the pain was sudden (acute), gradual, or ongoing (chronic) according to the patient.

Provocation

Provocational pain questions relate to the patient expressing if the pain symptoms become better or worse with any movement, pressure or palpitation, or other external factors such as resting or lying down or sitting up. Even if this information seems trivial, document it exactly as the patient describes the pain.

Quality

Quality of pain can be described in two ways. First, the patient should be asked an open-ended question such as "Can you describe this pain?" Patient responses could describe the pain as sharp, dull, aching, crushing, burning, tearing, traveling, throbbing, etc. Next, ask the patient about the duration of pain. Patient responses could include constant, intermittent, or occasionally severe, followed by a lesser pain. Be sure to document both types of quality of pain—by description and by duration.

Radiation

Radiation refers to how the pain exists in the body, and it is documented by region. Ask the patient if the pain moves to another part of the body or stays in one place. For example, in a myocardial infarction, the pain usually will move, or radiate, from the chest region to an arm or the jaw. Document where the patient states the pain is located. Then document if the patient states that the pain moves and include the body regions that the patient describes.

Severity

Severity of pain is usually assessed by asking the patient to identify the level of pain based on a scale of 1 to 10, with 1 being a small amount of pain and 10 being extreme pain. The pain can be documented as a Pain Score of _____. Documentation can be further based on comparative pain level (if the event has occurred before), or if the patient can relate the current pain to an unrelated prior event such as childbirth pain or pain from a prior accident or surgery. Additionally, ask the patient to describe the pain now in reference to the onset of this event's pain, or if there is any additional severity of pain with movement.

Time

Time refers to the pain condition now versus at the onset. Time can also be a measure of this event in reference to previous events. Ask the patient if the pain is better, worse, or the same since onset. Ask if the pain ever happened before. Finally, ask how long the pain had been occurring in the current event. Document the time pain assessment in minutes and or hours.

Documentation

There is no one plan that can completely assess the patient's subjective history. Three techniques were introduced to allow the learner to get insight into what the subjective patient history should include. Being skilled as an interviewer will come with practice. Culture does play a role in how patients will respond to particular questions. Sensitivity of the interviewer and adjusting questioning techniques in recognition of cultural diversity will create the best possible atmosphere for accurate patient diagnosis and treatment.

Box 5-6 is a sample patient intake form that contains various sections of additional information that is required of a patient when the person is able to respond and is not in a medical emergency. In a medical emergency, there may be nobody available to give the requested information, including the patient. However, the more information that can be obtained initially, the better the opportunity for a positive outcome. "Part 2—Insurance Information" has not been expanded upon here because the topic is beyond the scope of this text, but obtaining an insurance card will have much of the information to get started in this section. Often, the person obtaining the insurance information is not directly working in patient care because reimbursement for services is a distinct department within the administrative portion of the medical facility.

HIPAA Review

Insurance personnel do not normally need to know any information related to direct patient care except for the purpose of coding the procedures.

Box 5-6 Patient Assessment Questionnaire

Part 1—Demographics

- Name

- Address

- Age

- Ethnicity

Part 2—Insurance Information

Part 3—Patient History, Family History

Include Traditional Risk Factors for Cardiovascular Disease Listed Below

- Vital Signs

  Blood Pressure (ask about Hypertension—controlled by medications?)

  Weight (Obesity)

  Pulse Oximeter (Below 95%)

- Smoking

- Diabetes Mellitus (controlled by medications?)

- Laboratory (Elevated: Cholesterol Levels, A1C, BNP, HS-CRP?)

- Family History of Heart Disease

(Continued)

> **Box 5-6 Continued**
>
> **Part 4—Prior Testing (including ECGs, Stress Tests, other)**
>
> **Part 5—Previous Vital Signs**
>
> **Part 6—Today's Updates on History, Vitals, Any Testing Performed**
>
> - SAMPLE Assessment Answers
> - OPQRST Assessment Answers if presenting with Pain

Quick Check 5-8

Fill in the blanks.

1. The OPQRST assessment is a focused assessment used to evaluate patient _____ and is _____ in nature.

2. Quality in the OPQRST assessment refers to the _____ of pain and the _____ of pain.

3. Pain severity is rated on a(n) _____ of _____.

4. _____ can be used to measure this event in reference to _____ events.

5. _____ plays a role in how patients will respond to particular questions, so the interviewer needs to practice _____ and adjust questioning techniques accordingly.

SUMMARY

- The Health Information Portability and Accountability Act (HIPAA) provides patient protection in three areas, including patient privacy, security of patient information, and privacy in electronic transactions of medical records

- There are six primary vital signs: temperature, pulse, respirations, pulse oxygen level, weight, and blood pressure

- Primary hypertension develops over a period of time, is not curable, and has no known cause, but it may be linked to genetics, lack of exercise, obesity, or poor diet.

- Secondary hypertension may have a sudden onset due to an underlying medical condition, and it may be curable if the underlying conditions, such as diabetes, sleep apnea, or high alcohol intake, that caused a spike in blood pressure are addressed.

- A specialized type of blood pressure testing called the ankle brachial index (ABI) can be used to screen, diagnose, or monitor systemic blood pressure in a noninvasive manner. The problem with using the ABI as a routine test is that there is not a standardization of many variables, such as proper test administration, allowance for age of the patient, and allowance for underlying patient health issues.

- Diabetes is a disease caused by the body's inability to metabolize blood glucose.

- Type 1 diabetes is considered an autoimmune disease, and people with this type of diabetes must take insulin daily in order to survive because the body does not produce insulin in the pancreas.

- Type 2 diabetic people do produce insulin, but the body does not use the insulin effectively.

- Gestational diabetes occurs during the final trimester of pregnancy and usually disappears after the woman gives birth.

- Hypertension and diabetes cause numerous cardiac conditions to become critically worse. Lifestyle changes such as losing weight and becoming more physically active, along with drug therapy, can usually control diabetes and hypertension, but these two diseases are often called "silent killers" because people often don't know that they have either disease and they can remain asymptomatic for years.

- Many patients will have blood tests ordered prior to a specific diagnosis or treatment plan. No single test can accurately diagnose a particular condition but combined the blood tests can become a strong assessment tool.

- A lipid panel blood test measures cholesterol, triglycerides, and apolipoproteins found in the liver and plaque in the arteries.

- The HbA1C blood test measures the average glucose concentration in the blood over a period of time.

- Brain natriuretic peptide (BNP) is a brain hormone that is released by the body into the bloodstream, in an attempt to increase cardiac output when ventricular pressure changes due to stress.

- High-sensitivity C-reactive protein (hsCRP) is a blood test that detects inflammation within the body and is used to determine cardiovascular risk.

- It is important to document risk factors accurately while completing a patient assessment. Clinicians will consider risk factors and usually order additional tests such as the ECG to accurately diagnose potential heart conditions.

- Subjective assessments are responses from patients or patient representatives and are not always composed of reliable or accurate information.

- SAMPLE assessment gives patients an opportunity to actively provide relevant information concerning their signs and symptoms, allergies, medications, past medical history, last oral intake, and events that brought them to seek medical intervention.

- Patient pain assessment can be completed using OPQRST assessment. Usually, the OPQRST assessment is completed after the SAMPLE assessment, and the medical interviewer asks the patient to explain when, where, and what brought on the pain, how long the pain has existed, what level the pain is, and if the pain is radiating to other parts of the body.

Critical Thinking Challenges

5-1. Respond to the following scenario, citing at least three HIPAA violations. Explain how you would handle each HIPAA violation differently.

Scenario: A tall, handsome actor, who was in town shooting a movie, came to the clinic complaining of chest pain today. It wasn't hard to notice him, and several of the office personnel wanted to know why he was being seen, if he was still married, what his phone number was, and if he is going to be okay. Everybody was aware that the tabloids have stated that the patient was 6'6" tall, was having marital problems, but also stated that he is in perfect health. Your job is to complete the initial assessment, including taking the vital signs, and completing an ECG.

5-2. Explain the mnemonic for SAMPLE, and then write one or two sentences describing each section in the mnemonic.

5-3. Answer the following in a paragraph or less:

1. Explain why patient assessment is a valuable tool for clinicians.

2. When is a patient assessment completed?

3. Give three examples of open-ended questioning that could be used in patient assessment of chest pain.

Review Activities

5-1. Match the blood test with the proper definitions. Choices may be used more than once.

Blood Test Choices: BNP   HbA1C

                           HDL   hsCRP

                           LDL   VLDL

                           eAG   triglycerides

1. _____ detects inflammation within the body

2. _____ used to diagnose diabetes

3. _____ average glucose

4. _____ measured as a percentage of triglycerides

5. _____ protects the heart from stress

6. _____ indicates how open the arteries are

7. _____ analysis of glucose over the previous 120 days

8. _____ a high level indicates increased fluid or pressure in the heart

9. _____ measures plaque in the body

10. _____ indicates calories burned in relationship to food ingested

5-2. Match the term which goes with the acronym OPQRST with the correct description. Each description starts with "The patient …"

1. _____ identifies the level of pain

2. _____ identifies activities at time of the first sign of pain

3. _____ describes the duration of pain

4. _____ compares this pain to previous pain

5. _____ describes movement of pain

6. _____ explains what makes the pain worse

5-3. Complete an ABI on another person. Record your results in the spaces provided below.

Supplies needed: Doppler wand or probe
Correctly sized blood pressure cuff(s)
Ultrasound gel

Right arm systolic pressure _____

Right ankle—highest systolic pressure _____

Left ankle—highest systolic pressure _____

Left arm—systolic pressure _____

Higher systolic pressure of the two arms _____

ABI_R _____ ABI_L _____

Chapter Five Test

Part 1: Match the definitions found in the right column with a term in the left column. In the space provided, write only the letter used in front of the definition.

1. _____ SAMPLE

2. _____ BNP

3. _____ diabetes

4. _____ patient interview

5. _____ pulse oximeter

6. _____ Type 2 diabetes

7. _____ LDL cholesterol

8. _____ OPQRST

9. _____ hsCRP

10. _____ demographics

A) blood test that measures plaque in the arteries

B) measures arterial oxygen saturation and heart rate

C) blood test used to detect inflammation within the body

D) assessment tool that encourages active patient participation in the collection of patient history

E) assessment tool that is focused on pain

F) brain hormone that acts as a natural defense to relax blood vessels and promote excretion of sodium and water in urine

G) examples include name, address, age, and ethnicity

H) inability to metabolize glucose

I) thought to be caused by a combination of variables, including genetics, lack of exercise, obesity, and poor diet

J) dominant type of assessment

Part 2: Blood Tests: Fill in the Blank

1. The _____ provides an analysis of the patient's glucose control over a period of the last two or three months.

2. High levels of _____, measured as a percentage of triglyceride value, may indicate an increased risk of coronary artery disease.

3. _____ measure the calories burned in relationship to the amount of food ingested.

4. _____ are a combination of cholesterol, protein, and triglycerides.

5. _____ indicates how freely the blood is flowing in the arteries.

Chapter Five Quick Check Answers

Answer order is important except where noted otherwise (shown in parentheses).

When two correct answers are possible, both answers are given separated by the word "or."

5-1:
1. everything
2. administrator, staff
3. access, office protocol
4. confidentiality disclaimer
5. interactions, personal

5-2:
1. noninvasive, snapshot
2. arterial, heart rate
3. sufficiency, ventilation
4. load
5. artery disease

5-3:
1. cardiac cycle
2. diastole, systole
3. force, variance
4. increase, increase
5. Primary, secondary

5-4:
1. standardization
2. irregular, systolic
3. Doppler, pressure cuff
4. highest, foot
5. rise, fall

5-5:

1. 2, resistance
2. triglycerides, fat
3. glucose, prolonged or extended
4. stress, relaxing
5. heart disease

5-6:

1. open-ended
2. accurate, realistic
3. Objective, complete
4. subjective, objective (either order)
5. assessment, plan

5-7:

1. emergency
2. signs, symptoms
3. amount, frequency, dosage
4. medications, liquids, foods (any order)
5. preceding or before

5-8:

1. pain, subjective
2. type, duration
3. scale, 1–10
4. Time, previous
5. Culture, sensitivity

6

ELECTROCARDIOGRAM BASICS

OBJECTIVES

After reading the chapter and completing all Quick Check activities, the student should be able to:

1. Summarize the primary differences between a single-channel and multichannel ECG machine.
2. Differentiate between an ECG electrode and an ECG lead.
3. Interpret the theory of Einthoven's Triangle.
4. Summarize which leads look at each of the four heart walls.
5. List the anatomically contiguous and reciprocal leads.
6. Identify the placement of standard limb leads and precordial leads on a patient.
7. Describe lead placements for posterior and right sided ECGs.
8. Contrast placements of leads for 3-lead and 5-lead ECGs.
9. Define informed and implied consent.
10. Demonstrate performing and documenting a 12-lead ECG on a patient.

KEY TERMS

anatomically contiguous

augmented leads

bipolar lead

differential diagnosis

electrode

ground lead

implied consent

informed consent

leads

precordial leads

reciprocal

unipolar lead

vector (V)

INTRODUCTION

After the clinician obtains the patient assessment, an electrocardiogram (ECG) is routinely completed to add to the other assessment tools to aid in creating a diagnosis. The goal of a correctly completed ECG is to allow the clinician to obtain the most accurate picture of what is happening within the heart during the cardiac cycle, and to identify previous issues such as previous myocardial infarcts. This chapter begins by introducing the types of ECG machines and supplies such as electrodes and leads. An explanation of how leads and electrodes work is given, followed by an explanation of the six limb leads and six precordial leads. Views of the electrical activity of the heart through correct placement of these leads are identified. Proper placement of the leads is very important for an accurate reading. Informed and implied consent are also explained in this chapter. Documentation required before administering an ECG is reviewed followed by step-by-step instructions to perform an ECG.

ECG MACHINES

Many models of ECG machines are on the market today. The latest models used in clinics are handheld devices that can be connected to computers and print out and save the patient's current ECG. The software programs that accompany these powerful devices can provide overlays of several previous ECGs found in the patient's electronic medical record (EMR) to identify any current changes.

electrode
A small, self-adhesive pad used to amplify electrical current from a patient; contains a layer of conductive gel and an area to attach a lead wire to an ECG machine.

The purpose of an electrocardiogram is to measure heart muscle activity by magnifying the sound of the electrical signal through the chest wall muscles and recording graphic images of the amplified sound, shown as waves on rhythm strips. **Electrodes** are attached to the skin to help with the conduction of the sound. Electrodes have wires, called **leads**, that attach between each electrode and the ECG machine to transfer the sound. An ECG can detect previous myocardial events, enlargement of one side of the heart, abnormal rhythms and other heart abnormalities. The ECG does not measure the mechanical contraction of the heart and only records the blood pressure, without analyzing it. The ECG also does not identify cardiac output, nor can the ECG measure cardiac muscle hypertrophy.

leads
Insulated conductor wires that are attached to electrodes and measure voltage changes from different views or angles of the heart, as determined by the placement of the electrodes on the body.

The noninvasive ECG is typically obtained in one of three ways. First is the resting ECG, where the patient relaxes in a supine (lying down) position, or, if the patient is complaining of severe pain or discomfort while in the supine position, use the Fowler's (sitting) position and take an ECG using a standard or portable ECG machine. The second type of ECG is completed while the patient is exercising; this is called a stress test, which uses the ECG machine and a treadmill or stationary exercise bike, as shown in **Figures 6-1** and **6-2**.

The third type of ECG is obtained with a 24–48-hour monitoring ECG machine called a Holter monitor, which is shown in **Figure 6-3**. The Holter monitor is attached to the patient, and it is worn 1 to 2 days during the course of the person's everyday routine. Patients are instructed on how to maintain a diary of events while wearing the Holter monitor. Any time the patient feels a cardiac discomfort, they can press an event button on the Holter monitor. The Holter monitor contains only five or seven leads, as shown in **Figure 6-4**. The purpose of the Holter monitor is to capture any arrhythmias, heart irregularities, or patient events such as pain or chest tightness that occur during a 24-hour period versus the 10-second recording

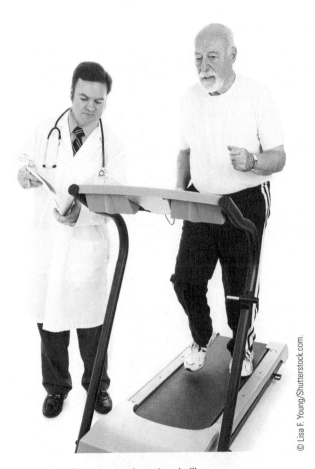

Figure 6-1 Stress test using a treadmill

© Lisa F. Young/Shutterstock.com.

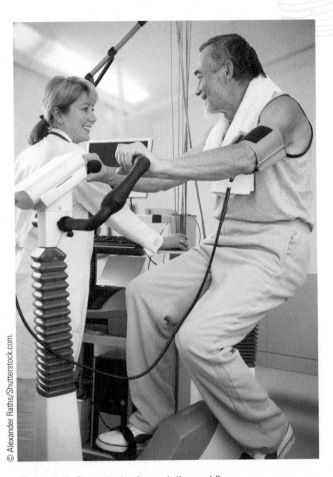

© Alexander Raths/Shutterstock.com.

Figure 6-2 Stress test using a stationary bike

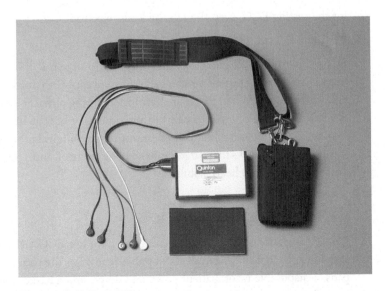

Figure 6-3 Holter monitor

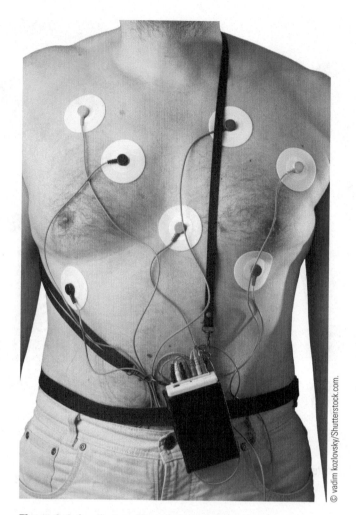

Figure 6-4 A patient wearing a Holter monitor

of the typical ECG. This chapter will primarily concentrate on preparation and performance for the resting ECG, even though the leads, electrodes, and theory are similar for all three devices.

differential diagnosis
Tests or procedures used by health care professionals to find potential causes for conditions with similar symptoms.

ECGs are used for diagnostic evaluations and to obtain a **differential diagnosis** because they are relatively inexpensive, can be performed easily in a doctor's office or clinic, and provide quick results. When ECGs are performed during physical exams, they are often used to develop a baseline of how the heart is functioning or how an implanted pacemaker is functioning. ECGs are also administered prior to many surgical procedures being scheduled, to identify potential risks that surgeons need to be aware of, and, after any heart-related surgical procedures, to verify heart stability.

ECG Testing Supplies

Before the patient comes into the room to have the ECG test performed, the technician should verify that they have all the supplies ready. For the patient, supplies include alcohol pads, a disposable razor, patient gown and drape, and a basket for the patient to put items from the patient's pockets such as change, cell phones, and belts, because these items can cause machine interference. Some clinics will provide a locker for the patient to put all his or her personal items, and then the person can lock up cell phones, purses, belts, or any other metal objects that he or she may have brought. Supplies for the ECG machine include having a minimum of 12 electrodes available, having lead wires in good condition, and having a working ECG machine. If the ECG machine is connected to a computer, check that there is paper for the printer (if results are to be printed).

If the ECG machine uses thermal paper, be sure that there is sufficient paper to run several ECGs in the machine. Never begin a new ECG if the thermal paper has a colored streak running along one side of the paper because that is an indication that the roll of paper is about to run out.

ECG machines come in two varieties: a single-channel machine that can record the ECG manually, one lead at a time, or the machine can be switched to an automatic mode, where the entire strip of leads is produced one lead after the other, producing a long "strip" of paper approximately 2 inches wide and often more than 24 inches long. When using a single-channel machine, the ECG "strip" will need to be cut and mounted on a special ECG patient record. The single-channel machine is time consuming and increases the chance of error while mounting the single leads because each lead needs to be cut individually and mounted on a chart.

Figure 6-5 shows a portable single-channel ECG machine with leads. Notice the ECG "strip" of paper.

Keys, belts, coins, cell phones, and other metal objects will usually interfere with the ECG machine. Instruct the patient to remove all such items before attaching the electrodes.

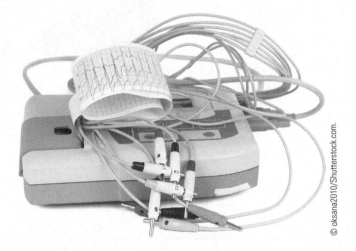

© oksana2010/Shutterstock.com.

Figure 6-5 Single-channel ECG machine

Most health care providers use the second type of ECG machine, called the multichannel machine. **Figure 6-6** shows an example of a multichannel ECG machine. A portable model is also available, which can be directly attached to a computer and electronic medical record for each patient. The multichannel ECG records all 12 views simultaneously.

The leads on a multichannel machine are typically recorded on a single 8 ½" × 11" paper or can be shown on a monitor. **Figure 6-7** shows an example of a three-channel printout. The three-channel machine does not require that the leads be cut and pasted into a chart. Older models of the multichannel machines may require the clinic to purchase specific 8 ½" × 11" ECG paper, but the newest multichannel machines use ordinary printer paper and save the ECG directly into the patient's EMR.

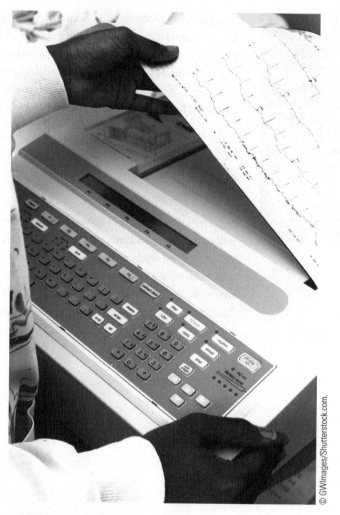

© GWImages/Shutterstock.com.

Figure 6-6 Multichannel ECG machine

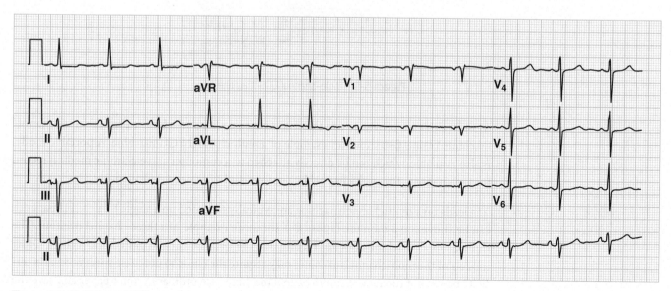

Figure 6-7 Multichannel ECG recording

Most three-channel machines also have a basic software program with additional modules available for purchase. The different modules can include computerized interpretation, multiple viewing choices, ECG overlays, a Holter monitor module, and a stress test module.

Electrodes

In 2011, the U.S. government issued a Guidance Document under the Food and Drug Administration (FDA) (21 CRF 870.2360) to regulate ECG electrodes used in the medical field for safety and effectiveness. Under the document guidelines, companies producing electrodes need to follow stricter packaging guidelines for electrodes. Some of the guidelines include identifying the risks to health, device description, performance characteristics, and labeling requirements. Identified risks of using the product, such as adverse tissue reaction through skin contact and the risk of electrical shock, must now be included on the packaging label. The product description must include the composition, as well as a listing of the features. Under the category of performance characteristics areas covered include the size, adhesiveness (or not), whether the electrodes are supplied as disposable (or not), and the expected shelf life.

Electrodes can be made as disposable products or as nondisposable products. Most health care facilities today prefer the disposable product, but if the product is a nondisposable item, the FDA requires that labeling explain handling, transport, cleaning, and biological decontamination of the electrodes. Electrodes can be made of foam, cloth, or wet gel and come in various sizes from neonate, infant, pediatric, and adult. In addition to the type of material, they can be made to snap on the leads in the center of the pad or clip onto the leads, usually to one side of the pad.

Electrodes are considered nonsterile by the FDA because the intended use is on a noncritical area of the body. Basic guidelines for disposable electrodes include keeping the electrodes in a sealed, airtight envelope so that they can retain the moisture on the pad needed for voltage conduction, and the electrodes should be used as soon as possible after the package has been opened. Electrodes have a shelf life of approximately two years when sealed, but the FDA suggests that shelf-life tests be performed at each medical facility to ensure quality.

Ordering electrodes should closely match the quantity used on a regular basis. If the electrode pad becomes dry, miscellaneous marks can appear on the ECG reading, giving inadequate or incorrect results. Electrodes usually come prepackaged in groups of 10 electrodes for the 12-lead ECG. Electrodes should be kept at room temperature with humidity at less than 80 percent, stored in the original packaging, and in an area that is well ventilated.

Leads

When studying electrocardiograms, there are two different meanings for the term "lead." In this section, the discussion identifies how a lead is used, packaged, and sold. In the next section, voltage from leads connected to electrodes that produce waves on graph paper will be discussed.

Leads attach to the ECG machine by a cable. The cable is normally reused, but the leads that are attached to the cable at one end and to the electrodes at the other end can be either disposable or reusable. The electrodes are attached by using clips, which also can be disposable or reusable. Some health care workers call the clips "alligator clips" because they are meant to tightly secure the lead much as a miniature clothespin would secure cloth. Each lead will attach to only one electrode. When purchasing leads, it is important to know the brand, model, and cable interface your ECG machine uses, in order to correctly replace new leads and clips. **Figure 6-8** shows an example of the electrode, lead, and clip. The color of the clips is usually irrelevant, but the leads are usually specifically identified by color and two or three letters that identify the location to place the electrodes. Placement of the leads and further description of colors and lettering will be discussed in detail later in this chapter.

Leads are usually packaged in sets of 10 because one set of 10 leads is needed to perform the standard resting ECG. Most often, it is the clips that attach to the leads that are replaced on a regular basis. If the leads and clips are reused from one patient to another, standard precautions for sanitizing the leads and clips need to be completed prior to use on the next patient.

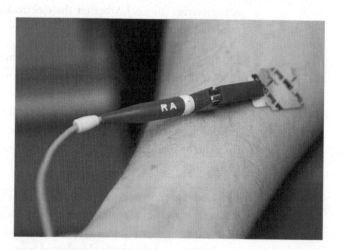

Figure 6-8 ECG electrode, lead, and clip

Quick Check 6-1

Fill in the blanks.

1. The ECG test cannot identify cardiac _____ and cannot measure cardiac _____.

2. _____ objects will usually cause interference with an ECG machine.

3. A continuous strip of paper that produces one lead after another describes a(n) _____ channel ECG machine, whereas 12 views recorded simultaneously describes a(n) _____ ECG machine.

4. The FDA regulates ECG _____ to ensure patient safety by requiring identification of the _____ that may occur with use, such as tissue sensitivity and electrical shock.

5. It is important to know the brand, model, and cable interface of your ECG machine in order to correctly replace supplies such as _____ and _____.

HOW ELECTRODES AND LEADS WORK

Electrodes are placed on the body to obtain different views or angles of each section of the heart. As mentioned earlier in the chapter, each electrode attaches to a lead, and each lead measures the direction and intensity of voltage being discharged by the heart at a specific time. Before learning to place the electrodes and the leads on a patient, it is important to understand how the leads measure electrical activity within the heart. The standard 12-lead ECG uses two groups of leads—the limb leads, which include the augmented lead views and ground lead, and the precordial leads. Stated another way, it is called a 12-lead ECG, but there are actually only 10 "wires" (leads) that attach between the machine and the patient. This is because there are only two sets of leads—the 4 limb leads and the 6 chest leads. Nine of the leads will show electrical activity of the heart from a different angle, and one lead, which is like a safety "wire" that carries no current, is called a ground lead.

Angles of the Heart

bipolar lead
Electrical voltage in a lead that has both a positive and a negative pole; limb Leads I, II, and II are all bipolar, shown from the frontal view.

unipolar lead
A lead that records electrical voltage in only one direction (from one pole); the augmented limb leads and all precordial leads are unipolar.

ground lead
A lead that carries no current.

Views of the heart are based on whether the lead is a bipolar, unipolar, or a ground lead.

Leads use the electrodes to monitor voltage changes in different directions or views, depending on whether the lead has both positive and negative poles, which is called a **bipolar lead**; whether the lead records the current in only one direction, which is called a **unipolar lead**; or whether the lead carries no current, which is called a **ground lead**. ECG machines are programmed to determine which electrodes will carry a positive current, a positive and negative current, or be used as a ground. The machine will come with the leads clearly marked. Electrode currents always flow from the negative electrode toward the positive electrode. This negative-to-positive current change is the period of time that the cardiac cells depolarize, which was covered in Chapter 3. The viewing angle will be discussed in greater detail in Chapter 7, when the direction of the current will be translated to waveforms that are recorded on graph paper.

Since the heart is a three-dimensional organ but the ECG only records in a two-dimensional format, many angles have to be viewed to see how the electrical impulse is being conducted to specific areas of the heart. There are four primary views of the heart, which are shown on a 12-lead ECG by the placement of the electrodes. They include a lateral wall view, inferior wall view, septal wall view, and anterior wall view. Each of the wall views shows different sections of the heart, as shown in **Figure 6-9**. Throughout the remainder of this chapter, unless noted otherwise, the same colors are used in the figures when referring to wall views, to help the learner begin to recognize the importance of referencing a particular lead view to a specific portion of the heart.

STANDARD LIMB LEADS

An important concept to aid in understanding leads has to do with lead placement. The limb leads are viewing electrical activity of the heart from the coronal or frontal plane. Chapter 1 introduced the coronal plane, which cuts the heart into a front half and a back half. Views of the leads are through the middle of the heart, looking at electrical activity from the top of the heart to the bottom of the heart. Included in the coronal views are six limb leads. The first three limb leads, called the standard limb leads, are identified as Lead I, Lead II, and Lead III and are all bipolar leads with a specific view, as identified next. When referring to the limb leads, use an uppercase L in the word Lead and a Roman numeral for the numbers I–III. The limb leads are normally placed on the arms and legs for standard 12-lead ECGs. There are several alternative sites that are also used, such as the wrists and ankles or on the torso below the clavicle and the leg leads placed on the lower abdomen within the rib-cage area.

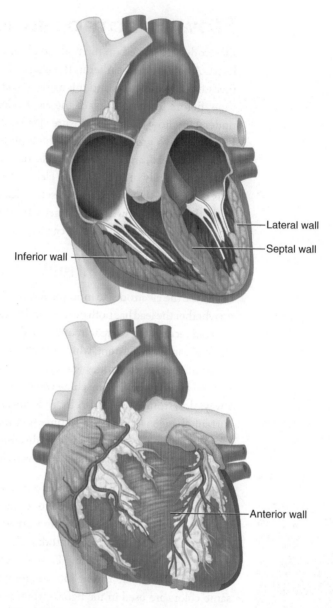

Figure 6-9 Views of the heart walls

For consistency, in North America, the American Heart Association (AHA) has identified the four limb leads using the following initials: RA (right arm), LA (left arm), RL (right leg), and LL (left leg). A second set of three limb leads is known as augmented leads and will be covered in the next section. All six limb leads view the heart's electrical activity from the anterior to the posterior axis of the coronal plane.

Einthoven's Triangle

In 1903, a Dutch scientist, professor, and physician named Willem Einthoven developed the first practical noninvasive recording of the heart with his premier string galvanometer ECG machine. In 1924, Einthoven won the Nobel Prize in Medicine for his work in electrocardiography. Einthoven used the concepts of the electrical flow from the first three leads caused by muscle contractions to produce a graphic image on paper, a theory that is still used today.

This theory is based on what direction the electricity passes through the heart. Since the view of the heart is always from the positive electrode, the electricity can be moving in an upward or downward direction, which is reflected on graph paper as a wave of electrical current. On a normal ECG, the electrical current in Leads I, II, and III are all moving upward (positive).

Energy flows from a negative pole toward a positive pole, so Einthoven's theory shows that each electrode is paired such that it has one positive and one negative pole. Taking his theory a step further, Einthoven used a triangle to show the potential difference between each of the three leads. In pairing the leads, Einthoven was able to explain how the different views of the heart are related to the placement of the three leads. Lead I shows the positive-to-negative pole (potential difference) between the left arm and the right arm. In Lead II, the potential difference is between the left leg and the right arm. Lead III shows the potential difference between the left leg and the left arm. Einthoven's triangle theory is shown in **Figure 6-10**. Notice that the triangle shows Leads I, II, and III, and each position of the electrodes is shown with a positive or negative current (and remember that the Lead III electrodes changed polarity). Collectively, Leads I, II, and III are all bipolar and are called the standard leads.

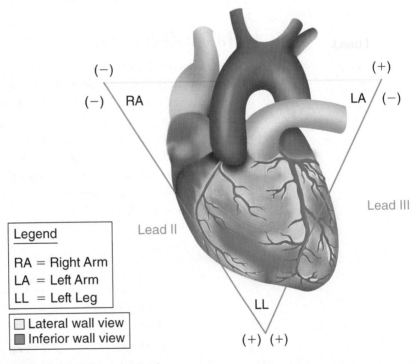

Figure 6-10 Einthoven's triangle

Einthoven's theory describes the potential difference between poles on Leads I, II, and III. The flow of energy for each lead is identified as follows:

Lead I = LA to RA

Lead II = LL to RA

Lead III = LL to LA

Lead I—High Lateral Wall View

As mentioned previously, two electrodes are placed bilaterally—one on the right arm and one on the left arm. Recall that the right arm electrode carries a negative charge toward the positive pole on the electrode placed on the left arm. The direction of the current through the heart is from right arm to left arm. The heart is viewed as if looking from the left arm; therefore, these two bipolar electrodes produces a coronal plane view of the lateral wall of the left ventricle and the left atrium. Collectively, these electrodes make up Lead I.

Lead II—Inferior Wall View

From the right arm lead, another electrode is placed 60° downward and to the left (usually placed on the left leg). Recall that the right arm electrode carries a negative charge, so the positive charge comes from the electrode placed on the left leg; therefore, the current flows from the right arm downward toward the leg, and the view of the heart is from the left leg. These two bipolar electrodes produce a coronal plane view of the inferior wall of the left ventricle, right ventricle, and apex of the heart. Collectively, these electrodes make up Lead II.

Lead III—Inferior Wall View

The first three electrodes, if placed correctly, form a triangle, with the three sides being composed of Lead I superiorly, being horizontal from the right arm to the left arm; Lead II, which is 60° downward and to the left of the electrode placed on the right arm, making this the right side of the triangle; and Lead III forms the third side, from the left arm downward, 120° to the right. The left arm electrode changes polarity in Lead III. The left arm becomes a negative pole, thus making the current flow downward toward the positive left leg electrode. The heart is viewed from the left leg. The bipolar electrodes making up Lead III also provide a coronal plane view the heart's inferior portion of the left and right ventricles. **Table 6-1** reviews the main concepts of the standard leads.

Table 6-1 Standard Limb Lead Charge & Views

	(−) Charge Electrode	(+) Charge Electrode	Heart Wall Being Viewed
Lead I	Right arm	Left arm	High lateral wall
Lead II	Right arm	Left leg	Inferior wall
Lead III	Left arm	Left leg	Inferior wall

Standard Limb Leads I, II, and III

- Provides three frontal plane views of the heart
- Are all bipolar, current flows from the negative pole to the positive pole
- Current flows from the limbs through the heart

Ground Lead

One might wonder, if you have placed the three standard leads on the body, one on the right arm, one on the left arm, and one on the left leg, what happens to the right leg? There is an electrode placed on the right leg, but this electrode does not view the heart's electrical activity. Instead, this electrode is considered the "grounding" electrode. The right leg electrode is also called the earth electrode. The purpose of the grounding electrode is to reduce electrical interference from outside of the body.

> In biopolar leads, the *current* flows from the negative pole through the heart to the positive pole, but the *view* is from the positive pole to the heart.

Quick Check 6-2

Fill in the blanks.

1. Leads measure _____ and _____ of voltage being discharged by heart muscles at a particular time.

2. Limb leads can be divided into two groups called _____ limb leads and _____ limb leads.

3. The 12-lead ECG machine contains _____ leads, of which _____ leads will identify heart electrical activity and one lead carries no current.

4. Limb leads view electrical activity from the _____ plane. The view of the heart is always from the _____ electrode.

5. All three limb leads view the left ventricle; however, the apex of the heart is normally viewed from Lead _____, while the left atrium is viewed from Lead _____.

AUGMENTED LIMB LEADS

augmented leads
Unipolar limb leads identified as aVR, aVL, and aVF. Leads are shown from the frontal view and are amplified by the ECG machine by 50 percent over the standard limb leads so that they are readable on an ECG strip.

The augmented limb leads give an additional three views of the heart from the coronal view. **Augmented leads** are leads that the ECG machine extends the signal size by 50 percent over the standard limb leads. The second set of limb leads are unipolar augmented leads named aVR, aVL, and aVF. The aV stands for augmented voltage, which means the voltage must be amplified in order to be able to view the waveforms on graph paper. The third letters R, L, and F stand for the positive electrode positions, which are the right arm, left arm, and left leg. To distinguish the augmented from the standard lead, the augmented F stands for foot, but the electrode is the same electrode that was placed on the left leg. The same electrodes used in Einthoven's triangle are used in the augmented limb leads, but the main differences are that the augmented leads use the heart in the center of the triangle, and the current flows outward from the heart toward the limbs.

Goldberger's Augmentation Leads

In 1942, Emanuel Goldberger was the first person to introduce augmented leads, which has led to the ECG graphic images as we know them today. The theory behind using an augmented lead is focused on using only one true positive sensor and exploring the heart from only one point, called a central point. In Einthoven's triangle, the two other limb leads were considered negative poles. As with the standard limb leads, the augmented leads are being viewed from the coronal plane. **Figure 6-11** shows Einthoven's triangle adapted to the direction of view from Goldberger's augmented leads.

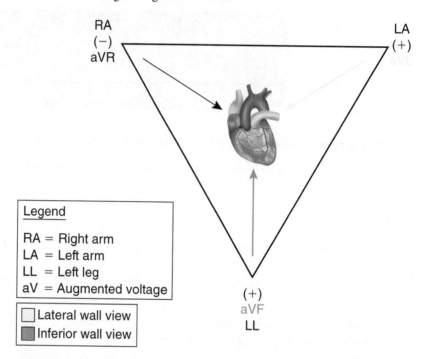

Figure 6-11 Views of the heart from the augmented leads

Lead aVR—No Specific View of the Heart Walls

Of all the limb leads, the aVR is the most underutilized, underanalyzed, and most often ignored lead. The aVR lead does not provide a specific view of the left ventricle of the heart as all the other limb leads do; instead, the aVR lead provides information on the blood outflow of the right ventricle, so it is potentially providing a coronal view from the center of the heart toward the right arm. The positive electrode is placed on the right arm; therefore, the negative pole is the average of the other electrodes where they come to a central point. However, most of the current is flowing away from this positive electrode because the normal heart depolarizes from right to left and from the top of the heart to the bottom (Chapter 3), so the summative change in an ECG tracing shows up as a negative waveform on the graph paper.

Lead aVL—Lateral Wall View

The aVL lead is oriented toward the left ventricle's high lateral and lateral walls. The positive electrode is placed on the left arm so that the coronal view is from the center of the heart through the lateral wall, toward the left arm. Again, the negative pole is the average of the other electrodes where they come to a central point.

Lead aVF—Inferior Wall View

The aVF lead is oriented toward the left ventricle's inferior wall. The positive electrode is placed on the left leg so that the coronal view is from the center of the heart through the inferior wall, toward the left leg. Once again, the negative pole is the average of the other electrodes where they come to a central point. **Table 6-2** shows a review of the important concepts for augmented leads.

> Augmented leads provide three views from a central point of the heart, but only two of the views (aVL and aVF) are of a heart wall.

Table 6-2 Augmented Limb Lead Charge and Views

	(−) Charge	(+) Charge Electrode	Heart Wall Being Viewed
aVR	Sum of LA and LL	Right arm	None
aVL	Sum of RA and LL	Left arm	lateral wall
aVF	Sum of RA and LA	Left leg	inferior wall

Augmented Limb Leads aVR, aVL, and aVF

- Provides three frontal plane views of the heart
- Are all unipolar
- Current flows from the heart toward the limbs

HEXAXIAL VIEW OF LIMB LEADS

The study of hexaxial views is often covered in advanced concepts books on ECGs. This book provides an introduction to hexaxial views by introducing the importance of what the lead is recording on an ECG based upon the placement of the lead and angle of view. Chapter 8 will provide examples of problems that the ECG technician will encounter when the leads identified by the machine are not placed in the proper location.

Later in this chapter, the correct placement of the leads and variations will be discussed. Learning to differentiate a normal ECG versus an arrhythmia is a process that begins by understanding hexaxial views. The hexaxial view is composed of the four limb leads, Einthoven's triangle theory, and Goldberger's augmentation theory of the electrical properties of said leads. The hexaxial view of the limb leads puts the study of angles (or views) of the heart into perspective. Another term for an angle or a view is a vector. A **vector** is a graphical record that is made up of lines showing the direction and strength of electrical forces. When thinking of the heart, the vector shows whether the electrical impulse is moving toward the limbs or toward the heart. Think of a typical 360° circle, with different "views" being identified. So far, we have covered the six views of the limb leads in this circle. If Figures 6-10 and 6-11 were superimposed into one new figure, Figure 6-12, it becomes more apparent that the straight lines for each limb lead are 30° apart. **Table 6-3** shows each individual limb lead and the corresponding degrees of the positive pole and opposite pole degrees.

vector (V)
A graphical record that is made up of lines showing the direction of electrical forces.

Table 6-3 Hexaxial Degrees of the Six Limb Leads

LEAD	I	II	III	aVR	aVL	aVF
DEGREES:						
Positive pole	0°	+60°	+120°	+30°	−30°	+90°
Opposite side of the pole	+180°	−120°	−60°	−150°	+150°	−90°

Understanding the degrees and the relationship to the areas of the heart being viewed is also important for future understanding of heart damages. Remember that the six limb views can be seen on one plane—the coronal (frontal) plane. Even though there are only four limbs, there are six views: three from Leads I, II, and III and three from the augmented leads, aVL, aVR, and aVF.

This information will be combined with the views found in the next section on precordial leads to give a three-dimensional picture of what you are looking at on an ECG tracing. Recall that you have one vector or line for each limb lead and one positive sensor on that line, so the degrees on the other end of the line will be exactly opposite. For example, Lead I has a positive pole at 0°; therefore, the opposite side of the vector is at 180°. **Figure 6-12** shows a hexaxial drawing of the six limb leads with the degree distance marked.

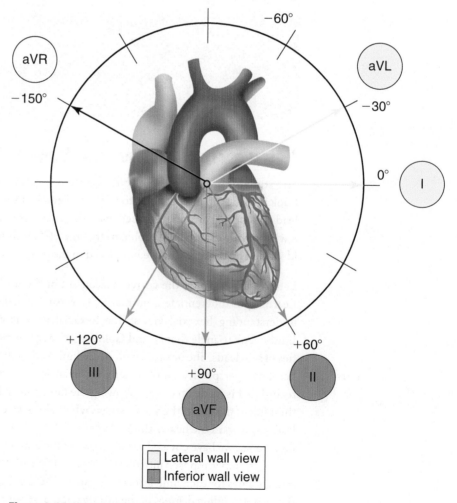

☐ Lateral wall view
■ Inferior wall view

Figure 6-12 Hexaxial view of limb lead vectors

Quick Check 6-3

Fill in the blanks.

1. When a lead is viewed with augmented voltage, the lead has been _____ for viewing.

2. Augmented leads are _____ leads, viewed from the _____ plane.

3. All limb leads view a wall of the heart *except* the _____ lead, which views blood outflow from the right ventricle. The lateral heart wall is viewed by Leads I and _____. The inferior heart wall is viewed by Leads II, III, and _____.

4. In augmented leads, current flows _____ the heart _____ the limbs.

5. A vector shows whether electrical impulses are moving toward the _____ or toward the _____.

PRECORDIAL LEADS

precordial leads
Chest leads that view the heart from a horizontal plane.

Precordial leads take a different approach to viewing the heart by using the transverse (horizontal) plane. Instead of looking from the coronal plane of the heart, the **precordial leads** are viewed from the transverse plane, which cuts the heart into two halves—a top half and a bottom half—and allows views of the heart to be recorded from a front-to-back and side-to-side perspective. The precordial leads are also called chest leads. There are six views created by placing six electrodes on the chest in specific locations as defined next, in order to obtain an accurate ECG. The precordial electrodes are labeled V1 through V6, with the letter V standing for vector.

Wilson Central Terminal

In 1934, Frank Norman Wilson and his colleagues were the first to describe using a central point of reference (which Wilson called a central terminal) to define unipolar potentials that would allow the measurement of unipolar leads. Wilson's theory found that the average potential over the body could be approximated by the potential average of the three limb leads, thus making the body a negative pole. All six precordial leads are considered positive unipolar leads, measuring electrical impulses in only one direction. By adding the six unipolar leads along with the limb leads, a three-dimensional picture of the heart's electrical activity could be accurately determined. Wilson is the one who first used the letter V for each of the six unipolar chest leads to stand for the word vector, along with the numbers 1–6. In the normal 12-lead ECG, the placement of the precordial leads is as described next.

Lead V1—Septal Wall View

The lead labeled V1 is the only precordial electrode placed on the right side of the chest for a normal 12-lead ECG. The lead is placed on the right side of the sternum in the fourth intercostal space of the ribs. This lead provides a transverse plane view of the interventricular septum of the heart.

Lead V2—Septal Wall View

Lead V2 is placed on the left side of the sternum in the fourth intercostal space of the ribs. The V2 electrode is placed on the chest opposite of the V1 electrode. Lead V2 provides another view of the interventricular septum from the transverse plane.

Lead V3—Anterior Wall View

Lead V3 is placed on the left side of the chest, but the electrode is not placed on the body until after lead V4 is placed because lead 3 will be positioned halfway between lead V2 and lead V4. Lead V3 provides a view of the anterior wall of the left ventricle from the transverse plane.

Lead V4—Anterior Wall View

Lead V4 is also placed on the left side of the chest, and like lead V3, it provides another view of the anterior wall of the left ventricle from the transverse plane. Lead V4 is positioned in the fifth intercostal space along a point of reference called the midclavicular line.

Lead V5—Lateral Wall View

Lead V5 is placed on the left side of the chest and provides a view of the lower lateral wall of the left ventricle. Lead V5 is also positioned in the fifth intercostal space at a point of reference called the left anterior axillary line.

Lead V6—Lateral Wall View

Lead V6 is placed on the left side of the chest at a point of reference called the midaxillary line. Lead V6 is the third lead that is placed in the fifth intercostal space of the ribs (the other two leads are V4 and V5), and it provides a view of the lower lateral wall of the left ventricle. **Table 6-4** reviews the main concepts on the normal placement of the precordial leads.

Table 6-4 Precordial Normal Placement and Views

	Placement	Heart Wall Being Viewed
V1	Right of sternum, fourth intercostal space	Septal wall
V2	Left of sternum, fourth intercostal space	Septal wall
V3	Left, between V2 and V4	Anterior wall
V4	Left, midclavicular line, fifth intercostal space	Anterior wall
V5	Left, anterior axillary line, fifth intercostal space	Lower lateral wall
V6	Left, midaxillary line, fifth intercostal space	Lower lateral wall

Precordial Chest Leads V1 Through V6

- Provides six transverse plane views of the heart
- Are all unipolar

PRECORDIAL VECTOR VIEWS

Recall that the transverse plane is used to show all precordial views. The same concept of vectors found with the coronal plane view in limb leads can be applied to the transverse plane view in the precordial leads. Using a 360° circle, and viewing from the transverse plane, the precordial leads would appear as shown in **Figure 6-13**. The precordial leads provide a picture of the direction of the electrical impulses of the heart during one cardiac cycle.

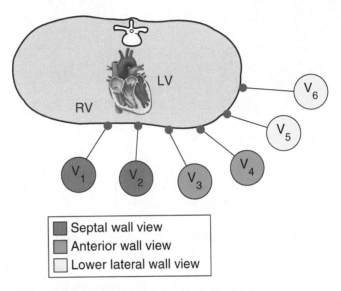

■ Septal wall view
■ Anterior wall view
□ Lower lateral wall view

Figure 6-13 Transverse view of precordial leads

ANATOMICALLY CONTIGUOUS AND RECIPROCAL LEAD VIEWS

anatomically contiguous
Describes leads that provide a different angle view but are located on the same wall of the heart.

All of the views are recorded by the placement of leads, and some leads provide more than one view. When the views are different angles but located on the same anatomical wall of the heart, the views are considered **anatomically contiguous**. In most cases, the left ventricle is the general area that the leads are viewing from various angles. For example, in the standard ECG, on the inferior wall, the aVF limb lead provides anatomically contiguous views with limb Lead II and limb Lead III. On the anterior wall, leads V3 and V4 provide anatomically contiguous views; on the septal wall, leads V1 and V2 provide anatomically contiguous views; and on the lateral wall, the aVL lead provides anatomically contiguous views with Lead I and the precordial leads V5 and V6. By identifying all the views as they would appear on a multichannel ECG tracing, **Figure 6-14** visualizes which leads are contiguous on a standard 12-lead ECG printout.

reciprocal
Lead views that can be interchangeable, used especially when acute injury is suspected but it is not showing on standard ECG lead views.

Two of the heart walls have reciprocal views. A **reciprocal** view means that the view of a particular wall can be viewed from more than one angle or that additional lead views will provide alternative views when a heart injury is suspected. Sometimes the ECG will not show elevation or depressions in the waves by looking at an acute injury, but by viewing the reciprocal angle, the injury becomes viewable. For example, the inferior wall of the heart is normally viewed on an ECG in Lead II or III or aVF. The reciprocal view for the inferior wall is Lead I and aVL. The lateral wall also has reciprocal views. The normal ECG would

Lateral wall	Inferior wall
Septal wall	Anterior wall

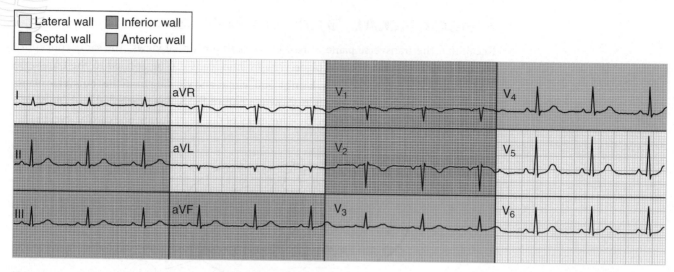

Figure 6-14 Heart wall views in a 12-lead ECG

provide information on Lead I, aVL, V5, and V6. Reciprocal views of the heart's lateral wall can be shown in Leads II or III and aVF. A review of the heart wall leads and reciprocal leads is found in **Table 6-5**.

Table 6-5 Heart Wall Reciprocal Views

	Lateral Wall of Left Ventricle	
	Normal Views	**Reciprocal Views**
Leads	Lead I, aVL, V5, and V6	Lead II, III, and aVF
	Inferior Wall of Left Ventricle	
	Normal Views	**Reciprocal Views**
Leads	Leads II, III, and aVF	Lead I and aVL

12-LEAD VECTOR VIEW ANALYSIS

All 12 views of the ECG have now been accounted for. It is time to combine the two planes for a combined view of the heart and check your understanding of the concept of vectors. When combining the hexaxial view of the limb leads (Figure 6-12) with the precordial vector views (Figure 6-13), the resulting view (Figure 6-15) is created. Notice that the inferior, anterior, and lateral heart walls have been identified in **Figure 6-15** so that you can reference which part of the heart is affected by each individual lead or group of leads.

Now that all of the leads have been identified and the views of these leads have been identified, the importance of understanding how the vector views provide information as the cardiac muscle becomes excited during the depolarization cycle (which was studied in Chapter 3) should aid in understanding the importance of correct lead placement. Additionally, in advanced studies, understanding vectors will aid in the interpretation of arrhythmias. Since the vector view shows both the strength and direction of the impulse, by understanding what lead or leads are showing a variance in wave patterns from a normal ECG, health care personnel can determine what area of the heart may have an injury, be blocked, or show necrosis.

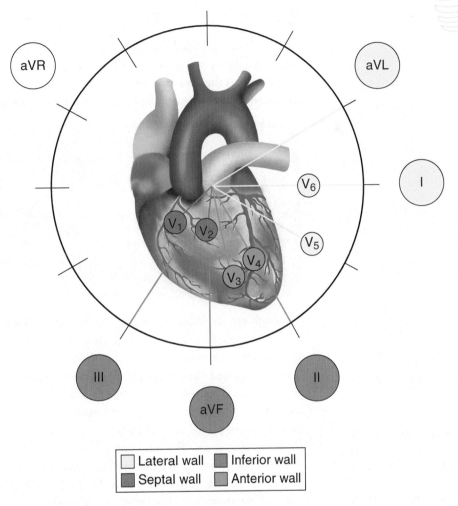

| Lateral wall | Inferior wall |
| Septal wall | Anterior wall |

Figure 6-15 Three-dimensional view of heart vectors

Quick Check 6-4

Fill in the blanks.

1. Precordial leads, which are also called chest leads, view the heart from the _____ plane.

2. Precordial leads create _____ views, and each lead begins with the letter V, which stands for the term _____.

3. The three heart walls viewed by precordial leads include the _____ wall, _____ wall, and the _____ wall.

4. Leads V1 and V2 are placed on the chest at the _____ intercostal space, while leads V4, V5, and V6 are placed on the _____ intercostal space.

5. The walls of the heart that do *not* share reciprocal views include the _____ wall and the _____ wall.

LIMB LEAD PLACEMENT ON PATIENT

The AHA has identified the colors of the limb leads as being white, with a secondary color that is usually shown as a colored ring on the white lead, or it may be shown in the writing that identifies the lead, or may be the listed color with a white ring. The North American limb lead color code is as follows: RA is white; LA is black; RL is green; and LL is red.

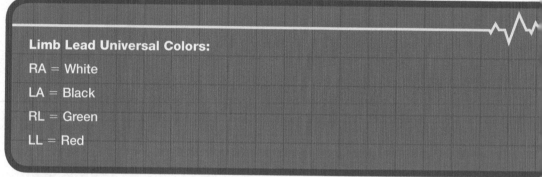

Limb Lead Universal Colors:

RA = White

LA = Black

RL = Green

LL = Red

Although modifications are made for hospital and emergency care and in cases when the legs are amputated or injured, the leads are typically placed as shown in **Figure 6-16**. Using the correctly colored lead is important because the machine will record the heart's rhythm and pattern based on where the lead is located. Incorrect placement can cause miscellaneous marks or false diagnostic interpretations, whereas proper placement of the leads can improve the detection of cardiac activity, both normal and abnormal. Recall that the limb leads LA and RA can be placed on the upper arm or the upper torso, or even on the wrists, but avoid thick muscular areas. The leads should be placed over the least muscular area because the signal will be strongest in a less muscular area. Also note that even though the leads can be attached in different areas, they must be equivalently placed on each side of the body. This means if placement is on one wrist, the other wrist should also be used; the lead should not be placed in a different location on the arm. The limb leads LL and RL can also be placed on the lower torso, legs, or ankles, so long as the leads are placed equivalently.

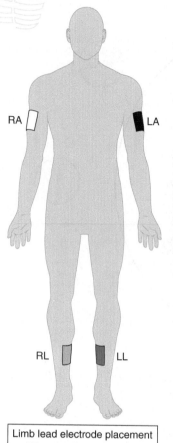

Limb lead electrode placement
☐ RA lead ☐ RL lead
■ LA lead ■ LL lead

Figure 6-16 Normal limb lead electrode placement on patient

PRECORDIAL LEAD PLACEMENT ON A PATIENT

Correct placement of the precordial leads is very important. Unlike the limb leads, there is little room to vary from the correct positions for an accurate ECG reading. Learning some imaginary anatomical lines may help in identifying the correct placement of chest leads. The imaginary lines use body areas such as bones as points of reference, which will be explained next. Recall that the heart is located in the thoracic cavity, under the sternum and slightly to the left.

With the exception of lead V1, be sure to affix all the electrodes on the left side of the sternum.

To correctly identify the imaginary lines on the body, use the following points of reference. First, identify the clavicle and sternum bones. The clavicle bone is often referred to as the collarbone, and the sternum is often called the breastbone. The sternum goes straight down the middle of the chest. Next, find the angle of Louis, which is also called the sternal angle. To find this angle, run your fingers over the skin from the throat down over the sternum until you feel a lump. The lump is the angle of Louis. Now move your fingers off the sternum at the angle of Louis, and you will feel the second intercostal space. Continue moving downward while counting the rib, and then the intercostal space, until you locate the fourth intercostal space. This is the position for leads V1 and V2.

Before you can actually connect the leads, you first attach electrodes over the correct chest position. The leads are then attached to the electrodes. The electrode for lead V1 is placed on the right side of the sternum at the fourth intercostal space, and the electrode for lead V2 is placed on the left side of the fourth intercostal space. Position those electrodes before continuing so that you have established your points of reference.

Go down one more intercostal space. You should now be on the left side of the sternum at the fifth intercostal space. Look back at the clavicle and find the approximate middle of the left clavicle, which will be the reference point for the midclavicular line. Creating an imaginary line, place the electrode for the fourth lead (lead V4) where the fifth intercostal space meets the midclavicular line. After placing the electrode for lead V4, go back halfway between the electrodes for leads V2 and V4 and place the electrode for lead V3. Lead V3, since it is halfway between the other two electrodes, may be attached to the skin over the fifth rib. This is the only lead where it is acceptable to place the electrode over a bone.

Continue along the left fifth intercostal space toward the side of the body. Identify a second imaginary line at the beginning of the axilla or anterior axillary line, commonly called the armpit. The electrode for the fifth lead, lead V5 is placed at the intersection of the fifth intercostal space and the anterior axillary line. After the electrode has been placed for lead V5, create one more imaginary line down the middle of the armpit. Keeping the fifth intercostal space landmark, place the electrode for lead V6 at the intersection of the fifth intercostal space and the midaxilla. After all six electrodes have been placed, verify that all electrodes are securely in place, and then attach the leads using the correct color for each lead. The precordial leads are brown and have another color, usually in the form of a colored ring, or else the letters that identify the lead are in a specific color. The colors are identified as follows: lead V1 is red; lead V2 yellow; lead V3 green; lead V4 blue; lead V5 orange; and lead V6 purple. **Figure 6-17** shows the correct color and placement. The imaginary lines that were mentally calculated for proper lead placement appear as dashes.

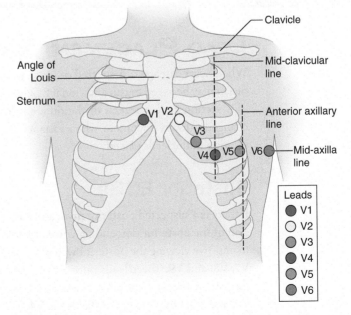

Figure 6-17 Normal precordial lead placement on patient

Precordial Lead Universal Colors:

V1 = Red

V2 = Yellow

V3= Green

V4= Blue

V5 = Orange

V6 = Purple

Quick Check 6-5

Fill in the blanks.

1. Correct placement of the colored limb leads is important to ensure that the ECG machine records proper heart _____ and _____.

2. Limb leads can be placed in various locations on the limbs, but the leads must be _____ placed on _____ side of the body.

3. Leads _____ and _____ are placed at the fourth intercostal space, on the right and left of the sternum.

4. Leads _____, _____, and _____ are placed along the fifth intercostal space at the midclavicular, axilla, and midaxilla.

5. Lead _____ is the only lead that may be placed on the skin over the fifth rib.

LEAD PLACEMENT VARIANCES

When heart damage is suspected or indicated from a standard 12-lead ECG, the ECG technician may be asked to run additional ECGs with the leads placed in various other positions. This section covers several of the different locations and describes which leads are interchanged. Always document when variance ECGs have been completed by identifying the location of the leads placed.

Posterior ECGs

If there is a suspected posterior myocardial infarction (MI), injury, or damage such as occlusion of the posterior descending coronary artery, the clinician may request additional leads to improve viewing the posterior wall of the heart. This can be accomplished by adding leads V7, V8, and V9. These leads mirror the location of leads V4, V5, and V6 but are placed on the patient's back, to the left of the spinal cord. **Figure 6-18** shows the placement of leads V7, V8, and V9. Only the precordial leads V4, V5, and V6 change positions; leads V1 through V3 remain in the standard position. Often an electrode is placed in the V6 position, but no lead is attached because it is only used for reference to place the three posterior leads. When correctly placed, leads V7, V8, and V9 will be in a horizontal line to the electrode placed for lead V6 on a normal ECG. V7 lead placement can be found by locating a posterior axillary line and using the lead labeled V4; the V9 lead is placed along an imaginary left paraspinal line using the lead labeled V6, and lead V8 is placed halfway between leads V7 and V9 using the lead marked V5, which will usually also be along the midscapular line and horizontal to V6. The ECG must be documented to indicate that V7, V8, and V9 were captured in place of leads V4, V5, and V6. The ECG should also be clearly documented and labeled "Posterior ECG."

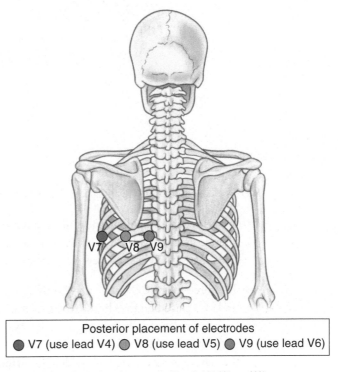

Posterior placement of electrodes
● V7 (use lead V4) ● V8 (use lead V5) ● V9 (use lead V6)

Figure 6-18 Posterior placement of leads V7, V8, and V9

Right-Sided ECG

If there is concern that the patient has right ventricular injury or damage such as a right ventricular infarction or occlusion of the right coronary artery, the precordial leads can be placed on the right side of the chest. Lead V1 is placed on the fourth intercostal space to the *left* of the sternum, lead V2 is placed on the *right* side of the fourth intercostal space, lead V4 is placed on the right fifth intercostal space along the midclavicular line, V3 is placed between V2 and V4, V5 is placed on the right anterior axillary line along the fifth intercostal space, and V6 is placed on the right midaxillary line of the fifth intercostal space. Remember to always document the right-sided ECG on the ECG strip when the leads have been mirrored. **Figure 6-19** shows the placement of a right-sided ECG. Be sure to document the right-side placement of this ECG test in the patient's record.

Three-Lead Placement

If you work in the emergency department, telemetry, or an area that offers day surgery, or where other medical procedures are performed in which the clinician may want to monitor the heart, the three-lead ECG may be used. The heart is monitored so that the clinician can watch for changes in rhythm. The three-lead ECG is sometimes called single-lead monitoring

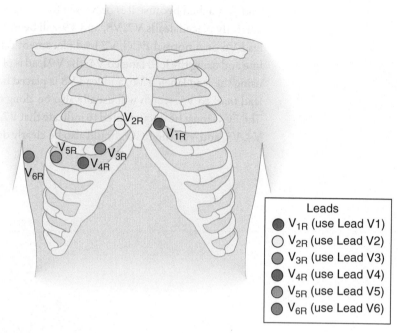

Leads
- V$_{1R}$ (use Lead V1)
- V$_{2R}$ (use Lead V2)
- V$_{3R}$ (use Lead V3)
- V$_{4R}$ (use Lead V4)
- V$_{5R}$ (use Lead V5)
- V$_{6R}$ (use Lead V6)

Figure 6-19 Right-sided ECG lead placement

because each lead will provide information for only the specific region being viewed, which often is from Lead II. When you print a recording of a three-lead rhythm strip, be sure to document which lead or view was being monitored.

The three-lead ECG uses only the right and left arm leads and the left leg lead. All three leads are placed on the chest to form Einthoven's triangle. In the three-lead ECG, two of the leads are polarized (have a negative or positive charge) and the third lead creates a ground. In the standard AHA placement, the white lead, labeled RA (right arm), is placed just below the clavicle near the right shoulder. The white lead always carries a negative polarity. Next, the black lead, labeled LA (left arm), is placed just below the clavicle near the left shoulder. The black lead changes polarity; in Lead I, the polarity is positive, but in Lead III, the polarity is negative. Finally, a third electrode, labeled LL (left leg) and colored red, is connected on the left, near the apex of the heart (which is approximately 2 inches below the left nipple). The red LL electrode carries a positive polarity in Leads II and III on the standard three-lead ECG. Often, the mnemonic "White = Right, Smoke over Fire" will remind students of the correct lead color and placement. Translated, the mnemonic means to place the white electrode on the right, the black electrode (smoke) on the left (both under the clavicle), and the red electrode (fire) down below the left nipple.

Three-Lead Placement Mnemonic

White = Right; Smoke (Black) over Fire (Red)

Recall that these electrodes are monitoring three views from the frontal wall. The views include from Lead I, the left lateral view of the heart; and from Lead II and Lead III, an inferior view of the heart. Using the three-lead ECG for monitoring will provide heart rate and regularity, as well as conduction time for the impulse to complete the cardiac cycle. This information can detect serious arrhythmias but cannot detect miscellaneous marks. **Figure 6-20** shows the placement of electrodes for a three-lead ECG.

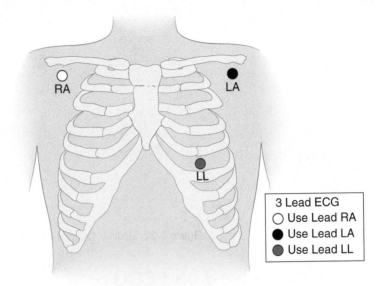

3 Lead ECG
○ Use Lead RA
● Use Lead LA
● Use Lead LL

Figure 6-20 Three-lead ECG electrode placement

Modified Central Lead (MCL) Placement

A variation of the three-lead monitoring ECG is called Modified Central Lead (MCL), and is often referred to as the modified chest lead. This variation will either use the precordial lead V1 or V6 to differentiate some clinical conditions. The negative pole is placed under the left clavicle, and the positive pole for MCL_1 is placed in the V1 position of the right, fourth intercostal space. A second variation uses the position of the V6 precordial lead and is labeled as MCL_6. MCL_6 is positioned on the left side, fifth intercostal space at the midaxilla area. **Figures 6-21** and **6-22** show the MCL_1 and MCL_6 lead positioning.

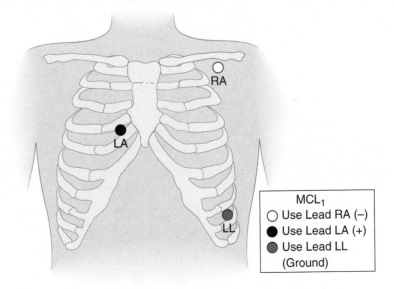

MCL_1
○ Use Lead RA (−)
● Use Lead LA (+)
● Use Lead LL
   (Ground)

Figure 6-21 Modified Central Lead (MCL_1) lead placement

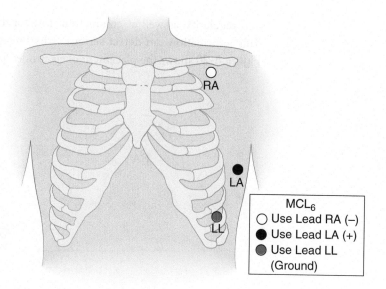

Figure 6-22 Modified Central Lead (MCL₆) lead placement

Five-Lead ECG

Another modification of the 12-lead ECG involves using only 5 leads. The 5-lead ECG uses the 4 limb leads plus the V1 lead. All 5 leads are located in the same positions as found on the 12-lead ECG. Five-lead monitoring is becoming much more accepted than the previous 3-lead model, and many newer model ECG machines will come with a 5-lead testing capability. The 5-lead ECG is primarily used to diagnose ventricular dysrhythmias—more specifically, to differentiate between supraventricular and ventricular tachycardia. This view uses a combination of electrodes to simulate a negative pole, while the positive pole is the V1 lead, which you may recall is located at the fourth intercostal space right of the sternum. The view of the heart is directly below the positive electrode, so it provides a more comprehensive electrical view of both sides of the heart as opposed to viewing it from Lead II, which primarily looks at just the apex of the left ventricle. **Figure 6-23** shows the common placement for the 5-lead ECG.

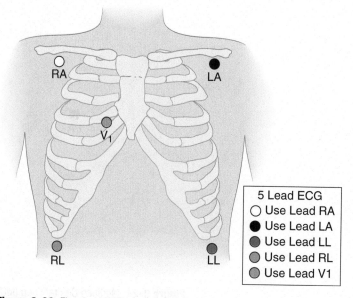

Figure 6-23 Five-lead ECG placement

Although there are several more variances, this book will concentrate on the standard limb and precordial leads as defined prior to this section.

Quick Check 6-6

Fill in the blanks.

1. Always document when variance ECGs have been completed by identifying the _____ of the leads placed.

2. In the posterior placement of leads, the leads V4, V5, and V6 are now identified as _____, _____, and _____.

3. When completing a right-sided ECG, the limb leads are kept in the same position as a standard 12-lead ECG, and the precordial leads are placed _____ of the standard 12-lead ECG.

4. The standard three-lead ECG uses the white lead labeled _____, the black lead labeled _____, and the red lead labeled _____.

5. In a five-lead ECG, use the four _____ leads and the precordial lead _____.

COMPLETING A 12-LEAD ECG

The following guidelines should be used in an ambulatory setting when the patient has come in for a routine or nonemergency ECG. Permission to touch a patient is always necessary under the Health Insurance Portability and Accountability Act (HIPAA), but there is more than one type of permission, as described next, and the type that is used depends upon the patient's circumstances.

Patient Rights

Before performing any patient testing, keep in mind the required legal guidelines health care providers must adhere to when working with people. Although an ECG is considered a non-invasive test and is a relatively safe procedure, there is always a chance that something could go wrong or that the patient could be injured; therefore, obtaining proper patient consent is one of the first steps in patient preparation.

Consent for Medical Treatment

Obtaining consent from a patient prior to the patient receiving medical care is based upon the common law concepts of personal autonomy and self-determination. A patient has a right to choose care or decline care based on his or her own personal decision. A patient also has the right to be informed of medical treatment plans in order to make decisions.

implied consent
Nonverbal consent, often used in emergency medical care if a patient is unable to provide informed consent but the patient's actions (such as seeking medical care) suggest that medical intervention is desired.

In health care, there are two types of medical consent. The first type, **implied consent**, occurs in a medical emergency, such as when a patient is brought into a medical facility for treatment, the treatment provided is of an emergency nature, and the patient cannot provide written consent. A signature of the patient might not have been obtained prior to medical care in an emergency or the consent might have been verbal, yet consent for emergency

informed consent
The legal doctrine that gives people the right to make decisions about their medical treatment by being informed of the medical procedure, the risks involved, the benefit of the procedure, possible alternatives, and consequences of choosing not to have a procedure.

treatment is implied because the patient was brought to the facility. When implied consent is obtained, written consent either by the patient or a patient representative is obtained as soon as possible. In a nonemergency clinical situation, informed consent to obtain medical treatment should always be obtained prior to the start of treatment. **Informed consent** means that the health care practitioner has discussed the procedure, the risks, and the benefits of the ECG and allowed the patient to ask questions to clarify any concerns. Possible alternatives and the consequences of not having the ECG should also be discussed so that the patient can decide what is best for him or her. Although the actual patient's consent (i.e., signature) to perform the ECG is usually obtained by a technician, it is the responsibility of the health care provider to discuss any procedures being considered so that the patient may make an informed decision on his or her own care plan.

> Implied consent = Not written; used in emergencies
>
> Informed consent = Written; patient understands the procedure, risks, benefits, and alternative treatments

After obtaining the necessary consent, the technician should review with the patient how the test will be performed. After identifying yourself, ask the patient if he or she has any questions before proceeding. Then explain that you (the technician) will be leaving the room so that the patient can disrobe from the waist up, remove shoes and belts, take cell phones, keys and other metal objects out of their pockets, and put on a gown with the opening facing to the front. Always provide the patient as much privacy as possible, and knock before reentering the room to start the ECG. Even though a patient may have had many ECGs previously completed, always obtain consent and explain the procedure prior to a new test being performed.

Step-by-Step ECG Procedures

After explaining the procedure to the patient, prepare for the ECG by first gathering your supplies and preparing the machine. Always start by washing your hands and gathering the supplies. Before calling the patient into the exam room, be sure that you have the following supplies ready:

- Disposable razor
- 4×4 sponges
- Two 10-packs of electrodes (one as a spare)
- Alcohol pads or other skin prep pack
- A patient gown and a drape

Next, prepare the machine. The machine should:

- Be turned *ON*
- Have the correct time, date, and patient information recorded
- Have clean or disposable leads and clips ready
- Have paper for the printer or ECG strip paper

Now you are ready to call the patient into the room.

After the patient is ready, position the patient in a supine position on the table. If the patient needs to be placed in any other position, document the position on the ECG or in the computer. Raise the pant cuffs to expose the lower legs. Complete the following procedures:

- Clean the skin where the electrodes will be placed with alcohol pads; let dry.
- Shave the area only if the electrodes will not stick. *Before* shaving any hair, be sure to explain to the patient why the hair must be removed. Remove as little hair as necessary to get the electrode to create a good bond to the skin.
- Attach all the electrodes before attaching the leads.

When the electrodes and leads have been attached correctly, ask the patient to breathe normally but do not talk, and then begin the ECG. After a short duration, check that the machine is recording the heart waves correctly (as will be explained in Chapter 7). Upon the completion of the exam, it may be clinic procedure to have the clinician review the ECG results before the patient is disconnected from the electrodes. If not, remove the leads, ask the patient if he or she prefers to remove the electrodes, and leave the room so the patient can redress. Appendix A includes a check-off style competency sheet for performing an ECG.

SAMPLE DOCUMENTATION

Documenting the ECG procedure is very important for health care reimbursement. With electronic medical records and claim processes, it is important to document the procedure as soon as possible after the completion of the test. In the medical record, some computer programs will automatically code the procedure as soon as the ECG has been entered into the system. In these systems, important patient information should be completed on the electronic ECG prior to submission to avoid unnecessary delay in reimbursement. All systems need at least the patient's name, age, physician's name, date of service, time of service, and any procedures that were completed in addition to the standard ECG. Other factors that may affect reimbursement include whether this was an emergency (STAT) ECG, a routine test, a follow-up test, etc.

Quick Check 6-7

Fill in the blanks.

1. When a patient has an ECG performed in an emergency situation, _____ consent is considered acceptable consent even though the consent is not written.

2. In a(n) _____ situation when an ECG is considered medically necessary, the health care clinician has the responsibility to inform the patient of the _____, benefits, and _____ treatments available.

3. A patient may need to have the hair on the chest or legs _____ so that the _____ will adhere to the skin.

4. In some clinics, the patient is allowed to remove the _____ after an ECG test.

5. _____ the ECG procedure is very important for correct reimbursement and should include whether the ECG performed was an emergency ECG, a _____, or a follow-up test.

SUMMARY

- An ECG is a recording of the electrical activity of the heart.

- The focus of the 12-lead ECG is to view the left ventricle during the depolarization stage.

- The views are manipulated to show a total of 12 different vectors. The vectors show the heart from the right to the left, from the superior to the inferior, and from the anterior to the posterior.

- A single-channel ECG test records the ECG manually, 1 lead at a time, whereas the multichannel ECG test records all 12 leads on a single 8 ½" × 11" paper or can show all 12 leads on a monitor at one time.

- Electrodes are first attached to the patient, and then the leads are attached to the electrodes in a specific order.

- Willem Einthoven used the concepts of the electrical flow from the first three leads caused by muscle contractions to produce a graphic image on paper, a theory that is still used today. This theory is based on what direction the electricity passes through the heart.

- A 12-lead ECG consists of 6 limb leads, identified as limb Lead I, Lead II, and Lead III, and the augmented limb leads, labeled aVR, aVL, and aVF, and 6 precordial leads identified as V1, V2, V3, V4, V5, and V6.

- There are four primary angles from which the ECG views the heart. The primary angle views include the lateral wall, anterior wall, inferior wall, and septal wall.

- Some limb leads and precordial leads provide anatomically contiguous views of the same wall. Those leads are located on the lateral and inferior walls.

- Standard limb leads are normally placed on the arms and legs. The precordial leads are positioned on the chest.

- ECG lead placement can be altered in certain situations when heart injury or disease is suspected. For example, leads may better view a suspected posterior MI, injury, or damage such as occlusion of the posterior descending coronary artery of the heart by being placed on the patient's back, or they can be placed on the right side of the chest to view a right ventricular injury.

- Three-lead ECGs use only the arm leads and will provide information for only a specific region of the heart that is being viewed.

- Five-lead ECGs use the arm leads and the V1 precordial chest lead to provide a better view of both sides of the heart.

- Implied consent is not written consent for treatment, but it is used in emergencies.

- Informed consent is written consent that the patient has given stating that the patient understands the procedure, risks, benefits, and alternative treatments.

Critical Thinking Challenges

6-1. Check your understanding of limb leads by completing the following table. The completed table can then be used as a review guide for future chapters.

LIMB LEADS

LEAD	Positive Electrode Location	What Part of Heart You See	Direction Voltage is Recorded	Which Heart Wall are You Viewing?
I				
II	Left leg			
III			From left arm down to left leg	
aVR				
aVL		Left ventricle		
aVF				Inferior wall

6-2. Check your understanding of precordial leads by completing the following table. The completed table can then be used as a review guide for future chapters.

PRECORDIAL LEADS

LEAD	Positive Electrode Location	What Part of Heart You See	Which Heart Wall are You Viewing?
V1	Right sternal wall, fourth intercostal space		
V2			
V3			
V4		Interventricular septum, left ventricle	
V5			Lateral wall
V6			

6-3. Using Figure 6-24, draw a hexaxial view of the limb leads. Be sure that your drawing includes the following:

A. Draw six lines, with degrees marked on each pole.

B. Identify each lead.

C. Color the lateral wall lead lines yellow.

D. Color the inferior wall lead lines orange.

Use colored pencils for C and D.

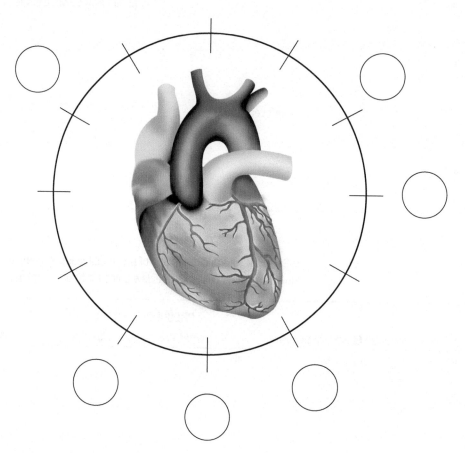

Figure 6-24

Review Activities

6-1. Using colored pencils, color the contiguous lateral walls yellow, contiguous septal walls pink, contiguous inferior walls orange, and contiguous anterior walls blue.

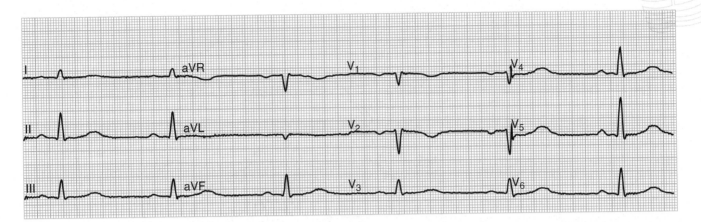

Figure 6-25

6-2. Correctly draw the standard location of the limb leads on Figure 6-26. Then using the colored pencils, choose the correct colors and color the limb leads on the body. Label the drawing with the correct abbreviations.

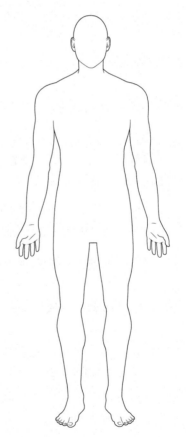

Figure 6-26

6-3. Using Figure 6-27, correctly place the precordial limb leads by drawing a circle in pencil, and labeling each lead correctly. Then, using AHA guidelines, color each circle with the correct limb lead color.

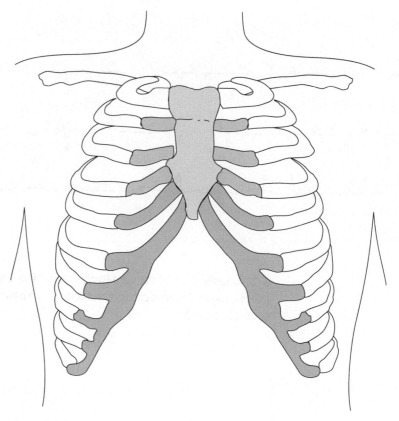

Figure 6-27

Chapter Six Test

Part 1: Fill in the blanks.

1. _____ are attached to the skin to amplify electrical current.

2. The ECG has a target viewpoint of the _____.

3–4. The movement of current through the heart is always from a(n) _____ pole to a(n) _____ pole.

5–6. In precordial leads, the current is flowing _____ the active _____.

7–8. _____ and _____ are bipolar modified chest leads that stimulate precordial leads V1 and V6.

9–10. The _____ reference system uses the six limb leads to determine the axis of the heart in the _____ plane.

11. Unipolar leads have a(n) _____ pole, whereas bipolar leads have a negative and a positive pole.

Part 2: Identify the anatomically contiguous leads for each heart wall.

1. Anterior wall _____

2. Inferior wall _____

3. Lateral wall _____

4. Septal wall _____

Chapter Six Quick Check Answers

Answer order is important except where noted otherwise (shown in parentheses).

When two correct answers are possible, both answers are given separated by the word "or."

6-1:

1. output, muscle hypertrophy
2. Metal
3. single, multichannel
4. electrodes, risks
5. leads, clips (either order)

6-2:

1. direction, intensity (either order)
2. standard, augmented (either order)
3. 10, 9
4. coronal, positive
5. II, I

6-3:

1. amplified
2. limb, coronal
3. aVR, aVL, aVF
4. from, toward
5. heart, limbs

6-4:

1. transverse
2. 6, vector
3. anterior, lateral, septal (any order)
4. fourth, fifth
5. septal, anterior (either order)

6-5:

1. rhythm, patterns (either order)
2. equivalently, each
3. V1, V2
4. V4, V5, V6
5. V3

6-6:

1. location
2. V7, V8, V9

3. opposite
4. RA, LA, LL
5. limb, V1

6-7:
1. implied
2. nonemergency, risks, alternative
3. removed, electrodes
4. electrodes
5. Documenting, routine test

7

WAVEFORMS, RATE, RHYTHM, AND ARTIFACTS

OBJECTIVES

After reading the chapter and completing all Quick Check activities, the student should be able to:

1. Measure duration and voltage on an ECG strip.

2. Describe the isoelectric line, and positive and negative wave reflections.

3. Explain Einthoven's waveforms.

4. Contrast the following terms: interval, segment, complex, and wave.

5. Calculate heart rate.

6. Analyze electrocardiogram rhythms.

7. Identify common artifacts.

8. Explain how to identify limb and precordial lead reversals.

9. Explain normal R wave progression.

KEY TERMS

amplitude

artifact

beats per minute (bpm)

biphasic

bradycardia

deflection

gain control

heart rhythm

interval

irregularly irregular rhythm

isoelectric line

morphology

normal sinus rhythm (NSR)

normal wave progression

regularly irregular rhythm

segment

sinus rhythm

somatic tremor

tachycardia

voltage

wave

waveform

INTRODUCTION

You have probably heard the saying, "To err is human," but now consider adding a second line: "Failure to identify or correct an error can be fatal." ECG technicians realize the importance of correctly administering an electrocardiogram (ECG) and obtaining accurate results in order to prevent errors, including potentially fatal errors. This chapter begins with the identification of waveforms on the ECG strip by using Willem Einthoven's graphic identification system. Examples are given of typical ECG tracings for the student to practice measuring the time and voltage of wavelengths. The isoelectric line and positive and negative deflections will be introduced, followed by an introduction to calculating heart rate and determining heart rhythm. The chapter concludes with identifying common errors that can occur with the patient, the machine, and the surrounding noise, as well as ECG technician errors, and offers solutions to correcting the errors.

THE ECG TRACING

Before discussing waveforms, an understanding of how to read the time and voltage on the ECG tracing will be demonstrated. When ECGs are recorded on paper, they are composed of little square boxes. It is irrelevant whether the paper begins as plain printer paper, commercial dot matrix paper, or proprietary pressure sensitive paper because all ECG tracings must be standardized with the meaning of each square that makes up a grid. Each little box is grouped into a matrix of 25 small boxes, five across and five down, to create one large box. Additionally, each little box is a square that measures 1 millimeter by 1 millimeter. **Figure 7-1** shows the standardized design of an ECG paper grid. Sometimes tick marks appear on the grid, which identifies each second of time along the horizontal axis. This figure shows an enlarged view of what a typical 6-second strip would look like in small and large boxes. The boxes represent two different measurements. The horizontal measurement describes the duration of time, and the vertical measurement measures both the height and the strength of the cardiac wave.

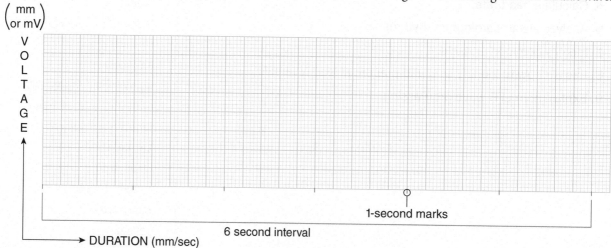

Figure 7-1 Standardized ECG paper

Measuring Time

The standard grid can be further identified by knowing that each light-colored vertical line along the horizontal axis is 1 millimeter (mm) from the previous light-colored line. A properly calibrated ECG machine records an ECG at a preset speed of 25 mm per second (25 mm/sec) along the horizontal axis, and records the wavelength from left to right. Each little box has a time value of 0.04 seconds in duration. Looking at the grid and doing the math, it is easy to see that each darker-colored vertical line comes after every fifth small box, so each large square is equivalent to 0.20 seconds in duration (5 boxes multiplied by 0.04). Therefore, to count 1 second using large squares, multiply 0.20 by 5 because one large square is only 1/5 of a second. The grid is designed to record an ECG over a period of time. Can you compute how many small boxes and how many large boxes would be found in a 6-second ECG strip?

Answer: One small box = 0.04 seconds

One large box = 5 small boxes, so one large box is 0.20 seconds

Five large boxes = 1 second, AND 25 small boxes = 1 second

So, in 6 seconds, there would be 30 large boxes: (5 * 6) or (0.20 * 30)

and 150 small boxes (25 * 6) or (0.04 * 150)

Being able to calculate the duration of each wave on the ECG strip is required knowledge in order to be able to calculate the heart rate (number of heartbeats) in 1 minute.

Remember that heart rate is calculated by using the horizontal axis. Count each waveform length by the number of small boxes, remembering that every five small boxes is equivalent to one large box. The cardiac cycle is also computed by using the horizontal axis and counting the waveforms over a period of time, typically counting the number of cycles that occur over a period of 6 or 10 seconds.

ECG Paper—Measuring Time

- Time is measured in seconds
- 1 small box = 0.04 seconds
- 1 large box = 0.20 seconds

Measuring Voltage

voltage
An amount of electrical stimulus or the difference in action potential created by cardiac cell movement within the heart.

amplitude
The strength or magnitude of the action potential as shown on an ECG recording.

In cardiac studies, **voltage** is the amount of electrical stimulus or the difference in action potential created by cardiac cell movement within the heart. Another term sometimes seen in lieu of voltage is **amplitude**. Amplitude is the strength or magnitude of the action potential.

Voltage is measured in millivolts (mV). It takes 10 mm (2 large boxes) to create 1 millivolt (mV), or 10 mm = 1 mV. Voltage measurement is important for the calibration of ECG machines and to be able to calculate the duration of voltage as the heart goes through each cardiac cycle. There are several reasons that a graphic view of the ECG may need to be enlarged or reduced in size. This can be accomplished by changing the amplitude at the beginning of the ECG recording. Some ECG machine manufacturers will put the calibration at the end of the test strip.

ECG Paper—Measuring Voltage

- Voltage is measured in millivolts (mV)
- 2 large boxes = 10 mm
- 10 mm = 1 mV

Figure 7-2 highlights a grid with one small box darkened, which can be stated as follows: 1 small box = 0.04 seconds; or 1 small box = 0.1 mV; or 1 small box = 1 mm.

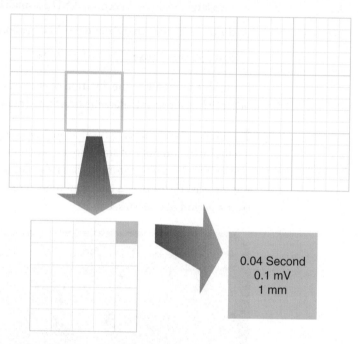

Figure 7-2 Value of one small square

Calibration Box

On an ECG machine, there may be a control feature known as **gain control**, where the wave height is adjusted so that the waves fit on the paper. Recall that the standard amplitude is 10 mm = 1 mV (2 large boxes shown vertically stacked), a large box is 5 small blocks wide by 5 blocks tall, and the speed is approximately 25 mm per second. If the waveform is too large for the paper, the gain control can be reduced to half-amplitude, or 5 mm (1 large box or a stair-step-shaped box). Similarly, if the waveform is too small, the gain control can be enlarged for better viewing to double amplitude and double speed, or an amplitude of 20 mm (2 mV) and an approximate speed of 50 mm/sec (4 large boxes stacked as a square, 2 boxes high by 2 boxes wide). **Figure 7-3** shows the gain control setting as it would appear either at the beginning or ending of the ECG strip, along the vertical axis. The standard setting is labeled (a), the half amplitude is labeled (b), and the double amplitude is labeled (c). It is unusual that the gain control needs to be adjusted, and technicians performing ECGs should document in the patient chart when it has been necessary to change the gain control.

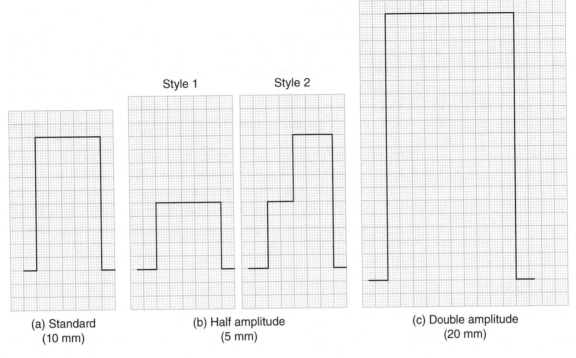

Style 1   Style 2

(a) Standard
(10 mm)

(b) Half amplitude
(5 mm)

(c) Double amplitude
(20 mm)

Figure 7-3 Amplitude setting on ECG

Quick Check 7-1

Fill in the blanks.

1. The ECG tracing measures _____ on the horizontal axis, and _____ and _____ on the vertical axis.

2. Properly calibrated ECG machines are set at an approximate speed of 25 mm per _____.

3. Calculate the number of large and small boxes on a 10-second ECG strip. Show your calculations.
   Answer: _____ large boxes and _____ small boxes

4. Calculate the number of seconds in a wave that is 7 small boxes wide and 3 small vertical boxes. Show your calculations. *Answer:* _____ seconds and _____ mV

5. Calculate the duration of a wave that is 2.5 small boxes wide by 3 large vertical boxes. Show your calculations. *Answer:* _____ seconds and _____ mV

THE ECG GRAPHIC IMAGE

wave
Electrical activity within the walls of the heart leading up to a ventricular contraction.

There are three different electrical activities that occur and create graphic images on the ECG strip. The activities create a **wave**, which identifies what is happening within the walls of the heart leading up to a ventricular contraction. This section will explain what each electrical activity stands for and provides a review of the electrical "loop" within the heart.

Isoelectric Line

When there is no electrical activity occurring within the heart, the ECG strip will show as a solid flat line. This flat line is called the isoelectric line. The isoelectric line is also referred to as the baseline because some waveforms will normally only occur above the isoelectric line, some waveforms normally occur only below the isoelectric line, and some waveforms normally occur both above and below the isoelectric line as part of one waveform. Therefore, movement away from the baseline in either an upward or downward direction makes up a waveform.

The difference in whether the waveform appears as a positive deflection (above the isoelectric line) or a negative deflection (below the isoelectric line) is determined by electrical current through the heart toward or away from the positive or negative pole in the lead. This concept explains why different leads point to different deflections on the ECG strip. To review information concerning positive and negative poles, please review Chapter 6. **Figure 7-4** shows an isoelectric line on an ECG strip.

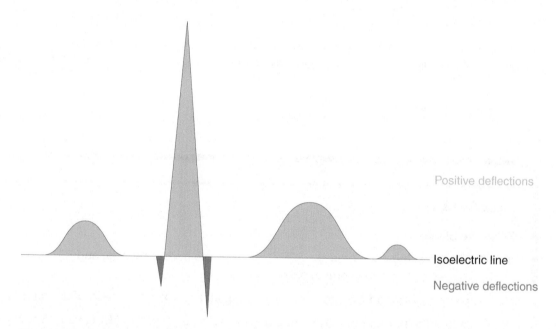

Positive deflections

Isoelectric line

Negative deflections

Figure 7-4 Isoelectric line and deflections

Positive Deflections from the Isoelectric Line

When the electricity is flowing through the heart *away* from a negative pole of the lead, a positive or upright deflection will occur as a pattern on the ECG strip. This information can also be considered as looking at the direction of flow as being through the heart *toward* the positive pole of the lead, therefore creating the positive or upright deflection.

Negative Deflections from the Isoelectric Line

Electrical current flowing through the heart *toward* a negative pole of the lead will create a negative or inverted deflection, appearing as a pattern on the ECG strip. This information can also be considered to be looking at the direction of flow as through the heart *away* from the positive pole of the lead, therefore creating a negative or inverted deflection.

Depolarization Loop

Recall from Chapter 3, one cardiac cycle includes depolarization through repolarization, and it is completed in approximately 0.08 seconds. Keeping this in mind, we begin by reviewing the wave of depolarization in a normal heart. First, a quick review. In the normal cardiac cycle, the sinoatrial node fires the depolarization impulse, which sends the depolarization wave through the internodal pathway to the atrioventricular node, where the intrinsic firing rate is slowed before the impulse continues through the bundle of His, along the interventricular septum via the bundle branches, and finally to the Purkinje network, which is located within the muscle walls surrounding the ventricles, where the ventricular contraction is initiated. This depolarization loop can be "viewed" by looking at the ECG printout of the 12 leads. The depolarization to repolarization cycle, then, is the electrical excitement or "wave" that occurs within the walls of the heart.

ECG WAVEFORMS

When Dr. Einthoven first developed recordings of the heart with the string galvanometer, he named the graphic images on the ECG with letters from the middle of the alphabet, starting with the letter P and continuing with Q, R, S, T, and U. All letters are written in uppercase Arabic letters unless abnormalities such as duplicate waves or missing waves are being pointed out. Each letter represents a specific action occurring within the heart during the normal cardiac cycle. This section covers the types of waveforms and then identifies each of Einthoven's graphic images.

Waveform Morphology

morphology
The structural appearance of a wave or waveform.

Morphology is the structural appearance (such as the size and configuration) of a wave or waveform. Morphology is the first of three core principles to understand to be able to read an ECG strip successfully. Waveforms can appear as curved, spiked, upright, inverted, biphasic, notched, fluttered, or fibrillated. Understanding what the normal morphology should look like and recognizing deviations will greatly enhance your ability to read the ECG strip. Curved waveforms can be either upright or inverted, but they appear rounded as opposed to spiked, where the waveform comes to a point. **Biphasic** waveforms cross the isoelectric line, with part of the waveform being upright and part of it being inverted. Biphasic waveforms can be either curved or spiked somewhere within the waveform. Notched waveforms appear as having an extra curve, sometimes referred to as a "hiccup" in the line.

biphasic
Waveforms with two distinct phases: one phase is above and one phase below the isoelectric line.

A waveform that appears to flutter is one that appears abnormally rapid and sometimes erratic. Fibrillation occurs when the heart muscle cells do not move as a coordinated wave; rather, the normal rhythmic ventricular contraction is replaced by rapid, uncontrolled, individual muscle fiber twitching. A heart in fibrillation mode can become deadly with the loss of blood circulation and pulse. **Figure 7-5** provides an example of what each

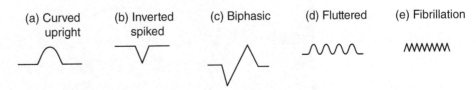

Figure 7-5 Waveform morphology examples: (a) curved upright; (b) inverted spiked; (c) biphasic; (d) fluttered; (e) fibrillation

type of morphology would appear as on an ECG strip. The shapes are labeled as follows: (a) curved upright; (b) inverted spiked; (c) inverted spiked and upright curved biphasic; (d) fluttered; and (e) fibrillation. A curved or spiked wave can present as either upright or inverted.

Deflection

deflection
The amount of deviation from the isoelectric line, determined by lead placement.

Deflection is the amount of deviation from the isoelectric line and is determined by the lead placement. When comparing the deflection of a wave, the leads will view the wave from different angles so that the deflection on each lead will be different, but several leads usually view the same waveform as a positive or negative deflection. At the end of the chapter, examples of placing the leads in the wrong position will be shown on ECGs.

Types of Waveforms

Now that the appearance and characteristics of a waveform have been discussed, it is time to identify the second core element to understanding how to read an ECG strip: that is, the type of activity of the waveform that should appear on an ECG tracing. In a normal ECG image, there are four types of wave activity that makes up the cardiac cycle, which is shown on the ECG strip. These activities include a wave, a segment, an interval, and a complex. A wave shows up as a curved or spiked line, either above or below the isoelectric line. When a wave connects with a second activity, it becomes known as a segment. The interval represents time between two waves, a segment, or a complex. A complex is a series of connected waves that all serve the same activity, such as depolarization of the ventricles. Diseases and a person's underlying physiology will determine variations in the appearance of heart activity on an ECG. Leads provide various views of the heart, and misplaced leads can hide or distort an electrical event.

Waveform Duration

Duration of waves is the third core element to understand in order to be able to read ECG strips. Each wave in the cardiac cycle should be of a particular duration on the ECG strip in order to be considered within normal limits. Being able to identify variances in the duration of the wave or waveform, either in time on the horizontal axis or in amplitude on the vertical axis, is the goal to understanding the graphic image of the heart. Duration is measured by counting boxes, either little boxes or large boxes, but always remember that the little box is 0.04 seconds and the large box is 0.20 seconds. The measurement of a wave starts when the wave departs from the isoelectric line. The measurement of the wave ends when the wave returns to the isoelectric line or levels off.

Three Core Principles of ECG Waveforms

1. Identify the normal structural appearance
2. Identify the type of activity (wave, segment, interval or complex)
3. Identify the duration of each cardiac cycle

Calipers

Duration can be measured with calipers. Before the use of computers, many health professionals used calipers to determine the duration of the waveform. Today, most ECG machines come with a software program that analyzes the ECG strip and identifies any variances from normal, so it is hard to find calipers still being used, even in a cardiologists' office. **Figure 7-6** shows a pair of calipers. For the student just beginning to analyze ECG strips, using calipers may increase their understanding and save time. Calipers can be purchased at many online medical supply companies.

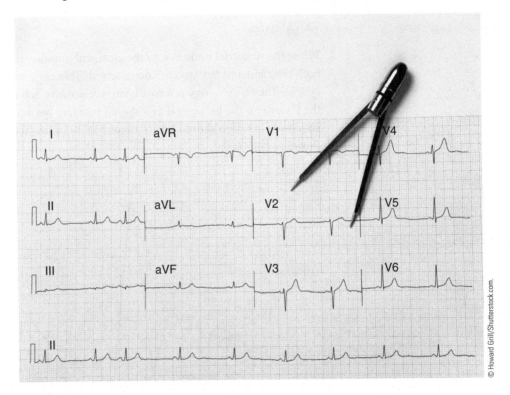

Figure 7-6 ECG calipers

© Howard Grill/Shutterstock.com.

Quick Check 7-2

Fill in the blanks.

1. The flat line on an ECG strip is called the _____ line and occurs when there is no _____ activity within the heart.

2. Movement away from the baseline in a(n) _____ or _____ direction creates a waveform.

3. _____ deflections of electricity away from the _____ pole of the lead create an upright deflection.

4. One cardiac cycle includes depolarization through _____ and is completed in approximately _____ seconds.

5. The three core principles of waveforms include _____, activity of the waveform, and _____ of waves.

EINTHOVEN'S GRAPHIC IDENTIFICATION SYSTEM

This section will identify the six waves that Einthoven used to identify graphic images on the ECG. The three core principles of morphology, type of activity, and duration on both the horizontal and vertical axis will also be explained. Additionally, identification of the heart phase from depolarization through repolarization will be identified.

P Wave

When the sinoatrial node begins the electrical impulse, the P wave is created on the grid as both the right and left atria are depolarized. This contraction phase is also known as atrial systole. The morphology is a small, curved, positive wave in Lead II. The time duration of the P wave on the horizontal axis should measure between 0.06 and 0.12 seconds, and the amplitude duration should be no more than 2–3 mm (0.02–0.03 mV). A normal P wave is shown in **Figure 7-7**.

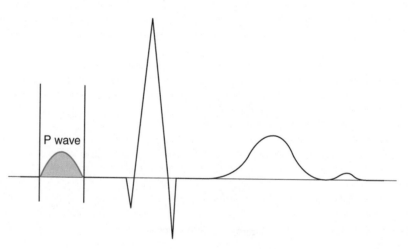

Figure 7-7 Normal P wave

Q Wave

As the electrical impulse continues down the interventricular septum toward the Purkinje fibers, a normal Q wave represents septal depolarization. The current flows downward from right to left through the septum. Morphology of the Q wave in Lead II, if present, should show itself as a small, negative, spiked deflection. The duration of the Q wave should be less than 0.04 seconds on the horizontal axis, and the amplitude on the vertical axis should be less than 2 mm (0.02 mV). The Q wave is the initial and lowest wave of the QRS complex. A normal Q wave is shown in **Figure 7-8**.

R Wave

In the R wave, the electrical impulse has traveled from the sinoatrial (SA) node through the atrioventricular (AV) node and is now going throughout the ventricular walls and represents

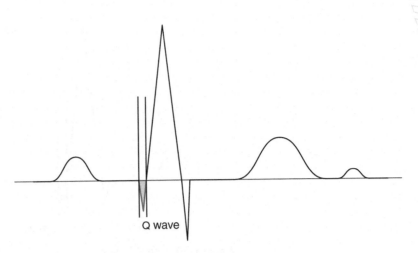

Figure 7-8 Normal Q wave

part of the ventricular depolarization cycle. The R peaks at the end of ventricular diastole and the start of systole. The morphology of a complete R wave is normally a large, positive, spiked deflection in Lead II. The R wave is the second wave in the QRS complex. The durations of time and amplitude of the R wave are usually given when the R wave is part of a segment or complex. **Figure 7-9** shows the normal R wave.

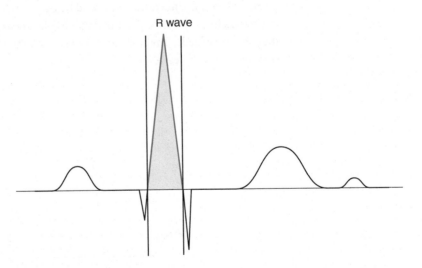

Figure 7-9 Normal R wave

S Wave

In a normal cardiac cycle, the impulse now depolarizes the Purkinje network of fibers. Recall that these fibers are spread throughout the ventricular walls, so the S wave covers the remaining portion of time needed for ventricular depolarization, also called ventricular systole. The morphology of a normal S wave is a small, negative, spiked deflection. The durations of time and amplitude of the S wave are usually given when the S wave is part of a segment or complex. **Figure 7-10** shows the normal S wave.

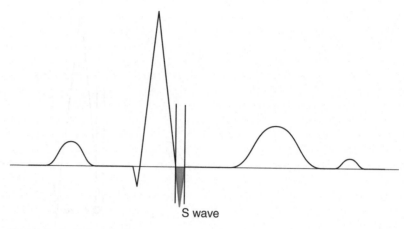

Figure 7-10 Normal S wave

T Wave

Ventricular depolarization is now complete, but before the cardiac cycle can begin again, the ventricles repolarize. The ventricular relaxation phase is also called ventricular diastole. The T wave represents the repolarization. Recall from Chapter 3 that repolarization is synonymous with the heart resting. The repolarization wave is from the apex toward the base of the heart and creates a morphology of a positive, deflected, curved wave in Lead II. In a normal ECG, the time duration would be between 0.04 and 0.08 seconds. Amplitude duration varies from less than 5 mm (0.05 mV) in the limb leads to less than 10 mm (1 mV) in the precordial leads. The normal T wave is usually symmetrical in appearance. **Figure 7-11** shows a normal T wave.

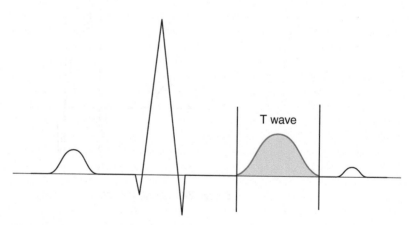

Figure 7-11 Normal T wave

U Wave

Uncommonly, there may be one additional wave shown on an ECG. This wave is called the U wave. The U wave is thought to represent the repolarization of the Purkinje fibers. It has been noted that the U wave sometimes appears as a result of certain antiarrhythmic drug effects, drug toxicity, or electrolyte imbalances. When the U wave appears, it is usually smaller in size and duration than the T wave. The morphology is a very small, curved, positive deflection. Typically, the amplitude will be less than 2 mm (0.02 mV) if normal, and inverted, spiked, or greater than 2 mm (0.02 mV) in height if abnormal. **Figure 7-12** shows the location of the U wave.

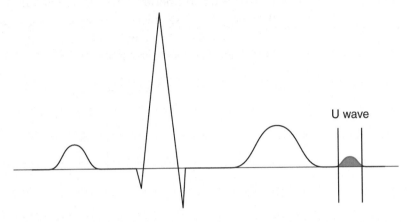

Figure 7-12 Location of the U wave

Quick Check 7-3

Fill in the blanks.

1. Positive deflections from the baseline would normally be found in the _____, _____, _____, and U waves.

2. Durations of time and amplitude of the _____ and _____ waves are normally given when the wave is part of a segment or complex.

3. It is thought that the U wave represents repolarization just as the _____ wave does, only the U wave is smaller in size and duration.

4. In a normal ECG, the _____ wave may not appear at all, or it will present as a small, _____, spiked deflection.

5. The two waves that represent ventricular depolarization include the _____ wave and the _____ wave.

INTERVALS, SEGMENTS, OR A COMPLEX

Many of the waves are combined to create intervals, segments, or a complex. In one normal cardiac cycle, there will be one complex named QRS, three intervals named P-R, Q-T, and R-R, and three segments named PR, ST, and TP. The following sections will explain the differences between these terms. Note that the waveforms can appear in more than one area, and the PR waves can be either a P-R segment or a PR interval (PRI).

QRS Complex

The normal QRS complex includes the Q wave, R wave, and S wave, but it is still called the QRS complex even if one of the waves is missing. QRS complex analysis is most important to determine the origin of rhythms.

If the Q wave is present, a normal complex will begin with a small, negative spike immediately preceding the large, positive, spiked R wave, followed by a small, negative, spiked deflection of the S wave. The normal total duration of time for the QRS complex should range from 0.06 seconds to just under 0.12 seconds. The QRS complex represents rapid ventricular depolarization of the AV node, bundle of His, bundle branches, and Purkinje fibers. A normal QRS complex is highlighted in **Figure 7-13**.

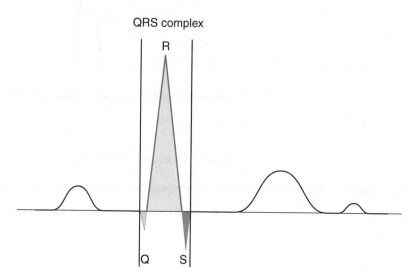

Figure 7-13 QRS complex

Intervals

interval
On an ECG image, the period of time between two waves that complete an event and includes time where no electrical activity is being recorded on the ECG.

Intervals are a time period between two waves that completes an event and includes time where no electrical activity is being recorded on the ECG. In the study of ECGs, two of the intervals when appearing consistently on an ECG signify atrial depolarization and ventricular depolarization, while the third interval can be used to determine the heart rate, even when it appears inconsistently. Intervals are recognized as events along the horizontal axis. Each event is further explained in this section.

P-R Interval (PRI)

The PRI morphology includes the P wave and a short duration of time on the isoelectric line before the start of the Q wave. The conduction delay accounts for the period of time after the P wave when there is no electrical activity being shown on the ECG tracing. The interval is named PRI, but actually it lasts only until the beginning of the Q wave, which is not always present on an ECG. The PRI signifies the period of atrial depolarization when the interval consistently appears before the QRS complex, and the normal delay found at the AV node. The normal duration of time for an adult is 0.12–0.20 seconds. **Figure 7-14** shows the PRI highlighted.

Q-T Interval

The morphology of the Q-T interval includes the QRS complex, the T wave, and the distance on the isoelectric line between the Q and T waves. The Q-T interval is important because it represents the entire ventricular depolarization and repolarization cycle. The Q-T

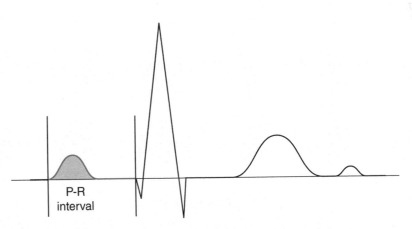

Figure 7-14 P-R interval

interval begins with the Q wave, continues until the end of the T wave, and corresponds to the ventricular action potential. It can be difficult to measure the Q-T interval because there must be several heartbeats showing the end of the T wave, and the interval changes with changes in heart rate. The normal Q-T interval duration should be less than 0.4 seconds for males and 0.44 seconds for females. A shortcut to measuring the Q-T interval is to measure the interval between two R waves and divide the answer by 2. The Q-T interval is highlighted in **Figure 7-15**.

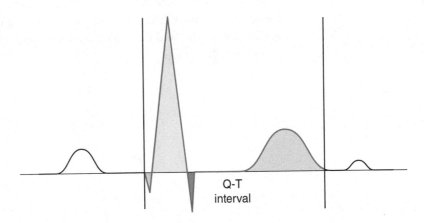

Figure 7-15 Q-T interval

R-R Interval

The R-R interval is a measurement between two cardiac cycles, whereas all other intervals, segments, the QRS complex, and the individual waves mentioned in this section all refer to the events of one heartbeat. It is important to understand that the R-R is an interval or period of time that is measured on the horizontal axis. The R-R interval is used to measure heartbeat rate and regularity. Calculating the heart rate and more detail on the R-R interval will be covered in greater detail later in this chapter. **Figure 7-16** shows the R-R interval measured from the point of the R wave in one cardiac cycle to the point of the R wave in a second cardiac cycle. The measurement is often characterized as "peak to peak."

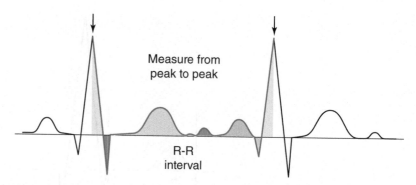

Figure 7-16 R-R interval

Segments

A **segment** on the ECG strip is a time period with no electrical activity occurring between waves, and, if normal, it looks like a flat line. A segment occurs three times on the normal ECG. The first event is the PR segment, the second event is called the ST segment, and the third event is called the TP segment.

PR Segment

The normal PR segment is located along the isoelectric line, meaning that no electrical activity is occurring during this event. Atrial depolarization occurs during a normal PR segment. The PR segment begins at the end of the P wave and ends at the beginning of the QRS complex. The difference between the PR segment and PRI interval is the exclusion of the P wave in a segment. The PR segment represents a conduction delay between the end of atrial depolarization and the beginning of ventricular depolarization. **Figure 7-17** highlights the normal PR segment.

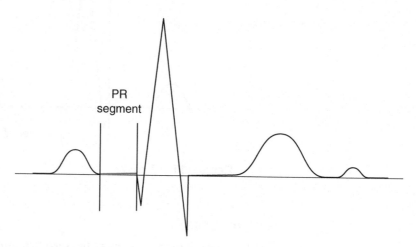

Figure 7-17 PR segment

ST Segment

As previously stated, no electrical current is flowing during the ventricular repolarization period that makes up the ST segment. For this reason, a normal ST segment should be on or very near and parallel to the isoelectric line. Recall from Chapter 3 that the ventricles are in the absolute refractory period when there is no electrical current, so the cells will not respond to stimuli as they are contracting in preparation for the next heartbeat. The ST segment is the early part of the repolarization of the ventricles, also known as early ventricular systole. The ST segment begins at the end of the S wave and ends at the beginning of the T wave. The ST segment represents a conduction delay between ventricular depolarization and ventricular repolarization. **Figure 7-18** highlights the normal ST segment.

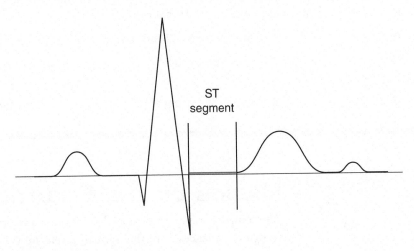

Figure 7-18 ST segment

TP Segment

During the TP segment, the atria and ventricles are relaxed, which means that the heart is in a diastolic state. When the heart is beating normally, the TP segment is on the isoelectric line; however, in times of a fast heartbeat (such as during exercise), the TP segment may be shortened or not seen at all because the T wave and P wave may seem to merge. The TP segment begins at the end of the T wave and ends at the beginning of the P wave. The TP segment is significant as a reference point in determining if the ST or PR segments are elevated or depressed. The TP segment has no known etiology that would cause the isoelectric line to be anything but straight. **Figure 7-19** shows the TP segment.

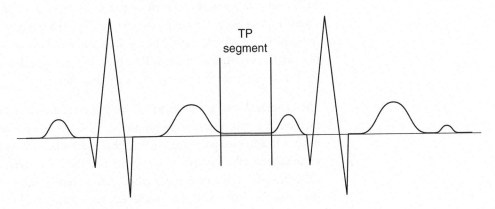

Figure 7-19 TP segment

Quick Check 7-4

Fill in the blanks.

1. The interval that can be used to determine heart rate is called the _____ interval.

2. The QRS complex can determine the _____ of rhythms and should be at least _____ seconds in duration to just under 0.12 seconds.

3. A(n) _____ is a time period with no electrical activity occurring between the _____.

4. No _____ is flowing during the _____ repolarization period that makes up the ST segment.

5. Arial _____ occurs during a normal _____ segment.

BASICS OF THE ELECTROCARDIOGRAM

After understanding the normal direction and size of waveforms, the next step is to learn to recognize variances from the normal waveform. We start by learning to identify the heart rate and heart rhythm. As was mentioned in Chapter 3, heart rate is defined as the number of heartbeats that occurs over a period of one minute. Most of the time the ventricular heart rate is being calculated, however, atrial heart rate can also be determined by the ECG. Heart rate is documented in **beats per minute (bpm)**. After computing heart rate, heart rhythm is identified, usually by visual inspection of the ECG strip, but it can also be calculated. Either method will be documented as being a regular rhythm or an irregular rhythm. When documenting from a 12-lead ECG, Lead II is most often used for calculating heart rate and heart rhythm.

beats per minute (bpm)
The number of heartbeats in 1 minute; used to calculate heart rate on a rhythm strip.

CALCULATING HEART RATE

It is important to recall that most of the characteristics of a normal ECG can vary in duration and amplitude and still remain within the normal limits. This is the reasoning behind always recording a patient's assessments (as mentioned in Chapter 5) and not just presenting the ECG results to a practitioner. Heart rate is an example of one important clinical tool found on the ECG. Heart rate can be determined by calculating an atrial rate, the ventricular rate, or both. The heart rate should be calculated as precisely as possible. In a normal heart, both the atrial and ventricular rates will be the same. When calculating heart rate, always measure the heartbeats from the horizontal axis or baseline.

This chapter shows several visual examination methods, as well as describing the calculation method. It is important to pick a method you are comfortable with that also is acceptable to your health care provider, and use that method consistently. There will be times when a more exact method of calculating heart rate than the quick visual method is needed. With either the visual or calculated method, always remember to check your work by measuring the pulse. The pulse will give you an estimate that should be approximately the same as the visual measurement. Heart rate calculations most often use the P-P interval or the R-R interval. Recall that the SA node creates an impulse 60 to 100 times per minute (Chapter 3). Now you should be able to conclude that the normal heart rate should be the same rate that the SA node releases the impulse, or 60–100 beats per minute (bpm), so be sure to always write "bpm" after your answer.

Atrial Heart Rate

Recall that the right atrium contains both the SA node and the AV node. Both are considered the heart's natural pacemakers. When the heart is working correctly, the electrical impulse begins in the SA node, moving quickly throughout the atria before exiting through the AV node. Many problems can and do occur when the atria do not complete the cycle as described. An irregular heartbeat may prevent the heart from pumping enough blood to the ventricles to meet the bodies' needs. Sometimes there may not be any symptoms, and the patient may not be aware that the heart is beating abnormally.

To calculate a normal atrial heart rate, look at the P waves on the ECG. Recall that the normal time duration of the P wave is between 0.06 and 0.12 seconds. There should be a P wave before every QRS complex, and all P waves should look the same in both length and height. The atrial and ventricular heart rate should be the same in a normal heart because the atrial rate is calculated on normal P waves.

Ventricular Heart Rate

The QRS complex determines ventricular heart rate and is measured by comparing the R to R intervals between consecutive QRS complexes. Recall that the normal QRS complex should begin with a small, downward, spiked Q wave and end with the S wave crossing the isoelectric line. One example of a ventricular disturbance in the QRS complex would be a premature ventricular complex (PVC), which originate in the ventricles and cause wider-than-normal QRS complexes. Recall that the normal QRS complex should be less than 0.12 seconds. Two other waves, the P wave and the T wave, are affected by PVCs. The P wave may not exist, and the T wave is opposite of the QRS complex along the baseline, meaning that if the QRS complex is upright, the T wave will be inverted, and the reverse is also true—if the QRS complex is inverted, the T wave is upright. PVCs are discussed in more detail later in the chapter.

> ### Formula to Calculate Heart Rate
>
> To find atrial heart rate: Measure the P to P intervals.
>
> To find ventricular heart rate: Measure the R to R intervals (peak to peak).

Visual Methods of Calculating Heart Rate

First, determine how many seconds are on the strip you are using. Typically, the strip is either 6 seconds in length or 10 seconds in length. As mentioned earlier, the majority of ECG strips are marked off in increments of 1 second or 3 seconds. If the strip you are looking at does not have seconds marked off on the strip, you will need to count boxes (as discussed in the next section), and then you can add the seconds mark.

10 Times Method

The 10 times method can be used for regular or irregular atrial or ventricular heart rates. The easiest way to determine the atrial heart rate is to count the number of P waves on a 6-second strip and multiply your answer by 10 (because a 6-second strip * 10 = 1 minute). If the atrial heart rate is normal, there should be the same number of squares between each heartbeat, and the duration in time of each P wave should also be the same over the period of a 6-second strip. Normally, only ventricular heart rate is calculated using this method when there is a visible P wave before every QRS complex. Also, ventricular heart rate is determined by using the R to R interval instead of the P to P. Be sure to count from the peak of one R wave to the peak of the next R wave. Refer to Box 7-1 for review of the 10 times method. This method is especially useful for counting two different rhythms on one 6-second strip.

Box 7-1 Determining Heart Rates Using the 10 Times Method

10 Times Method of Calculating Atrial Heart Rate

- Use a 6-second ECG strip
- Count the number of P waves on the strip
- Multiply the number of P waves by 10 = Atrial Beats Per Minute

10 Times Method of Calculating Ventricular Heart Rate

- Use a 6-second ECG strip
- Count the number of R waves on the strip
- Multiply the number of R waves by 10 = Ventricular Beats Per Minute

6 Times Method

Many computer ECG strips are 10 seconds in length. This method can also be used to determine atrial and ventricular, regular or irregular heart rates. To calculate heart rate using the 10-second strip, multiply the number of P waves by 6 to get a 1-minute atrial heart rate. Likewise, use the R waves to calculate the ventricular heart rate. Box 7-2 shows the guidelines for 10-second strips.

Box 7-2 Determining Heart Rate Using the 6 Times Method

6 Times Method of Calculating Atrial Heart Rate

- Use a 10-second ECG strip
- Count the number of P waves on the strip
- Multiply the number of P waves by 6 = Atrial Beats Per Minute

6 Times Method of Calculating Ventricular Heart Rate

- Use a 10-second ECG strip
- Count the number of R waves on the strip
- Multiply the number of R waves by 6 = Ventricular Beats Per Minute

To see how this looks on an ECG strip, **Figure 7-20** shows the P wave and formulas to calculate atrial heart rate. To find the ventricular rate, you would just count the peak of the R waves instead of the P waves.

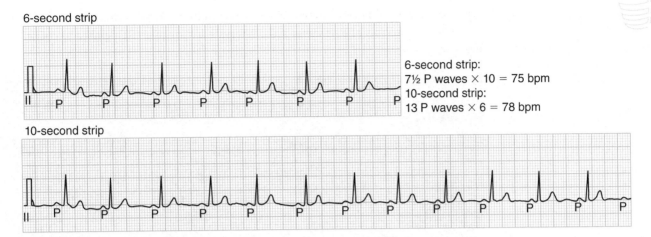

6-second strip

6-second strip:
7½ P waves × 10 = 75 bpm
10-second strip:
13 P waves × 6 = 78 bpm

10-second strip

Figure 7-20 Calculating atrial heart rate

Counting Grid Boxes Method of Calculating Heart Rate

The box counting methods listed next are more exact in calculating heart rate. Counting grid boxes takes longer, and for most applications, the visual method (counting P-P or R-R) is acceptable. Also recall that the heart rate is automatically calculated on computer-generated ECG 12-lead tests.

Calculating Heart Rates When No Seconds Markers Provided

This method will help you determine the heart rate on an ECG strip that does not have 1- or 3-second marks on it. Recall that you can determine the heart rate by counting P-P or R-R waves, but this method has one additional step. There are 30 large squares on a 6-second strip. To determine heartbeat using a 6-second strip, count the number of P or R waves and multiply the answer by 10. For example, using the visual method, if there are 8 P waves within 30 large squares, the heart rate can be estimated to be 80, because 8 * 10 = 80. With a regular rhythm, you can even estimate between the P-P and the R-R waves. For example, if there are 7½ R waves within the 30 large squares, you could estimate that the heart rate is 75 beats per minute (7½ * 10 = 75). The problem is that most patients seeing a cardiologist do not have a normal rhythm, so heart rate cannot be accurately determined with this method.

Calculating Heart Rate Using the Sequential Large Box Method

The sequential large box method is best used when there are irregular heartbeats to be counted. This method can be used for atrial or ventricular heart rates. Recall that 30 large boxes is equivalent to 6 seconds.

Look at the ECG. See if any R wave falls along the side of a large vertical box. If no R waves fall on a vertical line, you will need to estimate the number of large boxes by visual inspection, or remember if the R wave lands somewhere in the large box, but not on a large, dark, vertical line, just add the number of small squares to your total to estimate a large box. Recall that 5 small squares is equivalent to 1 large square. Now look at the tip of an R wave closest to a vertical line of a large box, and then count how many large boxes separate the tip of the first R wave from the tip of the next R wave. Use the chart in Box 7-3 to determine heart rate. Count at least three intervals of R-R waves if the intervals are irregular. Remember to count large boxes only.

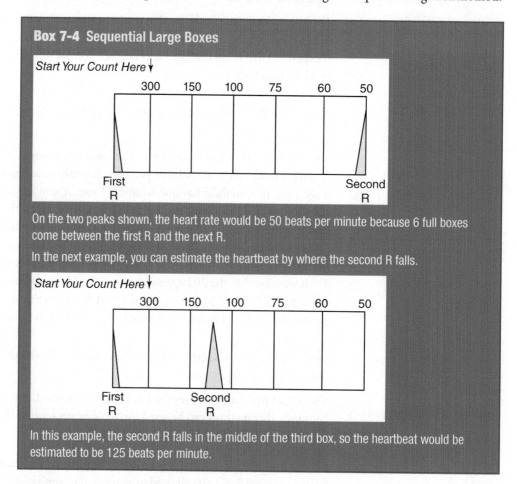

Box 7-3 Determining Heart Rate Using the Sequential Large Box Numbers

Number of Large Boxes	=	Beats per Minute
1 box		300 bpm
2 boxes		150 bpm
3 boxes		100 bpm
4 boxes		75 bpm
5 boxes		60 bpm
6 boxes		50 bpm

When using the sequential numbers, be sure to start the count at the end of the first large box. See Box 7-4 for an example of how to count the boxes using the sequential large box method.

Box 7-4 Sequential Large Boxes

Start Your Count Here

| 300 | 150 | 100 | 75 | 60 | 50 |

First R — Second R

On the two peaks shown, the heart rate would be 50 beats per minute because 6 full boxes come between the first R and the next R.

In the next example, you can estimate the heartbeat by where the second R falls.

Start Your Count Here

| 300 | 150 | 100 | 75 | 60 | 50 |

First R — Second R

In this example, the second R falls in the middle of the third box, so the heartbeat would be estimated to be 125 beats per minute.

Calculating Tachycardia Heart Rate

tachycardia
A consistent heart rate over 100 beats per minute.

Tachycardia occurs when the heart is consistently beating faster than normal (that is, faster than 100 beats per minute). Recall that normal is defined as 60–100 beats per minute. When the heart is beating more than 100 beats per minute, count the number of small boxes between the R-R intervals and memorize the scale shown in Box 7-5 to compute beats per minute.

Box 7-5 Determining Tachycardia Heart Rate		
Number of Small Boxes	**Heart Rate**	**Number of Large Boxes**
5	**300**	1
6	250	
7	214	
8	186	
9	167	
10	**150**	2
11	136	
12	125	
13	115	
14	107	
15	**100**	3

Precise Measurements—1500 Method

For the most precise heart rate calculation, count the number of small boxes between two R waves and divide by 1500 for a normal rhythm, and for an irregular rhythm, count at least three consecutive R-to-R wave small boxes. This is very time consuming, but there are ECG "rulers" and computer programs that also give precise measurements without the need to count.

Abnormal Heart Rates

bradycardia
A consistent heart rate slower than 60 beats per minute.

The heart rate does not remain constant at all times. It can vary by the activities that a person does during the day. Stress, exercise, general health, previous cardiac events, and even sleeping can all alter the heart rate several times a day. Recall when the heart rate is consistently faster than 100 bpm (tachycardia), the ECG strip will show the QRS complexes as being closer together. When the rate is consistently slower than 60 bpm, the rate is called **bradycardia**. In bradycardia, the QRS complexes will be spread out farther and there will not be as many QRS complexes on one 6-second ECG strip as the normal ECG strip. Bradycardia can be computed by the same methods used in tachycardia. **Figure 7-21** shows an ECG strip with a heart rate over 100. Compare Figure 7-21 to **Figure 7-22**, which shows a heart rate under 60 bpm. Then compare both Figures 7-21 and 7-22 to the normal heart rate shown in Figure 7-20.

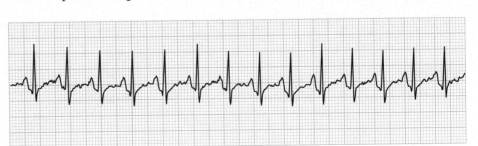

Figure 7-21 Sinus tachycardia

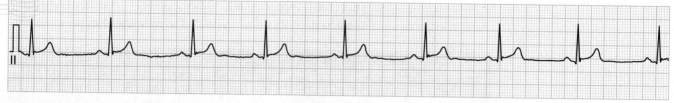

Figure 7-22 Sinus bradycardia

Quick Check 7-5

For each of the images shown below, first circle whether the heart rate is normal, tachycardia, or brady-cardia. (Be sure to recognize if the strip is a 6-second or 10-second ECG.) Then, using one method of your choice, calculate the heart rate in beats per minute.

1. Normal   Tachycardia   Bradycardia

_____ bpm

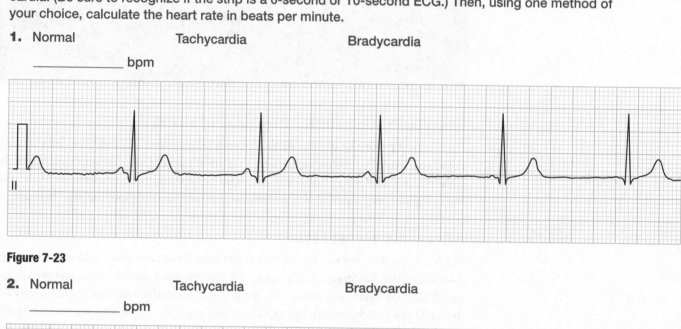

Figure 7-23

2. Normal   Tachycardia   Bradycardia

_____ bpm

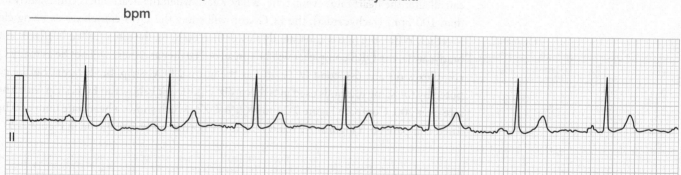

Figure 7-24

3. Normal   Tachycardia   Bradycardia

_____ bpm

(Continued)

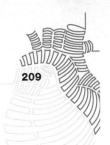

(*Continued*)

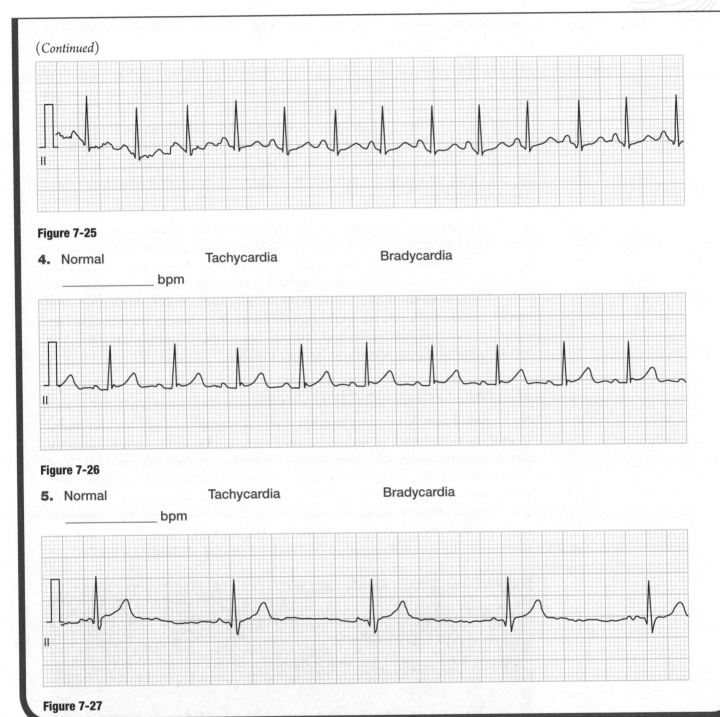

Figure 7-25

4. Normal   Tachycardia   Bradycardia

_____ bpm

Figure 7-26

5. Normal   Tachycardia   Bradycardia

_____ bpm

Figure 7-27

DETERMINING HEART RHYTHM

Heart rhythm may consist of rate disturbances or conduction problems. Rate disturbances include rhythms that are recorded as regular or irregular. Conduction disturbances refer to impulses that originate ventricularly instead of from the atria. Correctly identifying the rhythm is one of the harder aspects of analyzing the ECG because there are so many possibilities when correctly including consideration of heart rate, the regularity and morphology of the other waves that make up each cardiac cycle, and the relationship of the P wave to the QRS complex.

heart rhythm
A measurable, regularly recurring impulse of the heart.

As you have previously learned, electrical impulses cause the heart to beat. **Heart rhythm** is defined as a measurable, regularly recurring impulse of the heart. Heart rate should not be confused with heart rhythm. Just because the heart is beating, that does not mean that the heart is beating in a synchronized manner. Heart rhythm measures the beat whether it is synchronized or not. Some abnormalities to the heart rhythm can be deadly, while other irregular rhythms are just considered "abnormally normal" or a normal variant for a particular person based on genetics, age, prior medical history, and many other factors.

Recall from Chapter 4 that any rhythm that is abnormal or deviates from a normal rhythm is called a dysrhythmia. The abnormality can be of atrial or ventricular origin because depolarization occurs in both the atria and ventricles. When the heart rhythm or heart rate is consistently or predictably irregular, abnormal, or absent, it is known as an arrhythmia. When determining heart rhythm, regular rhythms can be determined by counting boxes and memorizing a formula, but irregular rhythms need to be determined by calculating the average of the widest and narrowest R-to-R intervals. This section covers basic types of rhythm that are important to note when they appear on an ECG.

Normal Sinus Rhythm (NSR)

normal sinus rhythm (NSR)
On an ECG, a group of characteristics that include a heart rate between 60 and 100 beats per minute; regular and uniform P waves before every QRS complex; a PR interval between 0.12 and 0.20 seconds; and a QRS complex of less than 0.12 seconds.

Since a normal heart rhythm has a heartbeat at regular intervals of 60–100 beats per minute (normal conduction) when the impulse is coming from the SA node, for the atria, that means there is a regular P wave rhythm as measured by the duration of time being between 0.12 and 0.20 seconds for the PR interval. For the ventricles, that means that there is a regular QRS complex rhythm, as measured by the duration of time of less than 0.12 seconds. A **normal sinus rhythm (NSR)** must have all the normal rhythm values, plus the P wave must be upright and uniform in Lead II and the rhythm must be consistent, with very little deviation. Refer to **Figure 7-28**, which shows a NSR. The rules to distinguish a NSR from other rhythms is highlighted in Box 7-6.

> **Box 7-6 Normal Sinus Rhythm Rules**
>
> - P wave is uniform before every QRS complex.
> - R-R intervals are all regular.
> - Heart rate is 60–100 beats per minute.
> - PRI is between 0.12 and 0.20 seconds.
> - QRS complex is less than 0.12 seconds.

A quick way to visualize whether a strip shows a normal rhythm is to take the side of a piece of straight paper and mark off two or three R peaks. Then compare your marked paper with the remaining strips on the paper. Normal rhythm strips will be the same distance apart.

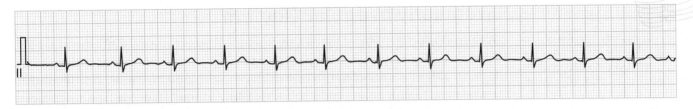

Figure 7-28 Normal sinus rhythm

Regularly Irregular Rhythm

regularly irregular rhythm
A heart rhythm that deviates from a normal rhythm on a regular basis and usually occurs as a patterned event.

A **regularly irregular rhythm** is a heart rhythm that deviates from a normal rhythm on a regular basis and usually occurs as a patterned event. For example, bradycardia is an irregularly slow rhythm and tachycardia is an irregularly fast rhythm. Look back at Figures 7-21 and 7-22. Do you see the regularity? Yes, they have all the waves in the correct order—they just come too fast or too slow. Is the rhythm normal? Yes, the P-P interval is the same in the atrial rhythms and the R-R rhythm is the same in the ventricular rhythms. The pattern on both of these regularly irregular rhythms is easy to spot on an ECG. Causes of a regularly irregular rhythm can be external, such as in dealing with the stresses of daily living, or can be internal, such as the body's reaction to thermoregulation on a very hot or cold day. Variations to the normal rhythm may also be a normal variant for some people with no other underlying health conditions. A regularly irregular rhythm would not be considered a NSR; rather, it would be called just a **sinus rhythm**. The rules for a sinus rhythm are the same as a NSR except for the rate, as shown in Box 7-7.

sinus rhythm
A rhythm that follows all the rules for a normal sinus rhythm except that the heart rate is too fast or too slow.

> **Box 7-7 Sinus Rhythm Rules**
>
> - P wave is uniform before every QRS complex.
> - R-R intervals are all regular.
> - *Heart rate is less than 60 beats per minute or more than 100 beats per minute.*
> - PRI is between 0.12 and 0.20 seconds.
> - QRS complex is less than 0.12 seconds.

Occasionally Irregular Rhythm

An occasionally irregular rhythm may be a normal variant for some people. Suppose that you notice on the ECG strip that the rhythm looks fine except for one or two events when the R-R interval is uneven or the QRS complex came too quickly, not leaving a consistent PR interval one or more times. This can occasionally happen when the right atrium does not have enough time for the atrial kick and the atrioventricular valve closes to begin the ventricular contraction cycle too early. Another example when this may occur is during atrial fibrillation (A-Fib). In A-Fib, the impulse from the SA node is occasionally disorganized, but the impulse may also be regular on the same ECG test. In both examples, the rhythm would be considered as an occasionally irregular rhythm. Occasionally irregular rhythms can also be easy to miss. To prevent missing occasionally irregular rhythms, take time to look at each P wave, PR interval, QRS complex, and QT interval to be sure they all maintain a consistent rhythm.

Irregularly Irregular Rhythm

irregularly irregular rhythm
A cardiac rhythm with no R-R pattern or similarity between the PR or QRS intervals.

With an **irregularly irregular rhythm**, there is no R-R pattern or similarity between the P-R intervals and QRS complexes. Irregularly irregular rhythms are due to abnormalities found in the atria. The three disorders that have an irregularly irregular rhythm are atrial fibrillation, a wandering atrial pacemaker, and atrial tachycardia. All three of these rhythms are discussed in detail in advanced books on ECG interpretation. For now, emphasis will be on noticing whether a rhythm is regular or irregular by looking at the P-P intervals for the atrial rhythm and R-R intervals for the ventricular rhythm using a visual inspection method. **Figure 7-29** shows atrial fibrillation with a ventricular rate (distance between the R-R intervals) that varies between 75 and 166 beats per minute, thus making the rhythm irregular; but additionally, the morphology of this ECG is irregular because there are no identifiable P waves.

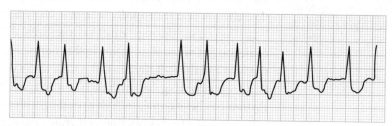

Figure 7-29 An irregularly irregular rhythm

Determining Heart Rhythm

Regular Rhythm: is consistently the same pattern between R-R intervals

Irregular Rhythm: has variations between R-R intervals

Quick Check 7-6

For each of the images shown below, first circle the term regular or irregular. Then determine the rate. (Be sure to recognize if the strip is a 6-second or 10-second ECG.)

1. Regular Rhythm   Irregular Rhythm

_____ Heart Rate

25.0 mm/s 10.0 mm/mV

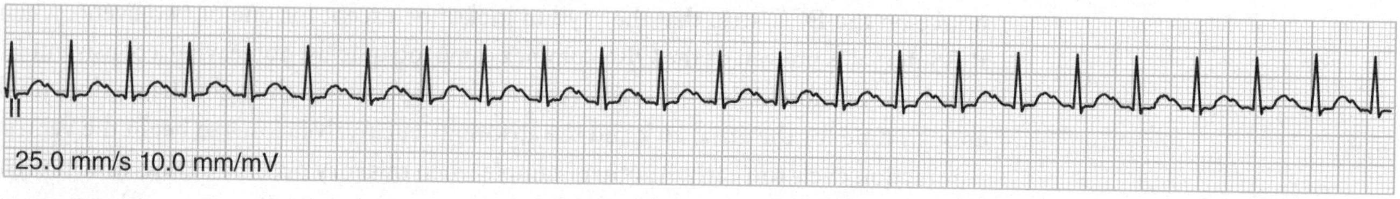

Figure 7-30

2. Regular Rhythm   Irregular Rhythm

_____ Heart Rate

(Continued)

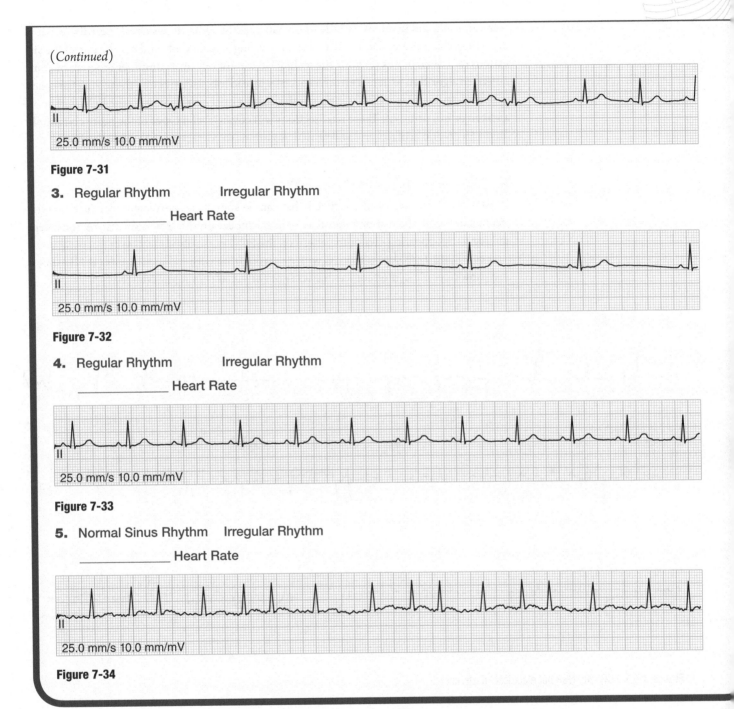

(Continued)

Figure 7-31

3. Regular Rhythm _____ Irregular Rhythm

_____ Heart Rate

Figure 7-32

4. Regular Rhythm _____ Irregular Rhythm

_____ Heart Rate

Figure 7-33

5. Normal Sinus Rhythm _____ Irregular Rhythm

_____ Heart Rate

Figure 7-34

RECOGNIZING ARTIFACTS

artifact

An unusual waveform that appears on the ECG but is not caused by the heart; rather, it originates from outside interference, technician or machine error, or patient movement.

An **artifact** can be defined as an unusual wave that appears on an ECG strip originating from an outside interference, machine or technician error, or patient movement. In any artifact, the indication of wavelength errors is *not* created by the heart. Artifacts that are not corrected can cause inaccurate test results by an untrained technician performing the ECG. Always observe the ECG as it is being recorded and correct any artifacts before running a new test. Also remember to document how the patient tolerated the procedure. If the patient is alert, able to communicate, and in relatively little or no pain, yet the ECG shows a major cardiac event is occurring, chances are that the ECG is not recording actual events and may be one of the situations described in this section. The technician cannot rely on a computer program or computerized algorithm to detect errors, especially in lead misplacement, so the technician needs to become aware of what looks different through a visual examination of the ECG, either on a screen or in a printout. These next sections will cover several types of the more commonly found errors and artifacts and will provide solutions to correcting the error or artifact.

Electrical Interference

Outside conditions can cause artifacts that can be sometimes corrected or reduced by the technician before the test or as soon as artifacts appear on the screen or strip. A consistent and regularly appearing sawtooth pattern on the ECG is usually indicative of electrical interference. **Figure 7-35** shows an ECG with a sinus rhythm within normal limits (WNL), but it also shows electrical interference that was not corrected throughout the test.

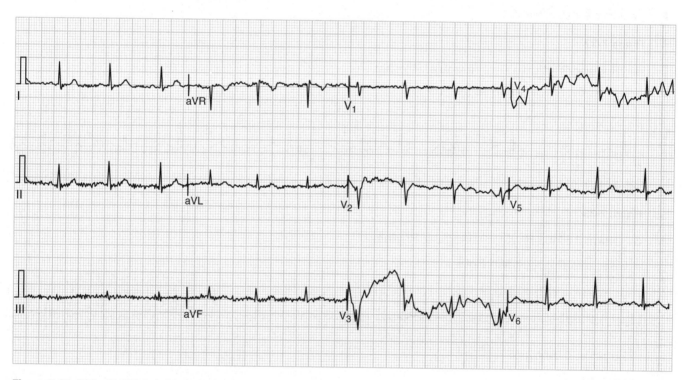

Figure 7-35 ECG with NSR but electrical interference

ECG machines come with filters to aid in the removal of artifacts, but some electrical interference can also be prevented by following a few simple guidelines. If the ECG is to be performed in a room with fluorescent lighting, simply turning off the light and using a lamp or other indirect lighting can be set up before the patient arrives. Another correctable electrical interference can be caused by cell phones. Ask patients if they have a cell phone on them. If they do, instruct them to remove it from their pocket at the same time as instructions for removing belts and other metal items are given, which can be part of the setup routine. Having a safe place for patients to temporarily store their cell phones will add to patient compliance, or ask patients to turn off their cell phones to prevent interference if they keep their phone in the testing room.

Taking the time to explain why you are asking patients to turn off the cell phone, instead of muting or putting the phone in vibration mode, will usually lead to better cooperation. Of course, staff should also turn off their own cell phones if they take them into the exam room. Radios and television sets can also cause electrical interference and should be turned off.

Machine Errors

When an ECG machine is correctly calibrated, the machine will operate at a standardized speed of 25 millimeters per second. Remember to check at the beginning (or ending) of each ECG strip for the machine calibration signal. The calibration test is shown on the strip in amplitude and in duration. Refer back to Figure 7-3 to review the amplitude settings. The earlier section explained how to manually set the gain control, which is the machine's calibration setting. In newer machines, the gain control is automatically set and self-adjusting so that the machine can actually recalibrate itself during the test if the ECG strip becomes unreadable due to tall waves or too small of waves. The technician may also readjust the calibration if waves are not being shown due to a lack of clarity on the strip (such as when a P wave seems to be absent, but after further review, at a higher calibration, the waves become visible).

Do not make the mistake of confusing the standardized speed with the calibrated amplitude signal. The normal amplitude setting is calibrated at 1 mV (or 10 mm), which is 2 large stacked squares or 10 small stacked squares, each being 1 large square or 5 small squares in duration. The calibration signal must be perfectly rectangular, and the standard is 10 mm high and 5 mm wide. The calibration limbs (vertical lines) should also be linear and form perfect 90° angles. If the speed of the ECG recording is adjusted to 50 mm/sec, the calibration symbol will change in width but not height, so the calibration symbol at 50 mm/sec is still 10 mm in height, but now it is 10 mm in width.

> Always document on the ECG test manually if you have changed the calibration or circle that the machine has recalibrated to a different calibration so it is not missed by the cardiologist.

Rewiring Error

On some older ECG machines, the lead wires may be replaceable. If your ambulatory care center uses this type of machine, and the leads have been recently replaced, always check the first time or two when you reuse the machine to see that the leads have been reconnected to the correct lead selector line into the ECG machine. Otherwise, the machine will be recording the wrong lead, but the leads will look like they are connected properly.

Technician Errors

Probably the most common technician error is attaching the leads incorrectly. Whether it is the reversal of the arm lead placements, arm-leg reversal, or reversal of the precordial leads, any of these common mistakes can lead to a misdiagnosis because leads that have been switched can mimic an infraction or other serious heart condition. Lead reversals can be spotted on an ECG by the trained observer, usually by the inversion of P waves. **Figure 7-36** shows a normal sinus rhythm ECG test from a multichannel ECG machine. This printout is what would be typically printed from most computerized ECG machines. While quickly scanning the ECG printout, notice the direction of the P and QRS waves. In all leads *except* aVR, aVL, V1, and V2, the P wave and QRS complex is upright (positive).

Recall that the direction and amplitude of the P wave represents atrial depolarization, and the QRS complex represents ventricular depolarization. Each lead recording will look slightly

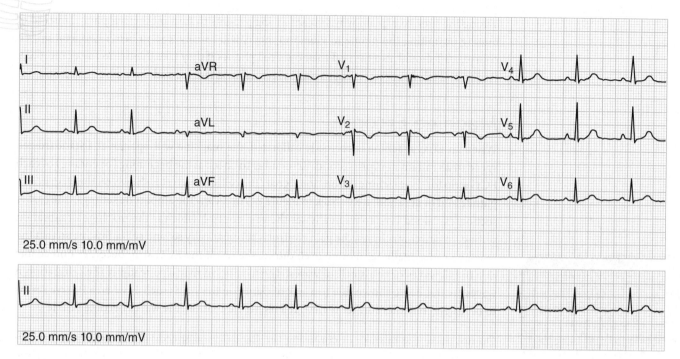

I   aVR   V₁   V₄

II   aVL   V₂   V₅

III   aVF   V₃   V₆

25.0 mm/s 10.0 mm/mV

II

25.0 mm/s 10.0 mm/mV

Figure 7-36 Normal ECG test

different because each lead is from a different view of the heart. It may be helpful to remember that the limb leads and augmented leads look at the heart from a vertical view, while the precordial leads look at the heart from a horizontal view. A "normal" ECG is not absolute—in other words, there can be many variations of a normal ECG even in healthy people. Common attributes of a normal ECG are identified in the following spotlight feature.

Common Normal Sinus Rhythm ECG Attributes

- There should be a P wave in front of every QRS complex. A missing P wave could indicate that the ECG is not a normal sinus rhythm.

- Amplitude in Lead I P waves should be smaller than the amplitude in Lead II P waves.

- Lead I will show opposite deflections from the aVR lead on the ECG because they are opposite in polarity.

- The P wave will be a small positive wave in Leads I and II if there is a normal sinus rhythm.

- Not every QRS complex will necessarily contain all three waves (Q, R, and S) in every lead.

- In the precordial leads (V1–V6), the R wave should get progressively larger in amplitude, while the S wave gets progressively smaller.

By recognizing these basic facts about the ECG recording, the technician can begin to understand what to look for when administering the ECG test.

Limb Lead Reversal Errors

The solution to all lead reversal errors is first, to recognize the error; second, to correct the error; and third, to re-administer the ECG test after the leads have been replaced correctly. The examples given in this section show how to pinpoint errors. In all the examples, the heart rate is 70 bpm and the corrected ECG should be a NSR. Additionally, in all examples, the pink striped arrow points to a reversed polarity or no polarity, and the green solid arrow points to waveform size differences from a NSR. One thing to remember when administering an ECG is to observe the patient. If the patient has a normal pulse and is in no apparent discomfort, and yet the ECG waveforms appear uncharacteristic, check the leads.

There are *many* variations to normal ECGs. These examples are designed to help students recognize that in Leads I, II, III, and aVF, the polarity of the P wave and QRS complex are normally positive, upward waveforms. The P wave and QRS complex in leads aVL and aVR are typically inverted, negative waveforms.

> ## Normal Sinus Rhythm Limb Lead Polarity
> Leads I, II, III, and aVF have positive polarity. Leads aVL and aVR have negative polarity.

Example One: Reversal of Left Arm and Right Arm Leads

Figure 7-37 shows an ECG with the arm leads reversed. The polarity in Lead I will be the opposite of normal, meaning that Lead I will show a negative deflection of the P waves and QRS complex. Also, notice the size difference in waveforms, which is most noticeable in leads aVR and aVL. To correct the problem, change the leads for the arms and administer a new ECG test.

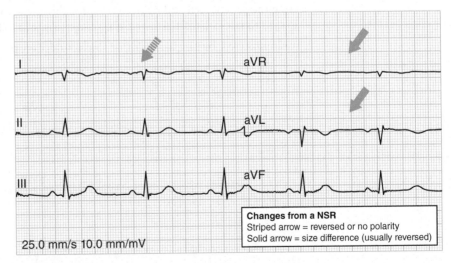

Figure 7-37 ECG showing reversal of arm leads

Example Two: Reversal of Left Arm and Left Leg Leads

Figure 7-38 shows the ECG with left arm and left leg reversal. The amplitude of the P waves in Leads I and II will be the opposite of normal, which means that in Lead I, the P waves will appear larger than in Lead II. Since the P wave is so small, sometimes it is easier to notice another common flaw in the ECG called a flat line. When the left arm and left leg lead is reversed, Leads I and II, and aVL and aVF, will show as opposites (in size). Additionally, reverse polarity changes are noted in Lead III, aVL, and aVF. To correct the problems shown in Figure 7-38, change the leads to the patient's left arm and left leg and repeat the ECG.

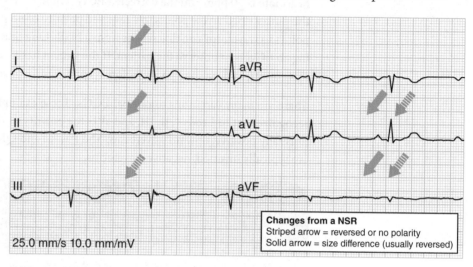

Figure 7-38 ECG showing reversal of left arm and left leg

Example Three: In Both Arms and Legs, Leads Are Reversed

Sometimes a difficult concept for the novice ECG student is that the ECG is being performed on another person, so don't make a beginner's mistake by attaching the limb leads to what looks like the left and right side to you (facing the patient), instead of the patient's actual left and right side! Study **Figure 7-39**. If you ever see an ECG with *all* the limb leads in reverse polarity, not using the patient's left and right sides is probably the culprit. All limb leads need the leads reapplied to the patient's left arm, left leg, right arm and right leg, then the ECG test should be readministered. Be sure to check that all electrodes are placed in the correct positions!

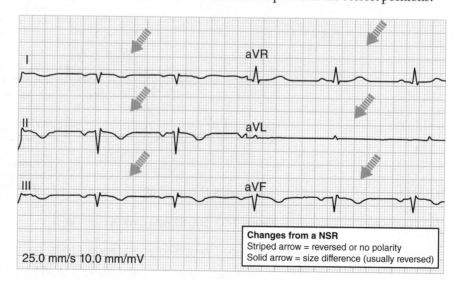

Figure 7-39 ECG showing reversal of all limb leads

Example Four: Reversal of Right Arm and Right Leg Leads

Since the right leg is the grounding electrode, placement can be anywhere on the body and no visible difference appears on the ECG tracing. What makes the ECG tracing in **Figure 7-40** noticeably different, though, is that Lead II shows up as an abnormal, almost flat line. When you see this pattern, check the right arm and right leg leads for potential reversal. Remove the leads and correctly replace them and readminister the ECG test.

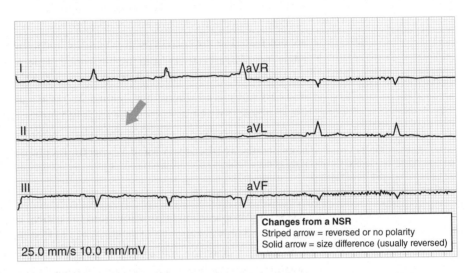

Figure 7-40 ECG showing right arm and right leg reversal

Example Five: Reversal of Left Arm and Right Leg Leads

Notice the similarity between Example Four (Figure 7-40) and Example Five (**Figure 7-41**). Example Four shows a nearly flat line in Lead II. The only difference in Example Five is that the nearly flat line is in Lead III. When Lead III is nearly flat, check for lead reversal between the left arm and the right leg. Remove these two leads and correctly replace them before readministering the ECG test.

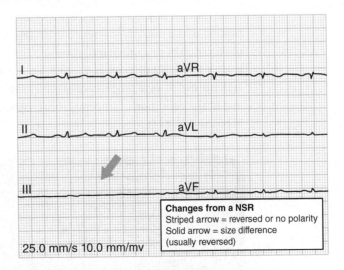

Figure 7-41 ECG showing reversal of left arm and right leg

Precordial Lead Errors

Recall that the precordial leads are V1–V6. There are two common types of errors in the precordial leads other than lead reversal. One error is the misplacement of the electrodes, and the other is rewiring the leads incorrectly.

Misplacement of Precordial Electrodes

Precordial electrodes can be placed too high, too low, or too close to each other. Additionally, if the electrodes are not attached to the skin so that they adhere properly or they are not placed in the correct position on the body, then the precordial leads cannot accurately record heart activity from the horizontal plane. Misplacement of the electrodes is the most common error occurring with the precordial leads. Obesity is the main reason that leads are not placed where they belong. To reduce obesity-related misplacement, always use anatomical markings, such as the angle of Louis and the medial left clavicle, to place the electrodes correctly. Another anatomy-related error occurs with female patients who have large breasts. To place the V4 and V5 electrodes properly, both should be placed under the breast fold.

If the electrodes do not properly adhere to the skin due to chest hair, shaving the area may be necessary. Always obtain permission from the patient or patient representative before shaving hair, and only cut enough of an area away so that the electrode can adhere firmly. There is no need to shave the entire chest or large sections of the chest. Finally, if the patient is sweating, wash the area where the electrodes need to be placed with alcohol, and then allow the area to dry before attaching the electrodes to obtain maximum adhesion.

normal wave progression
A concept associated with comparison of the precordial views of the ECG; V1–V6 show an amplitude change in each precordial lead, with V1 showing a small R wave and a large S wave progressing through V6, which shows a large R wave and a small S wave.

Normal wave progression is a concept associated with comparison of the precordial views of the ECG. In normal wave progression, when observing the precordial leads V1 through V6, lead V1 should consist of a small R wave and a large S wave, and the waves change in amplitude to where in lead V5, the R wave is large (has increased in amplitude) and the S wave is now small (decreased in amplitude in comparison to the R wave). Since V3 and V4 are approximately halfway between leads V1 and V6, the QRS complex deflections would be closest to the isoelectric line, which is especially noticeable in lead V3 in the sample ECG. There should be a smooth transition between each precordial lead in wave progression. The best way to observe if a precordial lead has been reversed is when you see an interruption of the smooth progression. Understanding normal wave progression will aid in the observation of precordial lead reversal. The most common reversal of precordial leads is in leads V1 with V2 or in leads V1 with V6. Look back at Figure 7-36 for what a normal ECG with normal R wave progression would look like. Remember that there are many variations that fit the definition of a normal sinus rhythm. The next two examples show lead reversals in precordial leads.

Normal Sinus Rhythm Precordial Lead Polarity

Precordial leads V3, V4, V5, and V6 show positive polarity. Leads V1 and V2 have negative polarity.

Example Six: Reversal of V1 and V6

Examine **Figure 7-42**. Reversal of the precordial leads V1 and V6 will show as reversed polarity in the two leads. They are also reversed in the expected size; V1 should be inverted and have a smaller R than that found in lead V6.

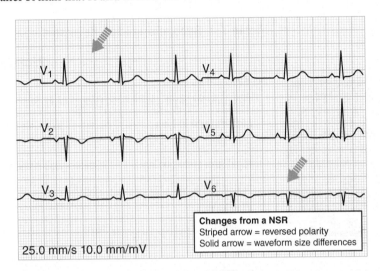

Figure 7-42 ECG showing reversal of V1 and V6

Example Seven: Reversal of V1 and V2

In **Figure 7-43**, the only difference between a normal sinus wave and the reversal of leads V1 and V2 occurs in the amplitude of the waves on V1 and V2. This makes this error much harder to detect. V1 should have the smallest amplitude among the precordial leads because it should be located on the right side of the chest. Notice that in the reversal, V2 shows the smaller waves. Polarity is not affected by the lead reversal.

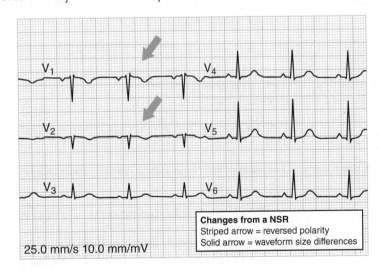

Figure 7-43 ECG showing reversal of V1 and V2

Review of Human Error Artifacts

A review of human errors due to lead reversals and how to correct these errors is presented in **Table 7-1**. The first column shows the error created by reversing the leads identified. The second column identifies which leads (if any) will show a reversed polarity or no polarity. Remember that no polarity equates to a straight line along the isoelectric line. The third column identifies waveform changes. These changes are often showing amplitude reversal changes or when there is no polarity, the waveform appears as a straight line.

Table 7-1 Recognizing Lead Reversals

	PROBLEM	
Reversal of:	Polarity	Waveform Size Differences
Left arm and right arm	Lead I—reversed	Leads aVR and aVL
Left arm and left leg	Lead III, aVL, aVF—reversed	Leads I and II, aVL and aVF
Both arms and both legs	All limb leads—reversed	N/A
Right arm and right leg	Lead II—NO polarity	Lead II—Flat line
Left arm and right leg	Lead III—NO polarity	Lead III—Flat line
V1 and V6	V1 and V6—reversed	V1 and V6
V1 and V2	N/A	V1 and V2

Always strive for accuracy when completing an ECG test. If you recognize an error, always correct it.

Quick Check 7-7

Fill in the blanks.

1. Artifacts that appear on the ECG tracing are not created by the _____ movement and will require the ECG technician to _____ the test.

2. ECG machines that are correctly _____ will show a symbol providing the amplitude and _____ on the ECG tracing.

3. The most common _____ error is attaching an incorrect _____ to a correctly placed electrode.

4. Using anatomical landmarks such as the _____ and the medial left clavicle will aid in correct placement of precordial electrodes.

5. In normal wave progression, correctly placed precordial leads will show a change in _____ in the R and S waves.

Patient Movement Errors

Patient cooperation is necessary for a good test. The technician should instruct the patient not to carry on a conversation while the test is going on, try to remain still, and to breathe normally during the test. However, not every patient will be able to cooperate fully by being still while the ECG test is being administered. Some diseases cause uncontrolled involuntary movements. A **somatic tremor** is muscle movement (either voluntary or involuntary) that shows up on an ECG as an artifact. In some cases, such as if the patient has Parkinson's disease, it is not easy to stay completely still. Another cause of a wandering baseline can be

somatic tremor
A muscle movement that shows up on an ECG as an artifact.

from patient respirations. Usually, this type of artifact can be reduced, but not eliminated. This section describes how to maximize the ECG output when there are uncontrollable muscle movements.

Patient instructions should include:

- No talking during the ECG test.
- Be as still as possible.
- Breathe normally.

Shivering and Patient Movement

This type of artifact may seem like common sense, but shivering can often be controlled by calming the patient down and providing a warm blanket to cover the patient. Patients can also cause muscle movement by moving their limbs, and even moving their fingers. Speaking to the patient in a calming voice and requesting that the person be as still as possible may help. **Figure 7-44**(a) shows an ECG with a somatic tremor. Notice the jagged erratic spikes. In comparison to an electrical artifact [Figure 7-44 (b)], notice that electrical interference shows small, regular spikes.

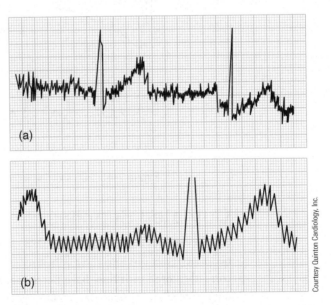

Figure 7-44 (a) ECG showing somatic tremor (b) ECG showing electrical interference

Parkinson's Disease

A patient with Parkinson's disease may have little control over muscle movement, but there are some things that the technician can do to help reduce artifacts. First, place the patient's hands under the buttocks. Second, change the limb electrodes to the hips and shoulders rather than the arms and legs. Third, place pillows under the head and knees. Be sure to explain to the patient why you are taking these extra steps to prepare for the ECG.

Wandering Baseline

If a patient moves while the electrodes are in place, the person may become tangled in the leads and cause the electrodes to lose good contact. If this happens, the electrodes will need to be replaced. A wandering baseline can also be caused by dangling cables. Be sure that the cables are not swaying or dangling from the bed. **Figure 7-45** shows an ECG with a wandering baseline.

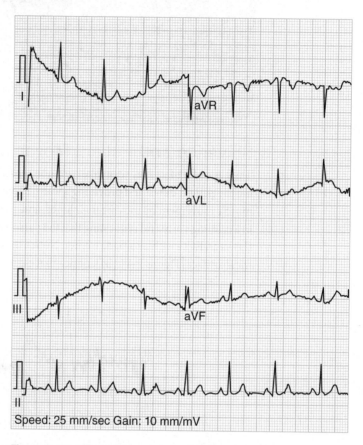

Figure 7-45 ECG showing wandering baseline

Outdated Supplies

Supplies such as electrodes should always be kept correctly stored and used in a timely manner. Electrodes can lose their adhesiveness even when not outdated if they have not been correctly stored or if they have been opened and not used quickly. Electrodes come vacuum-packed and should stay vacuum-packed until just before being used. Electrodes that lose the ability to provide good contact may cause artifacts. The technician should always check that electrodes are firmly attached on all leads and replace any electrode that will not stay adhered to the skin for the duration of the test. Loose electrodes can cause a wandering baseline, so if the baseline wanders, checking electrodes for good adhesion would be a first step to take.

Notable Patient Circumstances

Some patients will present with circumstances that merit special consideration by the ECG technician. Three of these types of situations are noted next.

Respiratory Distress Patients

Patients will not be as cooperative if they feel that their breathing will become more labored due to lying down for an ECG. The two options you have are to allow a patient to be in a sitting position and complete the ECG or place the limb leads on the shoulders and hips. If you administer the ECG while the patient is in the sitting position, document this fact as a comment on the ECG.

Sometimes patients equate holding still as the need to hold their breath. Be sure to instruct all patients to breathe normally during the procedure. If a patient takes a deep inspiration during the test, there is a possibility that Lead III may not show the small Q waves or inverted T waves.

Psychiatric Patients

A psychiatric patient may appear to be very anxious. The technician will want to take extra care to use a calming voice and smooth, quiet movements as they attach the electrodes. Reassure the patient that the test is painless and will be completed within a few minutes. Ask for the patient's cooperation during the test. Explain every detail, but do not use the term "electro" or "ECG" because those terms may be confused with electroconvulsive therapy (ECT), which is shock therapy.

Incarcerated Patients

Under the U.S. Constitution, all people being held against their will are entitled to receive free necessary medical care. Often, that care is given from within the local community. If your facility is located in an area in close proximity to a prison or jail, you may encounter an incarcerated patient that needs an ECG. Many times, an incarcerated patient will arrive in handcuffs, and some will also have leg shackles; and he or she will always be escorted by law enforcement. If your facility does not have an established protocol for providing care to an incarcerated patient, it is a common procedure to separate the incarcerated patient from the general population in waiting rooms by taking the person into an exam room and administering the exam as soon as possible. Law enforcement that accompanies the patient will normally not allow him or her to be left in an exam room alone. Treat incarcerated patients with the same dignity and respect as other patients, but also be aware that they may want to escape. Metal handcuffs and leg shackles cannot be left on while the ECG is being performed, but the plastic ties often used today can be applied by law enforcement if the patient needs to be restrained. To prevent artifacts, law enforcement officers will usually wait outside the door while the actual ECG is being performed because they may have a gun, taser, radio, cell phone, handcuffs, and numerous other items that can cause artifacts, attached to their body.

Female Patient Considerations

The most common three scenarios that the ECG technician needs to consider with female patients include bilateral breast implants, left breast mastectomies, and large breasts. Each scenario has a unique solution that will allow the ECG technician to obtain an accurate, clean ECG. With breast implants, always document any changes you make to lead placements due to this situation. The most common solution for a recent breast implant patient is to adjust the precordial leads V1 and V2 placed at the second or third intercostal space and complete the ECG as normal. Do not place the electrodes on the patient's breasts. The documentation of lead modification location should be written on the ECG test. Some computer ECG programs will allow the technician to document directly into the program. A patient who has previously undergone a radical mastectomy will have an ECG completed with the electrodes placed in the same positions and proper technique used in male patients. Remember that it is important to document that the patient has had a mastectomy and which breast has been removed. Be careful in placing the electrodes because the skin may be fragile or thin. Finally, special consideration is given to the patient with large breasts. Most important, be sure that the patient has removed her bra. The bra should not be on during a 12-lead ECG. Request assistance from the patient to hold the left breast up with her right hand so that the electrodes will firmly attach. She should hold the breast up the entire time the machine is running the test (less than 1 minute). Be sure to use the standard landmarks (V4 at the midclavicular line), and complete and record the test appropriately if any modifications have been made.

Review of Correctable Artifacts

The following spotlight feature lists artifacts that can be corrected, controlled, or reduced, which will therefore provide for a clean ECG.

Suggestions for Correcting Artifacts

- Reduce patient movement.
- Keep the patient comfortable and warm.
- Use new, current-dated electrodes.
- Be sure electrodes are securely fastened to the body.
- Explain to patients that they should breathe normally.
- Use a calming voice when speaking to patients.
- Turn off fluorescent lighting, and use indirect lighting or lamps.
- Turn off cell phones.
- Turn off radios, televisions, and other unnecessary electrical equipment.

Quick Check 7-8

Fill in the blanks.

1. Another term for muscle movement artifacts is a(n) _____.
2. Sometimes solutions to prevent muscle movements are as simple as speaking calmly to the patient and providing a(n) _____.
3. When electrodes lose good contact with the skin, they should be _____ so that the tracing does not show a(n) _____ baseline.
4. Electrodes may lose _____ if the _____ pack was opened days or weeks before the test.
5. If the ECG tracing looks normal except for Lead _____, the patient may be holding his or her _____.

Summary

- Time is measured along the horizontal axis of the ECG tracing in millimeters per second (mm/sec).

- Voltage is measured in duration along the vertical axis of the ECG tracing in millimeters (mm) or as millivolts (mV).

- Normal machine calibration is set to run at a standard speed of 25 mm/sec with an amplitude of 10 mm/mV. Machine calibration can be adjusted in order to better view the ECG strip by enlarging the waveform by increasing the speed of 50 mm/sec with an amplitude of 20 mm. The calibration can also be adjusted to half-height if the waves are too large for the strip.

- Three different electrical events occur during a cardiac cycle. No electrical activity is called the isoelectric or baseline, and this appears as a flat line on the strip. An upward or positive movement away from the isoelectric line is caused by electrical current flowing toward the positive pole of a limb lead. A negative deflection from the isoelectric line is caused by electrical current flowing away from the positive pole of a limb lead.

- The ECG waveform consists of graphic images of waves named P, Q, R, S, T, and U.

- Individual waves combine to create intervals, segments, and the QRS complex to signify the cardiac cycle of atrial and ventricular depolarization to repolarization. An interval is a period of time between two waves that completes an event, whereas a segment is a period of time with no electrical activity.

- In order to interpret an ECG, three waveform characteristics need to be understood including morphology, activity, and duration. Waveform morphology refers to the size and configuration of waves during each cardiac cycle. Activity refers to the actions of the waveforms. Duration involves recognizing variances from a normal sinus rhythm in either time or amplitude.

- Heart rate is calculated by measuring the distance between either the P-P or R-R intervals.

- To analyze an ECG tracing, record what is happening to P waves and the PR interval. Then calculate the R-R interval and heart rate. Finally, calculate the QRS complex.

- Interference on the ECG test is called an artifact.

- In normal wave progression, lead V1 should consist of a small R wave and a large S wave, and the waves change in amplitude to the point where in lead V5, the R wave is large (has increased in amplitude) and the S wave is now small (decreased in amplitude in comparison to the R wave).

- Lead reversal is the most common human error. Lead reversals require correct placement and retesting.

- Patients may need special consideration and sometimes electrode location modifications. When performing an ECG, modifications may be necessary for the following patients: patients with Parkinson's disease, incarcerated patients, patients in respiratory distress, psychiatric patients, and patients with breast implants, large breasts, or a mastectomy.

- Electrodes are packaged in vacuum packs and can cause artifacts if the technician does not use new electrodes and replace electrodes that will not remain adhered throughout the test.

Critical Thinking Challenges

7-1. Complete the following table. The completed table can then be used as a review guide.

	Normal Limits		
	Duration	**Amplitude**	
P Wave	_____	_____	
Q Wave	_____	_____	
T Wave	_____	Limb _____	
		Precordial _____	
QRS Complex	_____		
PR Interval	_____		
QT Interval	_____ (Males)		
	_____ (Females)		

7-2. On the following ECG tracings, first identify the rhythm as being either regular or irregular (circle one). Then classify the rhythm as being a bradycardia, tachycardia, or sinus rhythm (circle one). Finally, determine the ventricular heart rate. If the rhythm is irregular, compute the underlying rhythm range (for example 100-150 bpm).

1. Using the ECG strip in Figure 7-46, determine the following:

    A. Rhythm: Regular   Irregular

    B. Rhythm Classification: Bradycardia   Tachycardia   Sinus Rhythm

    C. Ventricular Heart Rate (or Range): _____ bpm

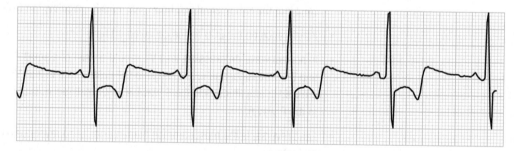

Figure 7-46

2. Using the ECG strip in Figure 7-47, determine the following:

    A. Rhythm: Regular   Irregular

    B. Rhythm Classification: Bradycardia   Tachycardia   Sinus Rhythm

    C. Ventricular Heart Rate (or Range): _____ bpm

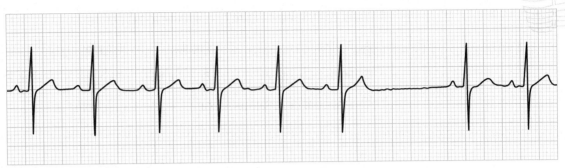

Figure 7-47

3. Using the ECG strip in Figure 7-48, determine the following:

   A. Rhythm: Regular   Irregular

   B. Rhythm Classification: Bradycardia   Tachycardia   Sinus Rhythm

   C. Ventricular Heart Rate (or Range): _____ bpm

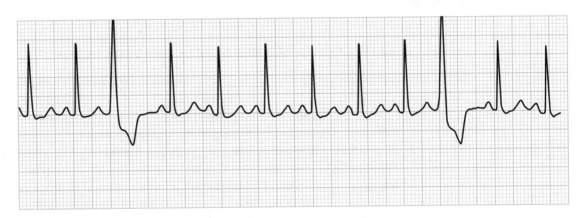

Figure 7-48

4. Using the ECG strip in Figure 7-49, determine the following:

   A. Rhythm: Regular   Irregular

   B. Rhythm Classification: Bradycardia   Tachycardia   Sinus Rhythm

   C. Ventricular Heart Rate (or Range): _____ bpm

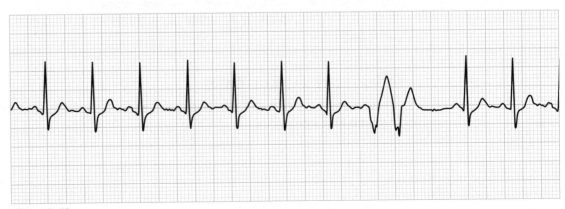

Figure 7-49

5. Using the ECG strip in Figure 7-50, determine the following:

   A. Rhythm: Regular   Irregular

   B. Rhythm Classification: Bradycardia   Tachycardia   Sinus Rhythm

   C. Ventricular Heart Rate (or Range): _____ bpm

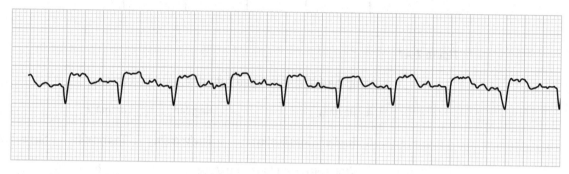

Figure 7-50

7-3. Fill in the blanks to this essay to create a review guide on artifacts.

Artifacts are wave length _____ found on an ECG tracing. Causes for artifacts usually originate from _____ interference, _____ or machine errors, or patient _____. Artifacts are not created by the _____. A sawtoothed pattern that is determined to be a regularly appearing artifact is usually indicative of _____ interference. Other forms of interference include _____ lighting, or _____ phones. Machine errors causing waveforms to be too tall or too small can be corrected by adjusting the _____ knob from the standard amplitude setting of 10 mm at the duration of _____ a second. The _____ symbol should always be _____ and come to perfect 90° angles. Attaching electrodes or _____ incorrectly is probably the most common _____ error. Limb lead reversal errors cause a change in _____. Always be sure to use the _____ right and left side when attaching the electrodes. _____ electrode placement may require shaving the patients' chest. In non-emergency situations, always obtain _____ consent before shaving the hair. Somatic _____ movement is a type of artifact that cannot always be controlled or _____. When completing an ECG on a female patient, bilateral breast _____, a left breast _____, and _____ breasts may require special considerations in the placement of electrodes or leads, or additional help by the patient. Be sure to always use _____ landmarks and complete and record the test appropriately if any modifications have been made.

Review Activities

7-1. For each wave, describe the morphology. In the second column, explain the part of the cardiac cycle the wave represents.

Wave	Normal Morphology	Representation in Cardiac Cycle
P Wave	_____	_____
Q Wave	_____	_____
R Wave	_____	_____
S Wave	_____	_____
T Wave	_____	_____

7-2. Label Figure 7-51 without referring back to the chapter.

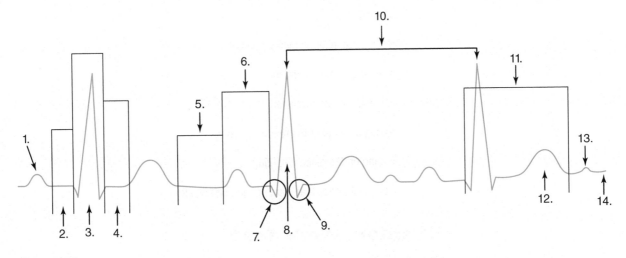

Figure 7-51

1. _____

2. _____

3. _____

4. _____

5. _____

6. _____

7. _____

8. _____

9. _____

10. _____

11. _____

12. _____

13. _____

14. _____

15. How many cardiac cycles are in Figure 7-51? _____

7-3. Matching: Using a letter from A to D, choose the artifact that best matches the error or error correction below. Some artifacts may be used more than once.

Artifacts:

A. outside interference   B. technician error

C. machine error   D. patient movement

Errors or Corrections:

1. _____ offering the patient a warm blanket

2. _____ speaking calmly to patient

3. _____ waveform is off the paper

4. _____ asking the patient to breathe normally

5. _____ turning off fluorescent lighting

6. _____ using electrodes that were opened last week

Chapter Seven Test

Fill in the blanks.

1. The standard ECG tracing is recorded at a preset speed of _____.

2. Heart rate is calculated on an ECG using the _____ axis.

3. _____ measures the strength or magnitude of the action potential.

4. If the ECG is not centered on the tracing, adjusting the _____ and documenting this on the tracing will enhance interpretation.

5. A(n) _____ identifies electrical activity on an ECG strip.

6. The _____ is a measurement between two cardiac cycles.

7. Computer ECG strips are recorded in either _____ or _____ seconds.

8. No electrical activity occurring in the heart is recorded as a(n) _____ on the ECG.

9. A(n) _____ is occurring after a P wave when there is no electrical activity shown on the ECG.

10. When determining heart rhythm, _____ are impulses that originate ventricularly instead of from the atria.

11. Heart rate is recorded in beats _____.

12. Another term for baseline is _____ line.

13. During a period of absolute refractory, there is no _____, so cells will not respond to stimuli.

14. Duration can be measured using a tool called _____.

15. The ventricular relaxation phase that is represented by the T wave is also called

_____.

Chapter Seven Quick Check Answers

Answer order is important except where noted otherwise (shown in parentheses).

When two correct answers are possible, both answers are given separated by the word "or."

7-1:
1. time, strength
2. second
3. 50, 250
4. 0.28, 0.3
5. 0.1, 1.5

7-2:
1. isoelectric, electrical
2. upward, downward (either order)
3. positive, negative
4. repolarization, 0.08
5. morphology, duration

7-3:
1. P, R, T (any order)
2. R, S (either order)
3. T
4. Q, negative
5. R, S (either order)

7-4:
1. R-R
2. origin, 0.06
3. segment, waves
4. electrical current, ventricular
5. depolarization, PR

7-5:
1. bradycardia, 53 bpm
2. normal, 75 bpm

3. tachycardia, 139 bpm

4. normal, 96 bpm

5. bradycardia, 44 bpm

7-6:

1. regular, 140 bpm

2. irregular, 70 bpm

3. regular, 35 bpm

4. regular, 72 bpm

5. irregular, 96 bpm

7-7:

1. heart's, re-administer

2. calibrated, duration

3. technician, lead

4. angle of Louis

5. amplitude

7-8:

1. somatic tremor

2. warm blanket

3. replaced, wandering

4. adhesiveness, vacuum

5. III, breath

8

RECOGNIZING ARRHYTHMIAS, PACEMAKERS, AND EMERGENCIES

OBJECTIVES

After reading the chapter and completing all Quick Check activities, the student should be able to:

1. Identify four major classifications of arrhythmias.

2. List four atrial arrhythmias.

3. Contrast a premature junctional complex to an accelerated junctional rhythm.

4. Identify the primary difference in the QRS complex between ventricular tachycardia and ventricular fibrillation.

5. Explain similarities between pulseless electrical activity and asystole.

6. Locate atrial and ventricular pacemaker spikes on an ECG tracing.

7. Describe three primary components of a synchronous pacemaker and an implantable cardioverter defibrillator.

8. Explain three pacemaker malfunctions.

9. Define the three stages of an acute myocardial infarction (AMI).

10. List emergency cardiac medications.

KEY TERMS

ablation

accelerated junctional rhythm

acute

agonal

asynchronous pacemaker

atrial arrhythmias

atrial fibrillation (A-Fib)

atrial flutter

atrial tachycardia

cardiac compromise

cardioversion

compensatory pause

crash cart

ectopic beat

electrophysiology studies (EPS)

escape beat

idioventricular rhythm (IVR)

implantable cardioverter defibrillator (ICD)

intrinsic rhythm

ischemia

junctional arrhythmias

junctional rhythm

junctional tachycardia

loss of capture

myocardial infarction (MI)

necrosis

P prime (P′)

pace

pacemaker

pacemaker spikes

pacing electrode

pathological Q wave

polymorphic

premature junctional complex (PJC)

pulseless electrical activity (PEA)

reflective lead

retrograde

sinus arrhythmia

sudden cardiac arrest

supraventricular arrhythmias

supraventricular tachycardia (SVT)

synchronous pacemaker

terminal rhythm

transcutaneous pacemaker (TCP)

underlying rhythm

ventricular asystole

ventricular fibrillation (V-Fib)

ventricular tachycardia (V-Tach)

INTRODUCTION

Chapter 8 is the capstone chapter in this book. All the previous chapters have explained the processes, provided explanations to what is normal, and examined common variances to normal. This chapter discusses how to detect abnormal waveforms, pacemakers, and emergency situations. When the disease process or accidents and injury affect the heart, a patient's life may be compromised. Although the electrocardiogram (ECG) technician is not normally the cause of the events that brings a patient to a life-threatening situation, fast corrective action by an observant and well-trained technician may make the difference of survival for the patient. Remember to always consider patient symptoms, such as chest pain, shortness of breath (SOB), fatigue, dizziness, or a rapid heartbeat in correlation to the rhythms observed on the ECG test. The purpose of this chapter is to recognize waveform changes, not to diagnose cardiac conditions.

This chapter begins with an introduction to major arrhythmias and is followed by an introduction to recognizing pacemaker spikes on the ECG tracing. The chapter uses numbered boxes to identify the rules for each arrhythmia and to quickly identify variances from a sinus rhythm. The next section of the chapter will describe waveform variances that may be caused by ischemia, injury, or infarctions. Also included in the final section will be an introduction to responding to cardiac emergencies.

INTRODUCTION TO ARRHYTHMIAS

An occasional arrhythmia occurs in almost everyone at some point in their life, and becomes more common with age, especially in people over age 60. Many of the arrhythmias are harmless, but all arrhythmias should be taken seriously until they have been diagnosed differently. Recall from Chapter 4 that an arrhythmia is an abnormal heartbeat that causes a disturbance in rhythm by altering the time, quality, force, or sequence of a waveform. A person may describe an arrhythmia as a "skipped beat," "palpitations," or "pounding in the chest," or a person may have no symptoms at all. Arrhythmias can occur after consuming too much caffeine, decongestant cold medications, drugs such as cocaine, smoking cigarettes, or they may have no known cause. A small group of people may have inherited an electrical conduction defect that may cause more severe arrhythmias, have other congenital heart defects leading to arrhythmias, or have other underlying health conditions that predispose them to arrhythmias. Many arrhythmias, especially the occasional arrhythmia, can be difficult to diagnose, but many health conditions such as uncontrolled hypertension, uncontrolled diabetes, sleep apnea, injury, or an overactive or underactive thyroid gland are all risk factors that increase the likelihood of arrhythmias occurring. Strong emotional stress or anger, lifestyle, smoking, and obesity are risk factors that people can try to control to reduce arrhythmias. Drug toxicity such as digoxin toxicity and amphetamines may also cause arrhythmias. Health care professionals can order many tests, which, when the results are combined, can lead to the diagnoses of an arrhythmia. Some of the tests include a stress test, holter and event monitoring, lipid profile blood tests, echocardiogram, chest x-ray, and the ECG.

Many entire ECG books are devoted to arrhythmias, but this text is designed to introduce the student to only the four major classifications of arrhythmias and the most common variations within each major category. The rules presented apply to the view of Lead II on the ECG because Lead II is the best lead for determining normal heart rhythm. The traditional format of an ECG test displays 2.5 seconds of each of the 12 leads in what is called a 4 x 3 view, with a rhythm strip of Lead II along the bottom of the page. Although arrhythmias should be recognized by the ECG technician, remember that the ECG technician does not have a license to practice medicine, so the ECG technician should not be explaining arrhythmias to patients without specific guidelines from the practitioner with a license, for whom the patient sought care.

The four major classifications of arrhythmias include sinus, atrial, junctional, and ventricular arrhythmias. A box at the end of each arrhythmia contrasts the normal sinus rhythm (NSR) to the changes found in each arrhythmia, so that variances from normal can be seen.

Sinus Arrhythmias

sinus arrhythmia
An electrical impulse that begins in the SA node and changes the heart rate with a person's respirations.

This text has previously discussed two of the rhythms found that originate in the sinoatrial (SA) node, which (as indicated in Chapter 3) is the heart's primary pacemaker. These normal rhythms were sinus bradycardia (normally regular, but a slow rhythm) and sinus tachycardia (normally regular, but a fast rhythm). A **sinus arrhythmia** refers to an electrical impulse that originates in the SA node; however, the rate changes with a person's respirations, and therefore the R-to-R interval changes. The P wave will be uniform in shape and will have a positive deflection (be upright). All the other rules for a normal sinus rhythm remain the same, as shown in Box 8-1.

> **Box 8-1** Sinus Arrhythmia Rules
>
> - P wave is uniform before every QRS complex.
> - *R-R intervals are irregular.*
> - Heart rate is 60–100 beats per minute.
> - PRI is between 0.12 and 0.20 seconds.
> - QRS complex is less than 0.12 seconds.
>
> (changes from a NSR are shown in italics)

Atrial Arrhythmias

atrial arrhythmias
The atrioventricular (AV) node overrides the sinoatrial (SA) node impulses, and the AV node becomes the heart's pacemaker.

In **atrial arrhythmias**, the atrioventricular (AV) node overrides the sinoatrial (SA) node impulses and the AV node becomes the heart's pacemaker. Recall that this means that the AV node initiates depolarization because the atrial impulses originated outside the SA node. This is sometimes caused by irritability, which causes the beat to come early, and sometimes is caused by escape beats, which causes the beat to come late and are identified by a prolonged R-R interval. The P waves can appear as being flattened, notched, spiked, biphasic, fluttered, or fibrillated (see Figure 7-5 in the last chapter), or hidden behind the T wave. When the heartbeat originates outside the SA node, it is called an **ectopic beat**. An ectopic beat can occur just once, it can be several beats, or it can continue throughout the entire rhythm. In atrial arrhythmias, the most notable change on the ECG occurs with the P wave. Left untreated, some atrial arrhythmias can cause blood clots to form in the heart. The treatment for controlling atrial arrhythmias is to first control the heart rate, then use of anticoagulation therapy to return the atria to a sinus rhythm. This section describes four atrial arrhythmias including atrial tachycardia, premature atrial complex (PAC), atrial flutter, and atrial fibrillation (A-Fib).

Atrial Tachycardia

Earlier in this book, we learned that tachycardia is a heart rate over 100 beats per minute with a regular rhythm for more than three successive heartbeats. The primary difference between the sinus tachycardia and atrial tachycardia is found in the appearance of the P wave. The P wave of a normal (sinus) tachycardia is smooth and upright, but in **atrial tachycardia**, the P wave can present as being flattened or hidden behind the T wave. Atrial tachycardia heart rate is usually in the range of 150 to 250 beats per minute and with a regular rhythm. The conduction (PRI and QRS complex) should be within normal limits with atrial tachycardia. A noticeable apical or peripheral pulse rate is usually the only outward sign that a patient has atrial tachycardia. Some of the complications resulting from atrial tachycardia include the loss of atrial kick and a reduced cardiac output, which will cause organs and tissues to receive less oxygen-rich blood. The rules to remember for an atrial tachycardia are shown in Box 8-2.

> **Box 8-2 Atrial Tachycardia Rules**
>
> - *P waves are different from sinus P waves; they can be flattened, notched, or hidden.*
> - *R-R intervals are all regular.*
> - *Heart rate is more than 100 beats per minute, typically between 150 and 250 bpm.*
> - PRI is between 0.12 and 0.20 seconds.
> - QRS complex is less than 0.12 seconds.
>
> (changes from a NSR are shown in italics)

Premature Atrial Complex (PAC)

A premature atrial complex (PAC) occurs when there is an ectopic beat originating in the atria, which means the P wave in a PAC will have a different morphology than the sinus P wave. The P wave in a PAC may have characteristics of being flattened, notched, spiked, or hidden. PACs do not carry through the entire rhythm; they commonly appear as one ectopic beat among several normal beats. Because the P wave may come prematurely, the rhythm may appear to be irregular. When the rhythm appears irregular, first look for an **underlying rhythm**—that is, review the overall rhythm on the ECG without including the area that shows the abnormal ectopic beat, and try to determine if the rhythm is otherwise a normal rhythm. If the underlying rhythm is regular (normal), label the rhythm as regular, with the exception

ectopic beat
A heartbeat that originates outside the sinoatrial (SA) node.

atrial tachycardia
The atrioventricular (AV) node overrides the sinoatrial (SA) node impulses, and the AV node becomes the heart's pacemaker. Heart rate is over 100 beats per minute.

underlying rhythm
A review of an overall rhythm on the ECG when an abnormality is not included in the rhythm; for example, a review of the ECG without including an ectopic beat to see if it is otherwise a normal rhythm.

of the PACs. The conduction (PRI and QRS complex) should be within normal limits on a PAC. PACs commonly have no outward signs or symptoms and can occur frequently in a normal heart. If symptoms do occur, they may include dizziness, anxiety, or palpitations. In people who have been diagnosed with heart disease, PACs can lead to more serious arrhythmias such as atrial flutter or atrial fibrillation. Box 8-3 identifies the rules for PACs.

Box 8-3 Premature Atrial Complex Rules

- *P wave is usually premature and can be flattened, notched, spiked, or hidden.*
- *R-R intervals depend on the underlying rhythm, interrupted by PAC.*
- *Heart rate depends on the underlying rhythm.*
- PRI is between 0.12 and 0.20 seconds.
- QRS complex is less than 0.12 seconds.

(changes from a NSR are shown in italics)

Atrial Flutter

atrial flutter
The atria become very irritable due to a rapid reoccurring ectopic impulse, causing the heart to beat at 250–350 beats per minute.

A major change to heart rate occurs with **atrial flutter** because the atria become very irritable due to a rapid reoccurring ectopic impulse that creates a reentry circuit within the right atrium. The typical heart rate with atrial flutter falls between 200 and 350 beats per minute. The ECG will show this fluttering with numerous P waves, which makes the PR interval impossible to compute. Often, the term used for describing atrial flutter P waves is "sawtooth" flutter waves. **Figure 8-1** shows what sawtooth atrial flutter waves present as.

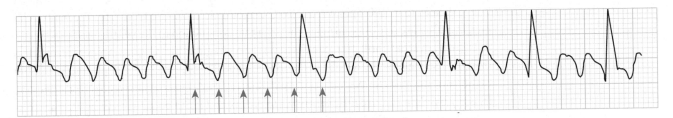

Figure 8-1 Atrial flutter sawtooth waves

Recall that the AV node is designed to naturally slow the wave of depolarization, which in turn causes a slower ventricular rate. Sometimes the impulse gets through to the ventricles more rapidly than not, and can cause ventricular conduction to be as high as 150 beats per minute. For beginners, it may be difficult to determine the difference between atrial tachycardia and atrial flutter. The difference can be noticed by observing the isoelectric line, which is absent in atrial flutter but usually present in atrial tachycardia. When viewing an ECG with atrial flutter, expect to see numerous P waves, but if the AV node is able to block many of these P waves, the QRS complex should remain normal (less than 0.12 seconds in duration) in appearance and in regularity, as shown in the R-R interval when the AV node conducts impulses through the continuing conduction path. Like atrial tachycardia, atrial flutter can cause a loss of atrial kick, which can cause blood left in the atria to create blood clots, which can lead to embolisms. Recall that the loss of atrial kick also decreases cardiac output. Unstable atrial flutter that is less than 48 hours old is an emergency rhythm

cardioversion
A process of using chemical (antiarrhythmic drugs) or timed electrical (shock) procedures to restore a normal sinus rhythm (NSR).

that may be addressed with cardioversion by a licensed professional. **Cardioversion** is a process of using chemical (antiarrhythmic drugs) or timed electrical (shock) procedures during depolarization to restore a normal sinus rhythm. Atrial flutter is often a condition found after cardiac surgery or may indicate other intrinsic health conditions including heart disease, or chronic liver or lung disease. Box 8-4 highlights the rules found in atrial flutter.

Box 8-4 Atrial Flutter Rules

- *P waves are numerous and fluttering.*

- *R-R intervals are usually regular; however, they can be irregular.*

- *Heart rate is 200–350 beats per minute.*

- *PRI cannot be computed.*

- QRS complex is less than 0.12 seconds.

(changes from a NSR are shown in italics)

Atrial Fibrillation (A-Fib)

atrial fibrillation (A-Fib)
Electrical impulses that are not regular, causing the heart to contract in a disorganized pattern.

A heart in **atrial fibrillation (A-Fib)** is depolarizing repeatedly in the atria, causing the heart to contract in a disorganized, chaotic manner. The P wave becomes very close to the isoelectric line, therefore considered nonexistent because it is too numerous to count. The morphology of the P wave is considered fibrillated much like useless twitching or very fast chaotic motions. The heart rate is greater than 350 beats per minute for the atrial rate but is much lower in the ventricles (normally under 100 beats per minute). However, if the ventricular rate is greater than 100 bpm, the major therapeutic goal will be to control the ventricular rate. Impulses are so disorganized in the atria that conduction to the ventricles varies greatly. This is why in atrial fibrillation, the rhythm is very irregular. The QRS complex measures less than 0.12 seconds wide, which is of a normal width; however, QRS complexes are seldom of the same duration for two consecutive R-R intervals. A-Fib is usually recognized easiest by its wavy baseline and irregular ventricular rhythm, and it can occur in both healthy and diseased hearts. In healthy individuals, emotional stress or excessive alcohol consumption can bring on temporary A-Fib. Symptoms of A-Fib may include dizziness or nausea. In people with inflammation, hypertension disease, coronary heart disease, or rheumatic heart disease, A-Fib can become a serious condition by further damaging the heart's electrical system and it may be a precursor to a person developing a CVA, **myocardial infarction (MI)**, embolisms, or a renal infarction. A myocardial infarction occurs when the coronary arteries are blocked, which prevents oxygenated blood from circulating in the heart. The heart tissue that loses oxygenated blood can cause permanent damage to the heart muscle tissue within minutes. Box 8-5 highlights the rules found in atrial fibrillation.

myocardial infarction (MI)
An occlusion of the coronary arteries that prevents oxygenated blood from circulating within the heart, causing permanent heart muscle tissue damage.

Box 8-5 Atrial Fibrillation Rules

- *There is no P wave.*

- *R-R intervals are irregular.*

Box 8-5 Continued

- *Atrial heart rate is greater than 350 bpm; ventricular heart rate is usually less than 100 bpm.*

- *PRI cannot be computed.*

- QRS complex is less than 0.12 seconds.

(changes from a NSR are shown in italics)

Quick Check 8-1

Fill in the blanks.

Review the rules for a normal sinus rhythm and the atrial arrhythmias. Then, using the ECG strips below, classify the rhythm and calculate the heart rate. (Be sure to recognize if the strip is a 6-second or 10-second ECG.)

1. Rhythm classification _____

  Heart rate _____ bpm

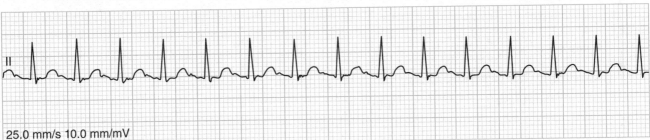

25.0 mm/s 10.0 mm/mV

Figure 8-2

2. Rhythm classification _____

  Heart rate _____ bpm

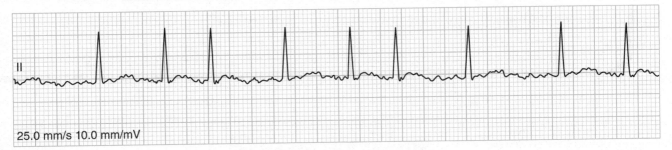

25.0 mm/s 10.0 mm/mV

Figure 8-3

(Continued)

(*Continued*)

3. Rhythm classification _____

     Heart rate _____ bpm

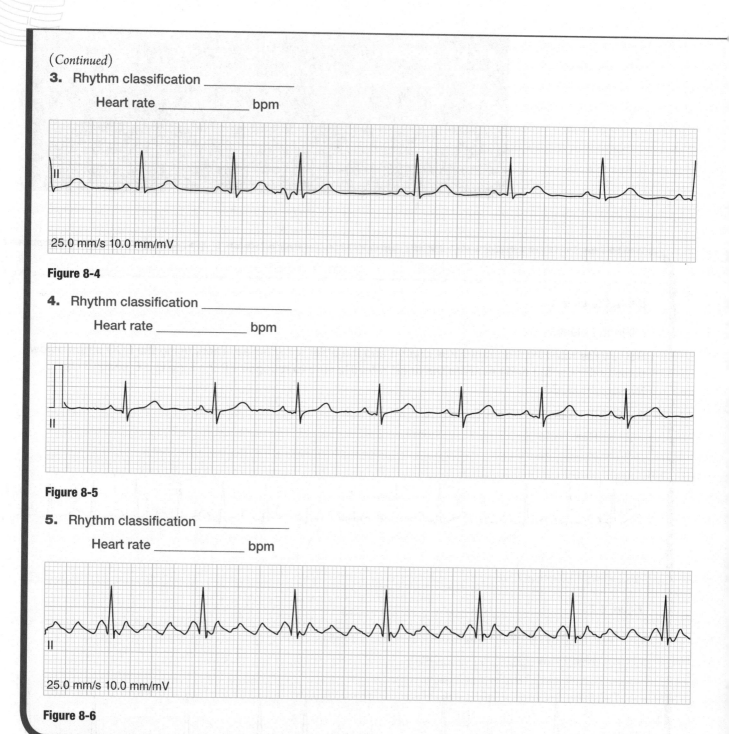

25.0 mm/s 10.0 mm/mV

Figure 8-4

4. Rhythm classification _____

     Heart rate _____ bpm

Figure 8-5

5. Rhythm classification _____

     Heart rate _____ bpm

25.0 mm/s 10.0 mm/mV

Figure 8-6

junctional arrhythmias
Instances that occur when the sinoatrial (SA) node either fails to conduct an impulse or there is a blockage of the impulse so the impulse originates in the atrioventricular (AV) node.

Junctional Arrhythmias

Junctional arrhythmias can occur when the SA node either fails to conduct an impulse or there is a blockage of the impulse within the AV node. The rhythm of junctional heart-beats can deliver the impulse before the ventricles are ready, or the impulse can originate

escape beat
A junctional beat that originates in the bundle of His, or a ventricular rhythm that takes over supraventricular pacing.

somewhere other than the SA node (ectopic beats); or the impulse can be an **escape beat**, which originates in the bundle of His. The escape beat comes after a delay of the cardiac cycle due to the origin of the impulse being from a junctional rhythm. Junctional escape rhythms can be identified on the ECG with a rate of 40–60 bpm. Like atrial arrhythmias, probable causes of junctional arrhythmias may include caffeine, smoking, alcohol, or drug induced by digitalis, electrolyte imbalances, or could be due to ischemic heart disease or hypoxia. A person may be asymptomatic with junctional arrhythmias, but if they do have symptoms, the symptoms may mimic a multitude of potential conditions because typical symptoms include dizziness, hypotension, or confusion due to low cardiac output. This section begins with an introduction of junctional rhythms and is followed by three common junctional arrhythmias, including junctional tachycardia, a premature junctional complex (PJC), and an accelerated junctional rhythm.

Junctional Rhythms

retrograde
An impulse that goes backward in the conduction path.

P prime (P′)
A term used to represent a P wave that originated from anywhere other than from the sinoatrial (SA) node.

Junctional rhythms originate in the area of the AV node and the bundle of His. From the SA node, the AV node is the next pacemaker, but in junctional rhythms, the impulse that originates in the junction may go back toward the atria to depolarize the atria. If an impulse goes backward, it is known as a **retrograde** impulse. When a retrograde impulse occurs, one ectopic impulse splits; half goes back into the atria and the other half of the impulse continues to the ventricles following normal conduction paths. This action can cause the ventricles to be depolarized before the atria. The P wave, written as **P′ (P prime)**, will also be inverted when the atria receive a retrograde impulse because the P wave did not receive the impulse from the SA node. The ECG of a junctional rhythm can show the P wave coming before or after, or being hidden by the QRS complex (therefore not appearing at all) in Lead II. **Figure 8-7** identifies the sinus P wave and possible P prime (P′) wave presentations.

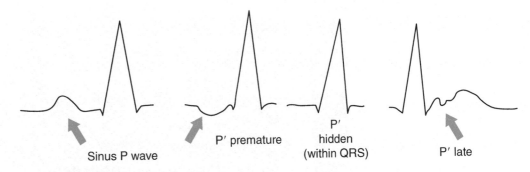

Sinus P wave   P′ premature   P′ hidden (within QRS)   P′ late

Figure 8-7 Possible P wave presentations

junctional rhythm
A pacemaker impulse created in the bundle of His.

Recall that the AV node is the backup pacemaker for the heart and the normal conduction of the AV node is 40–60 beats per minute. If the AV node is blocked, a pacemaker impulse can be created in the bundle of His and is called a **junctional rhythm**. Junctional rhythms have a normal QRS complex, so the rhythm will be normal, but notice the P′ wave activity. Junctional rhythms can easily be confused with atrial arrhythmias when atrial impulses include retrograde depolarization and inverted P waves. In these cases, the PR interval is used to determine the rhythm. Recall that a normal PR interval originates in the atria and is 0.12–0.20 seconds in duration. In a junctional rhythm, the PR interval will be less than 0.12 seconds because it originated in the AV junction and not in the atria. Box 8-6 identifies the rules for a junctional rhythm.

> ## Box 8-6 Junctional Rhythm Rules
>
> - *P' wave has a downward deflection and can appear before, within, or after each QRS complex, but the appearance is the same throughout Lead II.*
> - R-R intervals are regular.
> - *Heart rate is 40–60 beats per minute.*
> - *PRI is short (0.10 seconds or less) and visible only when P' comes before the QRS complex.*
> - QRS complex is less than 0.12 seconds.
>
> (changes from a NSR are shown in italics)

Junctional Tachycardia Rhythm

junctional tachycardia
A junctional rhythm with a rate of 100–140 beats per minute.

Junctional tachycardia occurs when the junctional rate is 100–180 beats per minute. Recall that because it is a junctional rhythm, the impulse occurs in the junctional area when the SA node either fails to conduct an impulse or there is a blockage of the impulse within the AV node. In junctional tachycardia, the rhythm is normal but the ventricular rate is over 100 beats per minute. Recall that the hallmark of junctional rhythms is the P', which provides a short PRI when the P' is before the QRS complex. Junctional tachycardia complications may include the loss of atrial kick and the possibility of compromising cardiac output. Patients may be asymptomatic but will normally observe heart palpitations or fluttering. Junctional tachycardia can be life threatening to patients who have had a recent MI or other cardiovascular event. Box 8-7 identifies the rules for junctional tachycardia rhythms.

> ## Box 8-7 Junctional Tachycardia Rhythm Rules
>
> - *P' wave has a downward deflection and can appear before, within, or after each QRS complex, but the appearance is the same throughout Lead II.*
> - R-R intervals are regular.
> - *Heart rate is greater than 100 beats per minute.*
> - *PRI is short (0.10 seconds or less) and visible only when P' comes before the QRS complex.*
> - QRS complex is less than 0.12 seconds.
>
> (changes from a NSR are shown in italics)

Premature Junctional Complex (PJC)

premature junctional complex (PJC)
Heart rhythm disturbances; occur when there is one or more ectopic beats originating in ventricles.

PJCs have many of the same characteristics as the PAC rhythms studied earlier. A **premature junctional complex (PJC)** occurs when a single ectopic beat originating in the AV junction begins a new cardiac cycle and creates what appears as an irregular rhythm. Like with a PAC, look for an underlying rhythm first. One hint that it is junctional in nature comes from the inverted P' wave, if it is present, but be aware that the PJC does not always have a retrograde impulse. If the P wave is a sinus P wave, it will be upright and the PRI will be consistent. When observing the ECG, record the PJC rate as that of the underlying rhythm. PJCs rarely provide signs or symptoms for the patient unless they experience hypotension due to numerous (more than 4–6) PJCs in 1 minute, which may indicate a more serious condition. The rules for PJCs are shown in Box 8-8.

Box 8-8 Premature Junctional Complex (PJC) Rules

- *If sinus P wave, PRI will be consistent.*

- *If there is a P wave, PRI is short (0.10 seconds or less) and visible only when P' comes before the QRS complex.*

- *P' wave appears prematurely, has a downward deflection, and can appear before, within, or after each QRS complex, but the appearance is the same throughout Lead II.*

- *R-R intervals depend on the underlying rhythm, interrupted by PJC.*

- Heart rate depends on the underlying rhythm.

- *Premature QRS complex, is less than 0.12 seconds.*

(changes from a NSR are shown in italics)

Accelerated Junctional Rhythm

accelerated junctional rhythm
A rhythm between 60 and 100 beats per minute; originates in atrioventricular (AV) junctional area and contains P' waves.

When thinking of the term accelerated, normally one might think of a tachycardia rhythm, but in an **accelerated junctional rhythm** the junctional rhythm is between 60 and 100 beats per minute. This is the ventricular rate, so coming from the AV junction area, this rate would be considered fast or accelerated because the normal AV node fires an impulse at 40–60 beats per minute. The rhythm is normal, so the accelerated junctional QRS complex would resemble the normal sinus rhythm QRS complex. As with other junctional rhythms, the P wave will show as P' (inverted), when it appears. Box 8-9 identifies the variances of the accelerated junctional rhythm in comparison to a normal sinus rhythm.

Box 8-9 Accelerated Junctional Rhythm Rules

- *Regular P wave may be present.*

- *P' wave, if present, has a downward deflection and can appear before, within, or after each QRS complex, but the appearance is the same throughout Lead II.*

- R-R intervals are regular.

- Heart rate is 60–100 beats per minute.

- *PRI is short (0.10 seconds or less) and visible only when P' comes before the QRS complex.*

- QRS complex is less than 0.12 seconds.

(changes from a NSR are shown in italics)

In addition to the P′ waveform, the major differences among junctional rhythms is directly related to the rate of each rhythm. The spotlight feature identifies the normal junctional rate and rates for the three common junctional arrhythmias, including junctional tachycardia, a PJC, and an accelerated junctional rhythm.

Junctional Rhythm Rates

Normal junctional rhythm rate is 40–60 beats per minute.

Accelerated junctional rhythm rate is 60–100 beats per minute.

Junctional tachycardia rhythm rate is 100–180 beats per minute.

Premature junctional complex rhythm rate is the rate of the underlying rhythm.

Quick Check 8-2

Review the rules for junctional rhythms and junctional arrhythmias. Then, using the ECG strips below, classify the rhythm and calculate the heart rate. (Be sure to recognize if the strip is a 6-second or 10-second ECG.)

1. Rhythm classification _____

   Heart rate _____ bpm

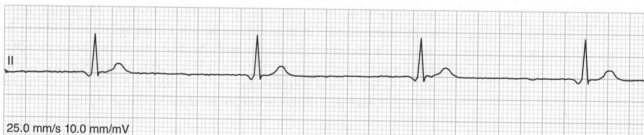

25.0 mm/s 10.0 mm/mV

Figure 8-8

2. Rhythm classification _____

   Heart rate _____ bpm

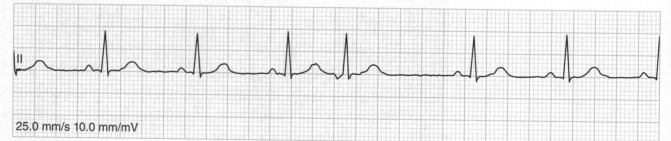

25.0 mm/s 10.0 mm/mV

Figure 8-9

(*Continued*)

3. Rhythm classification _____

Heart rate _____ bpm

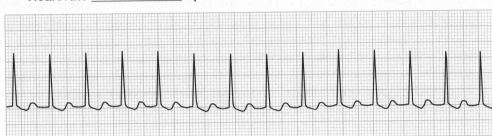

Figure 8-10

4. Rhythm classification _____

Heart rate _____ bpm

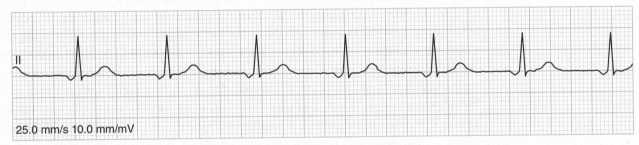

Figure 8-11

5. Rhythm classification _____

Heart rate _____ bpm

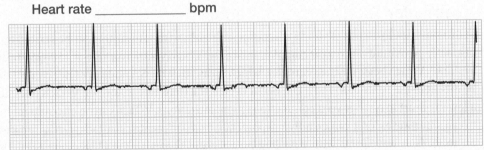

Figure 8-12

Ventricular Arrhythmias

Ventricular arrhythmias can be the deadliest of all arrhythmias because when the abnormal waveforms originate in the ventricles, it is an indication that the heart has run out of options to correct the problem with an impulse in the normal conduction path. Recall the SA node is the primary pacemaker. When it fails, the AV node can take over, which slows the heart rate, but the heart can still reasonably compensate for the SA node. If the SA and AV nodes

supraventricular arrhythmias
Arrhythmias that originate above the ventricles.

supraventricular tachycardia (SVT)
Occurs when the electrical system above the ventricles sends abnormal impulses that interfere with sinoatrial (SA) node impulses, creating a very fast heart rate that begins and ends suddenly.

are blocked, the bundle of His can generate the impulse and create a junctional impulse. All of the arrhythmias that occur above the ventricles are called **supraventricular arrhythmias**. When all supraventricular arrhythmias fail to continue to send the conduction impulse to the ventricles, the ventricles must work in retrograde from the bottom of the heart, which is not very efficient, to take over the heart's pacemaking role. **Supraventricular tachycardia (SVT)**, also called paroxysmal supraventricular tachycardia (PSVT), occurs when the electrical system above the ventricles sends abnormal impulses that interfere with SA node impulses, creating a very fast heart rate that begins and ends suddenly. SVT heart rates occur between 150 and 250 beats per minute and occur more commonly in infants, children, and young adults who are anxious or extremely fatigued. In addition to typical symptoms of a fast pulse, dizziness, and heart palpitations, SVT symptoms can also include shortness of breath (SOB) or syncope (fainting) and can cause complications for the patient if the abnormal impulses cause the ventricular heart rate to increase excessively.

A quick review of supraventricular waveforms will show that many of the arrhythmias will have a P wave, which, even if irregular, represents atrial depolarization, and a QRS complex, which represents ventricular depolarization. So far, all the rhythms and arrhythmias studied also show the QRS complex to be a relatively normal width of less than 0.12 seconds, which signified that when the impulse reached the ventricles, the heart had compensated for the irregular impulse and ventricular depolarization was normal. In ventricular arrhythmias, the QRS complex will always be 0.12 seconds or more because the impulse originated from the ventricles. Additionally, except for ventricular tachycardia, in the other ventricular arrhythmias, the P wave is nonexistent, so there is no atrial depolarization, no atrial contraction, and no atrial kick. The loss of these processes will result in a noticeable loss of cardiac output. This section covers six of the most common ventricular arrhythmias, including ventricular tachycardia, premature ventricular complex, ventricular fibrillation, idioventricular rhythm (IVR), pulseless electrical activity (PEA), and ventricular asystole. It is very important that the ECG technician save all rhythm tracings, especially when a patient has ventricular arrhythmias.

Ventricular Tachycardia (V-Tach)

ventricular tachycardia (V-Tach)
A high ventricular heart rate of 150–250 beats a minute.

Ventricular tachycardia (V-Tach) can occur suddenly, without warning, or be started by a distinctly premature ventricular complex and causes a high ventricular rate of 150–250 beats a minute. V-Tach begins in the ventricles, which means that the SA node does not control the heartbeat of the ventricles, and it can occur even if the sinus rate is normal. V-Tach does not allow the heart to rest between contractions (depolarization). V-Tach can be intermittent between sinus waves, or it can be polymorphic. **Polymorphic** ventricular tachycardia presents on an ECG as waveforms with changing polarity and shapes in the QRS complexes. The QRS complex will often appear as a sawtooth waveform when the ventricular rate is very high (250 beats or more), commonly called bizarre, but is still uniform and measurable. The amplitude of the QRS is usually increased and the duration of the QRS is unusually wide—greater than 0.12 seconds. Polarity in the T wave will be opposite of the QRS complex. The atrial rhythm and rate cannot usually be determined. When only ventricular tachycardia is shown on the ECG as the dominant rhythm, it should be described as sustained ventricular tachycardia. The rhythm is considered a dominant rhythm when three or more PVCs occur in a row or it lasts more than 30 seconds. Ventricular tachycardia is considered a very unstable rhythm that is usually a precursor to ventricular fibrillation or sudden cardiac death. Ventricular tachycardia does not allow the ventricles to fill with blood adequately,

polymorphic
Waveforms with changing polarity.

thus causing reduced cardiac output. If the ECG technician observes a V-Tach waveform on the ECG test, they should immediately obtain a licensed practitioner for emergency intervention because this rhythm cannot be sustained for very long and the patient may quickly become unresponsive. Unresponsive patients require initiation of an emergency protocol and cardiopulmonary resuscitation (CPR). Patients may require immediate resuscitation or synchronized cardioversion, if the patient is responsive and has a pulse. V-Tach has many documented causes such as coronary artery disease, myocardial ischemia, acute MI, congestive heart failure, and even electrolyte imbalances. Complications of V-Tach include ventricular fibrillation and asystole. Box 8-10 highlights the rules for ventricular tachycardia.

Box 8-10 Ventricular Tachycardia Rules

- *P waves are usually absent, but if present, they are calculated with underlying rhythm.*

- *R-R is calculated with underlying rhythm, and is usually regular.*

- *Ventricular heart rate is between 100 and 250 bpm.*

- *PRI usually cannot be calculated; if P is present, calculate it with underlying rhythm.*

- *QRS complex is wide (and usually bizarre), 0.12 seconds or more in duration, calculated with underlying rhythm, and can show as a sawtooth appearance.*

- *T wave, if shown, presents as opposite polarity from QRS complex.*

(changes from a NSR are shown in italics)

Premature Ventricular Complex (PVC)

Premature ventricular complexes (PVCs) are the most common ventricular arrhythmias and are caused by an early ectopic impulse within the ventricles. A normal heart can occasionally create a PVC; what makes the PVC significant is the number of occurrences that the patient experiences. The occurrences of PVCs are called "runs" or "episodes" and in serious cases, usually come before ventricular tachycardia or ventricular fibrillation. PVCs are typically named by their location. They can occur after a sinus P wave before a normal QRS complex, below the bundle of His, which extends depolarization resulting in wider QRS complexes that are often bizarre in shape, or between two consecutive sinus beats. PVCs that begin within the intraventricular conduction system are called narrow complex PVCs. PVCs present in many different morphologies and names, with many being identified by the number of ectopic occurrences on the ECG. The most dangerous patterns of PVCs include PVCs that occur more than six times in a minute, multifocal or multiform (each PVC is of a different morphology in the same lead), bigeminy and trigeminy (every other or every third beat is a PVC), and the R on T phenomenon (PVC occurs on the downward slope of the T wave). A PVC will normally show on an ECG as having a premature QRS complex, may have an underlying sinus rhythm, and the T wave may slope in the opposite direction of the ST segment and QRS complex. When a PVC comes early, a **compensatory pause** may be created. A compensatory pause can be found on an ECG between two QRS complexes showing a PVC and a duration twice the distance of other R-R intervals that do not have a PVC. There are many causes thought to create a PVC including hypertension, hypoxia, electrolyte imbalances, and myocardial ischemia, but these conditions can be

compensatory pause
On an ECG, the duration is twice the distance between two R-R intervals that have the underlying rhythm disturbance caused by a premature ventricular complex (PVC).

related to a multitude of diagnoses. The ECG is usually one of the diagnostic tools to confirm PVCs. The technician should be able to highlight any PVC, document any patterns, and determine the frequency of occurrences. The patient may be asymptomatic or may feel as though their heart is skipping beats, they also may have a weaker pulse after a PVC. Patients may complain of dizziness or syncope if they have a lowered cardiac output. If the patient complains of cardiac pain, the licensed practitioner will often order oxygen, nitroglycerin and morphine, and antiarrhythmic therapy. Box 8-11 shows the general rules for premature ventricular complexes.

Box 8-11 **Premature Ventricular Complex Rules**

- *P waves, unremarkable in sinus waves, are calculated with underlying rhythm.*

- *R-R, calculated with underlying rhythm, usually is regular.*

- *Ventricular heart rate is between 100 and 250 bpm.*

- *PRI usually cannot be calculated; if P is present, calculate with underlying rhythm.*

- *QRS complex is premature, wide (and usually bizarre), 0.12 seconds or more in duration, and calculated with underlying rhythm which has differing morphologies.*

- *T wave and ST segment present as the opposite polarity from an underlying QRS complex.*

(changes from a NSR are shown in italics)

Ventricular Fibrillation (V-Fib)

ventricular fibrillation (V-Fib)
Chaotic, indistinguishable waves caused by multiple ectopic and reentry patterns originating from many different areas in the ventricular walls.

terminal rhythm
A continuous rhythm that cannot reverse to a normal rhythm without medical intervention.

Ventricular fibrillation (V-Fib) is a **terminal rhythm**, meaning that V-Fib cannot reverse to a normal rhythm without intervention and it is continuous versus intermittent. V-Fib presents on the ECG as chaotic, indistinguishable waves caused by multiple ectopic and reentry paths originating from many different areas in the ventricle walls, and yet V-Tach has no recognizable rhythm or pattern. The arrhythmia is very serious because there is no cardiac output and no cardiac contraction, and the patient will not have a pulse. Since there is also no blood pressure, the person will lose consciousness within 30 seconds and are considered in full cardiac arrest. In V-Fib, the ventricles quiver and cannot contract to pump the blood out of the ventricles. V-Fib can begin without notice, or can follow V-Tach or PVCs. Imbalanced amounts of cardiac electrolytes (potassium, calcium, and magnesium), certain medications, and electrical injuries can cause V-Fib in hearts that are already weakened due to structural abnormalities, congenital heart disease, or after a severe MI. ECG technicians must be able to identify V-Fib, which is considered one of the easier ECG tracings to recognize because of the lack of distinguishable waveforms. Once a licensed clinician has confirmed V-Fib by checking other leads and pulses, and observing the patient, immediate CPR and defibrillation is necessary, which is why most people who are not in a hospital at the time of the occurrence do not survive. V-Fib can be mimicked by artifacts such as muscle tremors, patient movement, patient shivering, or can be caused by using old supplies such as dried electrodes. Always check for a pulse and consciousness, because if either exists, the condition is not V-Fib. Patients who are known to have a weakened heart can sometimes qualify (healthwise) for an implanted automatic defibrillator. Box 8-12 describes the rules for the waveforms found in ventricular fibrillation.

Box 8-12 Ventricular Fibrillation Rules

- *Waveforms are chaotic with no regularity.*
- *No distinguishable P wave.*
- *R-R intervals are not distinguishable and have no rhythm.*
- *No heart rate.*
- *No PRI interval.*
- *No distinguishable QRS complex.*

(changes from a NSR are shown in italics)

Idioventricular Rhythm (IVR)

idioventricular rhythm (IVR)
An impulse originating in the ventricles, produces a rhythm of 20–40 beats per minute.

When all of the heart's supraventricular pacemakers have failed to provide a rhythm either because of a blockage along the conduction path, or sinus arrest, the third pacemaker in the heart- the ventricles, can produce a very slow impulse and rhythm called an **idioventricular rhythm (IVR)**, or ventricular escape rhythm. The rate of the impulse will only be at the ventricular rate of 20–40 beats per minute. This rhythm may function as an escape rhythm and is usually regular. There is no P wave because the higher pacemakers failed to produce an impulse. An IRV may occur in short runs and the heart may self correct from the rhythm, but in a continuous run of ventricular beats, the IRV is not very reliable as the heart rate decreases. If the heart rate drops below 20 bpm, the QRS pattern loses uniformity and becomes an irregular terminal rhythm called an **agonal** arrhythmia. The ECG technician will want to bring IRV rhythm ECG tracings to the attention of a licensed professional as soon as possible so that treatment to increase the heart rate can begin if the run of ventricular beats is continuous. Box 8-13 identifies the rules for an idioventricular rhythm.

agonal
An irregular terminal rhythm that occurs when the heart rate drops below 20 beats per minute and the QRS pattern loses uniformity.

Box 8-13 Idioventricular Rhythm Rules

- *No P wave.*
- R-R intervals are regular.
- *Heart rate is 20–40 beats per minute, and sometimes less.*
- *No PRI.*
- *QRS complex is wide, bizarre, and 0.12 seconds or more.*
- *T wave is usually the opposite deflection of QRS complex.*

(changes from a NSR are shown in italics)

Pulseless Electrical Activity (PEA)

pulseless electrical activity (PEA)
A condition where the heart muscle cannot contract, even though electrical activity appears on the ECG.

Pulseless electrical activity (PEA) is not really an arrhythmia but rather a condition, where the heart muscle cannot contract even though electrical activity appears on the ECG. The condition may also be referred to as electrical mechanical dissociation because the heart is deprived of adequate mechanical function. In PEA, the ECG may show a sinus rhythm or any of the arrhythmias; however there is no palpable pulse, no blood pressure, no cardiac output, and the patient is unresponsive, which means that the patient is in cardiac arrest. A few reasons that PEA may occur include a massive pulmonary embolism, massive MI, extreme electrolyte imbalance, a drug overdose, or blunt force trauma. PEA may or may not be reversible—much depends on the underlying reason for the rhythm, and the condition is always treated as an emergency situation. When the ECG technician notices this event, a licensed practitioner needs to be notified immediately to begin lifesaving CPR and emergency drug intervention.

Ventricular Asystole

ventricular asystole
The absence of any ventricular activity.

Ventricular asystole is the absence of any ventricular activity—no depolarization, no pulse, no blood is flowing through the heart, and no cardiac output. It is commonly just called asystole. The patient is unresponsive, and this is an emergency situation. The ECG tracing may show a P wave for a while or when CPR is administered, otherwise the waveform is nearly a flat line. Asystole is always confirmed in two leads to confirm lack of response to drug intervention or CPR. A patient in asystole is not defibrillated as this is a terminal condition.

There are many more arrhythmias that are beyond the scope of this book. In advanced ECG courses, the student will go into these abnormalities in greater detail along with other arrhythmias such as heart blocks, conduction defects, heart chamber enlargement, and perfusion deficits.

Quick Check 8-3

Review the rules for ventricular arrhythmias. Then, using the ECG strips below, classify the rhythm and calculate the heart rate. (Be sure to recognize if the strip is a 6-second or 10-second ECG.)

1. Rhythm classification _____

Heart rate _____ bpm

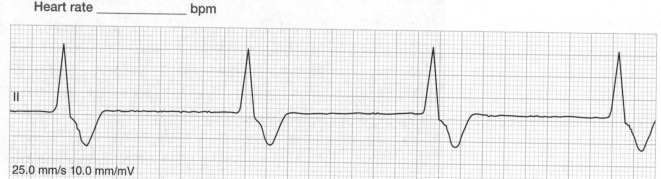

25.0 mm/s 10.0 mm/mV

Figure 8-13

(Continued)

(*Continued*)

2. Rhythm classification _____

Heart rate _____ bpm

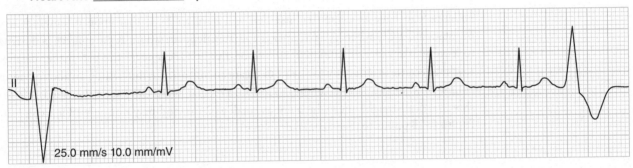

25.0 mm/s 10.0 mm/mV

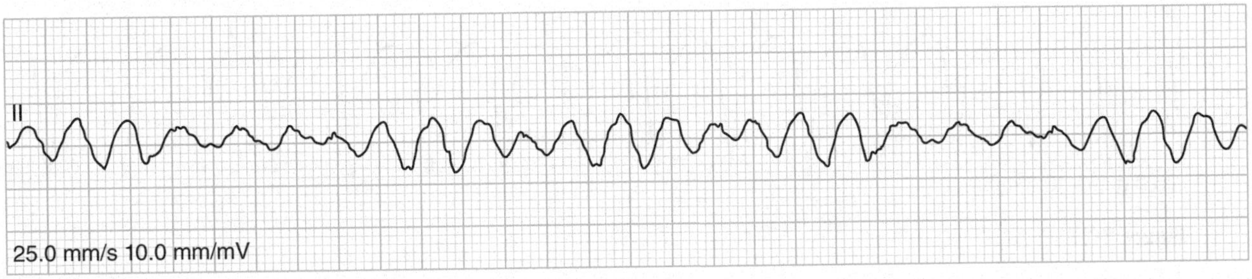

Figure 8-14

3. Rhythm classification _____

Heart rate _____ bpm

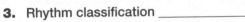

25.0 mm/s 10.0 mm/mV

Figure 8-15

4. Rhythm classification _____

Heart rate _____ bpm

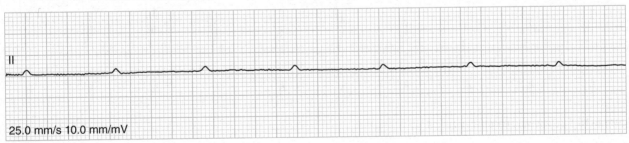

25.0 mm/s 10.0 mm/mV

Figure 8-16

(*Continued*)

(*Continued*)

5. Rhythm classification _____

Heart rate _____ bpm

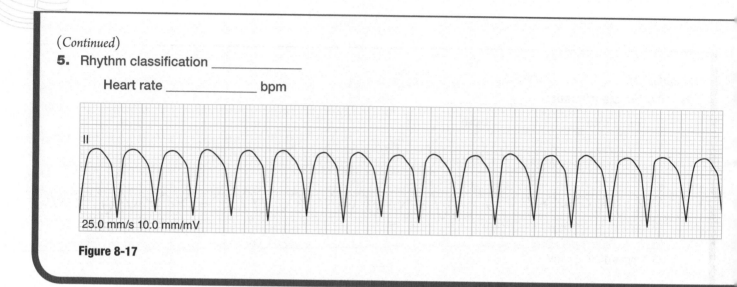

Figure 8-17

PACEMAKER ECGS

Patients who have a pacemaker installed will have an ECG that appears different from the standard ECG when the pacemaker initiates depolarization. A pacemaker is designed to leave marks called **pacemaker spikes** on the ECG whenever the pacemaker creates a rhythm because of failure by the heart to create an intrinsic rhythm within an allotted period of time or when the pacemaker fires to restore a regular heartbeat. Pacemaker spikes are very short vertical straight lines which are as small as 2 ms, and may not be visible in all leads. **Figure 8-18** points to the pacemaker spikes in an ECG.

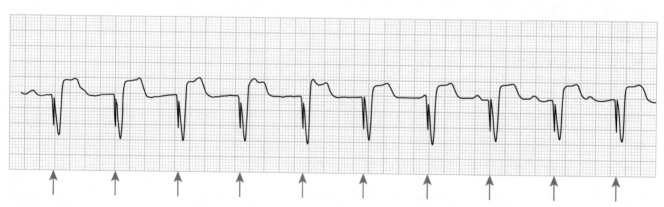

Figure 8-18 ECG showing pacemaker spikes

Pacemaker patients are administered an ECG like other patients; however, be sure not to place an electrode over the pacemaker. Some clinicians prefer that the limb leads be placed on the torso instead of the appendages so that the ECG may show less artifacts from noise or patient movement. If the ECG machine provides a "detect pacing mode," be sure to select this option. The patient should be carrying a card with important pacemaker information that the ECG technician will record in the patient's record. Record the type of pacemaker—brand, model, functions, and magnet mode. This information will be necessary if the patient is ever taken to surgery, if the pacemaker malfunctions, or if the pacemaker needs the batteries replaced. The clinician will monitor the ECG results more attentively to see if the pacemaker is working as it was designed to work.

How Pacemakers Work

pacemaker
A device that measures the movement of electricity in the heart, designed to provide an electrical stimulus in the event that the heart does not provide a normal heartbeat.

pace
To follow or track a heartbeat or rhythm.

transcutaneous pacemaker (TCP)
An external pacemaker with two parts that include electrodes that are placed in a special pad attached to the skin, and a power source.

People who have a condition where the heart cannot maintain a normal intrinsic rhythm may have a pacemaker installed. **Pacemakers** measure the movement of electricity in the heart and provide electrical stimulus in the event that the heart does not provide a normal heartbeat so that the myocardium can depolarize, thus creating a contraction. Pacemakers are designed to **pace**, or track, the electrical activity. Pacemakers are sometimes referred to as pulse generators. Pacemakers are implanted under the skin below the clavicle if they are permanent, or they can be a temporary external device called a **transcutaneous pacemaker (TCP)**. The TCP attaches to a person by a special pad that contains the electrodes to deliver an electrical current through the skin, and a power source. Temporary external devices may be used for patients for an extended period of time (even years sometimes), but permanent pacemakers are usually installed for the life of the patient. **Figure 8-19** shows an internally implanted pacemaker. Note the flexible electrodes. External pacemakers have specific locations for the placement of the TCP special pads, as shown in **Figure 8-20** for both the male and female patient.

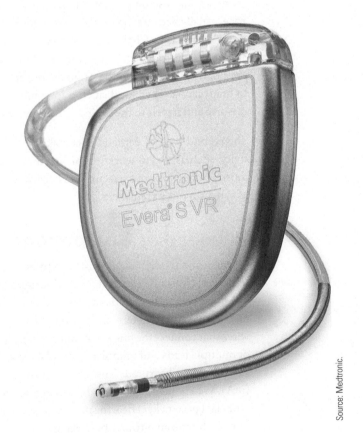

Source: Medtronic.

Figure 8-19 Internal pacemaker

asynchronous pacemaker
A pacemaker that generates a continuous current at a preset rate.

synchronous pacemaker
One type of this device sets the heart rate at a preprogrammed pace and the second type changes the rate according to patient activity; also called demand pacemaker.

There are two main classifications of pacemakers, each of which stimulates the heart differently. The **asynchronous pacemaker** generates a continuous current at a preset rate. Asynchronous pacemakers are installed in patients who do not have a reliable intrinsic heart rhythm. The second category, the **synchronous pacemaker**, has two subcategories; both are often referred to as a demand pacemaker. One category of the demand pacemaker will

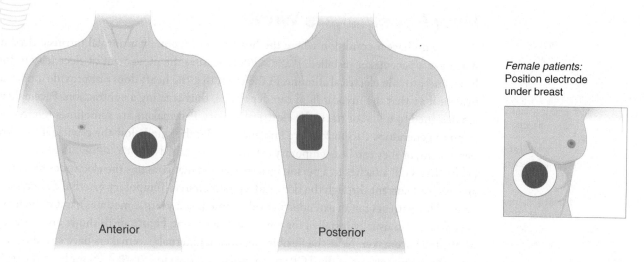

Female patients:
Position electrode
under breast

Anterior

Posterior

Figure 8-20 Transcutaneous pacemaker pads

create an impulse only when the patient's heart rhythm does not keep a preprogrammed pace, usually because the rhythm is too slow (bradycardia). Bradycardia can be just as deadly as tachycardia. In Chapter 2, a cerebral vascular accident (CVA), the medical term for a stroke, was introduced. Recall that a CVA is caused by reduced or blocked blood flow to the brain. Expanding on the original concepts, embolic strokes often form in the heart due to bradycardia. The blood sits too long in the atria and clots form. When the clot does not dissolve and travels to the brain, a stroke occurs when the coronary arteries become blocked.

The second type of demand pacemaker is able to change the rate according to patient activity, such as a gym workout, or inactivity, such as sleeping. The following sections refer mostly to synchronous pacemakers because asynchronous pacemakers are not used as much as synchronous pacemakers.

Pacemaker Components

pacing electrode
Single or multiple leads that can be unipolar or bipolar leads and can provide the electrical stimulus in a pacemaker.

A synchronous pacemaker consists of three main components: a pulse generator, at least one lead, and at least one electrode that is located at the tip of the leads, called a **pacing electrode**. The pulse generator includes a power source, a battery, microchips used to program the pacemaker and set parameters, and a magnetically activated timer. The leads are flexible insulated wires that connect the pulse generator to the electrodes. The pacing electrode can have single or multiple leads and unipolar or bipolar leads, and they provide the electrical stimulus and sense intrinsic heart rate. The current provided by the pacemaker is measured in milliamps (mA). When the heart fails to maintain a set rate, the timer starts the process of creating an artificial (pacemaker) heartbeat. If the heart *does* maintain a predetermined rate, the timer is reset each time an intrinsic beat occurs.

Pacemaker Functions

intrinsic rhythm
A heart rhythm created by a person's own heart rather than by an artificial means.

Synchronous pacemakers have three functions: they have the ability to sense a patient's own heart rhythm, called an **intrinsic rhythm**; they capture the chamber being paced; and they fire an electrical impulse if the heart did not provide one. The basic way a pacemaker works is shown on the flowchart in **Figure 8-21**.

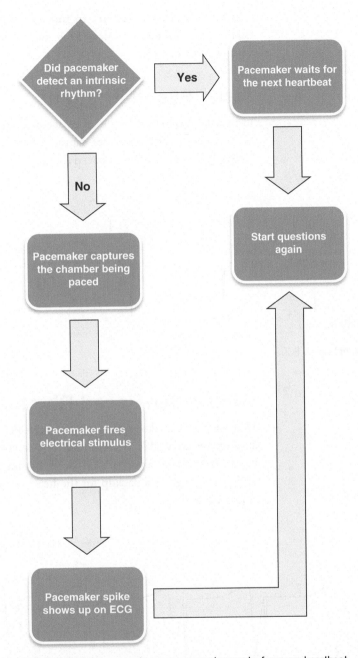

Figure 8-21 How a synchronous pacemaker works for every heartbeat

It is important to understand that an ECG tracing from a patient with a pacemaker may have wide or bizarre QRS complexes if the pacemaker captures the chamber that it is pacing. The pacemaker can pace particular chambers—either the atria or ventricles, or both atria and ventricles (dual).

Pacemaker ECG Features

There is much more to the study of pacemakers than what is introduced in this chapter, but as an ECG technician, it is important to be able to recognize a pacemaker ECG and potential malfunctioning pacemakers. It takes time and practice, and it helps to be able to learn from a cardiologist while you are administering ECGs, if they will explain various waveforms and malfunctions. In this section, an atrial-paced rhythm, ventricular-paced rhythm, dual-paced rhythm, and loss of capture are shown on an ECG to familiarize you with what to look for.

Atrial-Paced Rhythms

In an atrial pacemaker rhythm, the pacemaker spike may be seen before an abnormal P wave because the of atrial chamber capture. The QRS complex can be normal in appearance. **Figure 8-22** shows an atrial-paced rhythm.

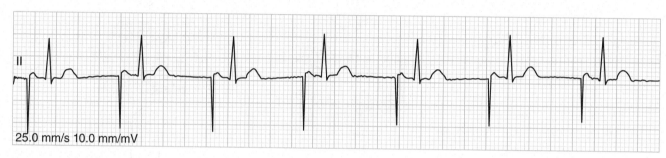

Figure 8-22 Atrial-paced ECG

Ventricular-Paced Rhythms

Ventricular pacemaker spikes may be seen before each QRS complex, and normally, no atrial spikes are visible. P waves may not be visible, except possibly in precordial lead V1. **Figure 8-23** shows a ventricular-paced rhythm. Atrial and ventricular pacemakers are typically considered as a backup for the heart in case the intrinsic heart rhythm pauses on a consistent basis.

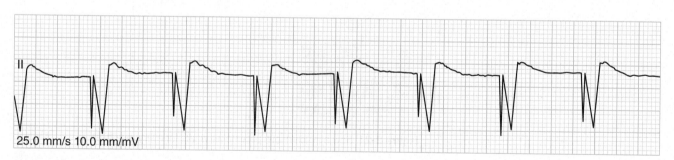

Figure 8-23 Ventricular-paced ECG

Dual-Chamber Pacing Rhythm

The pacemaker spikes in dual pacing may appear before only the P wave, only in front of the QRS complex, or they may appear in front of both the P wave and the QRS complex. There may also not be any pacing spikes if the heart is able to produce its own electrical current during the ECG exam. In **Figure 8-24**, notice that two spikes appear—one before the P wave and a second before the QRS complex. Dual-chamber pacing is usually the type of pacemaker that is used on people who suffer complete heart blocks.

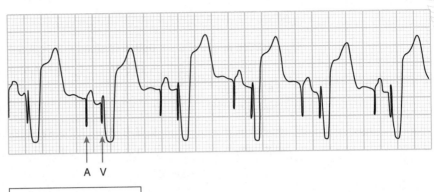

A = Atrial capture
V = Ventricular capture

Figure 8-24 Dual-chamber pacing ECG

Quick Check 8-4

Fill in the blanks.

1. Pacemakers measure the movement of _____ in the heart and can provide stimulus if necessary to cause the myocardium to _____.

2. Synchronous pacemakers are usually programmed to correct _____ rhythms.

3. A synchronous pacemaker has three main components including a pulse _____, a flexible _____ and one or two _____.

4. _____ chamber pacing may show two visible _____ on an ECG tracing.

5. _____ and _____ pacemakers are typically considered as backup rhythm generators used in case the heart pauses between waveforms.

Pacemaker Codes

There are five classifications, or modes, that pacemakers are set to operate; however, there are typically only three of the classifications identified in a pacemaker code, including the chamber that is being paced, the chamber that is being sensed, and the type of pacing that the pacemaker has been set to operate. **Table 8-1** identifies each code with an uppercase letter for each of the classifications.

After the three letters, in synchronous pacemakers, there will be a number that stands for the programmed heart rate. For example, if the code is VVI 60, it would be read as ventricular chamber pacing, sensing for intrinsic rate of ventricles, inhibits pulsing if intrinsic electrical activity is noted at more than 60 bpm.

The code that mimics the natural intrinsic heartbeat and rhythm of a normal heart is DDD, which stands for dual pacing and sensing of the atrium and ventricle, and an intrinsic P wave or QRS complex inhibits pacing.

Table 8-1 Pacemaker Codes

Location in Code	Option Choices	Action
First letter	A, D, O, V	Chamber being paced
Second letter	A, D, O, V	Chamber being sensed
Third letter	D, I, O, T	Response to Sensing
Fourth letter	C, M, O, P, R	Pacemaker's programmability or rate modulation
Fifth letter	D, O, P, S	Tachycardia response

Legend for option choices:

A = atrium

C = communication function (i.e., telemetry)

D = dual chambers (both atria and ventricles)

I = inhibits pacing

M = multiprogrammable

O = none

P = pacing ability (overrides tachycardia rhythm)

R = rate responsive (adjusts to patient's metabolism)

S = shock (pacemaker provides defibrillator action)

T = triggers pacing

V = ventricle

With the asynchronous pacemaker, the codes are AOO, VOO, or DOO because there is no sensing for intrinsic rhythms and the pulse cannot be inhibited because the pacemaker is set to produce a paced beat at a fixed rate.

Pacemaker Malfunctions

There are three types of pacemaker malfunctions the ECG technician should be able to identify. First, the pacemaker may fail to capture a paced chamber. Second, the pacemaker has failed to pace, which is noticeable by missing pacemaker spikes. Third, timing problems occur with synchronous pacemakers when the pacemaker creates an impulse prematurely or late. The main problem with asynchronous pacemakers is that they can actually cause pacer-induced tachycardia because there is no timer, so when an intrinsic rhythm occurs, the pacemaker still creates a preprogrammed rhythm.

Loss of Capture

loss of capture
On the ECG, two pacemaker spikes with no waveforms between the spikes.

A capture of a chamber can be identified on an ECG by the presence of a P wave, the QRS complex, or both the P wave and a QRS complex after a pacemaker spike appears. If a spike appears by itself with no P wave and no QRS complex, then it is called a **loss of capture**.

Visualizing loss of capture is probably the most recognized malfunction. Notice in **Figure 8-25** the flat line between abnormal beats. The pacemaker should have captured the chamber being paced but did not do so, resulting in two pacemaker spikes with no waveforms between the spikes.

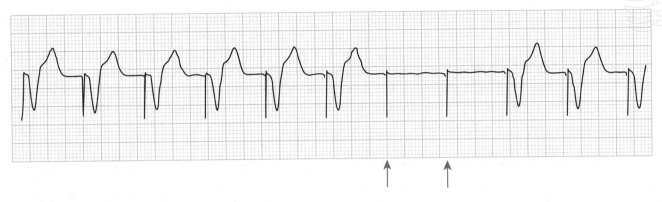

Figure 8-25 Loss of capture ECG

A loss of capture on an ECG should be given to a clinician for review as soon as possible because the pacemaker may be malfunctioning.

Failure to Pace

When the malfunction is a failure to pace, the ECG will show no pacemaker spikes on the ECG tracing. The first thing to check with this malfunction would be the batteries. It seems that manufacturers could have coined another phrase for weak batteries, but unfortunately, manufacturers have created a code named "end of life mode," meaning the battery's life is dead. A battery on the pacemaker will last anywhere from 5 to 12 years, but the patient needs to keep regular cardiology appointments and have the pacemaker checked at least annually. When a battery's life is almost over, the entire pacemaker's pulse generator containing new circuits is replaced. The leads and electrodes are not normally replaced if the malfunction is just the battery.

Oversensing or Undersensing

Oversensing or undersensing pacemakers can be detected on an ECG when the pacemaker fails to sense intrinsic P or R waves. This situation must be handled by a trained professional who will have to reprogram the sensitivity of the pacemaker. For the ECG technician, take care to notice pacing spikes or the lack of pacing spikes in people who are known to have a pacemaker, and bring the situation up to the clinician as soon as possible.

IMPLANTABLE CARDIOVERTER DEFIBRILLATOR (ICD)

implantable cardioverter defibrillator (ICD)
A device implanted into patients who need two levels of heart stimulus; one level is designed to correct ventricular tachycardia, and a stronger level of shock is designed to correct ventricular fibrillation.

electrophysiology study (EPS)
A study performed on an implanted cardioverter defibrillator (ICD) to determine if the ICD is working correctly.

When medication no longer controls tachycardia, especially ventricular tachycardia or ventricular fibrillation, an **implantable cardioverter defibrillator (ICD)** may be implanted into the patient to control these life-threatening arrhythmias. They can also be used to prevent sudden cardiac arrest or bradycardia. ICDs are very similar to pacemakers, but they are a little larger and can be implanted anywhere at or above the waist, but are normally implanted in the same location (below the clavicle) as the pacemaker. They have the same three main components—the pulse generator, flexible leads, and electrodes. ICDs require an **electrophysiology study (EPS)** after implantation to confirm correct heart monitoring. The difference between a pacemaker and the ICD is that the ICD can deliver two levels of electrical stimulus. Tachycardia can be corrected with small electrical impulses like a pacemaker would deliver, but fibrillation may require the ICD to deliver a high-energy shock to the heart to get it back into correct rhythm. The ICD will record any events as they occur, along with the action used to correct each situation. Batteries in the ICD usually last 4–8 years. There are also additional limitations for patients to stay away from strong magnetic fields and to keep cell phones at least 6 inches away from the ICD implanted site.

Quick Check 8-5

Fill in the blanks.

1. In a pacemaker code of VVI 60, a normal ventricular _____ restarts or resets the _____ if the event occurs at or after 60 bpm.

2. In a pacemaker code of AAI 60, an intrinsic _____ wave _____ atrial pacing.

3. Loss of capture on an ECG tracing can be identified by a(n) _____ between abnormal heartbeats.

4. The primary difference between the ICD and the pacemaker is that the _____ has two levels of _____.

5. Ventricular fibrillation usually requires a(n) _____ shock to get the heart back into a normal rhythm.

RECOGNIZING ISCHEMIA, INJURY, AND INFARCTIONS ON ECGs

necrosis
Tissue death.

ischemia
A decrease in oxygenated blood flow to the heart muscle.

Heart damage to **necrosis** (tissue death) occurs in three stages: first **ischemia** occurs, which is defined as a decrease in oxygenated blood flow to the heart muscle. A person suffering from ischemia will usually present with symptoms of chest pain, tightness or pressure, burning pain, or a squeezing of the heart. The symptoms have usually lasted for at least 20 minutes and are not lessened by resting. Untreated ischemia then causes injury to the myocardium. Injury can occur within the first hour after symptoms appear. If no treatment is provided, the injured myocardium progresses to a myocardial infarction (MI), usually within 2 to 24 hours, and resulting necrosis of myocardial tissue. The ECG is the primary tool used for initial assessment along with blood analysis and monitoring patient symptoms.

Role of Coronary Arteries

acute
A sudden or recent event, usually an event of less than 24 hours' duration.

Blockage of one or more coronary arteries that supply blood to the left ventricle is usually the cause of an **acute** (which means sudden) myocardial infarction (AMI). Those arteries include the septal branch and diagonal branches of the left anterior descending (LAD) coronary artery; branches of the left circumflex (LCx) coronary artery; and branches of the right coronary artery (RCA). **Figure 8-26** highlights these arteries.

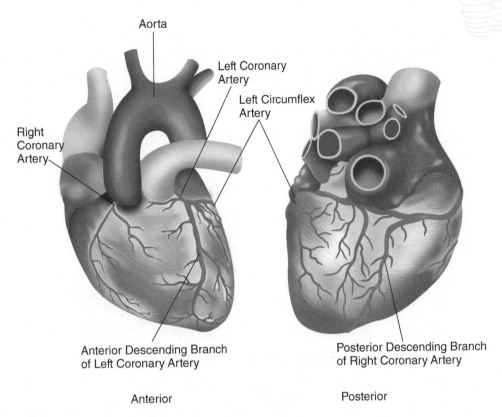

Figure 8-26 Coronary arteries

Locating Heart Damage

The location of heart damage can often be determined by understanding the views of the heart walls, along with changes in specific leads. The walls of the left ventricle are most commonly the area damaged. Recall from Chapter 6 that the walls of the left ventricle can be viewed anteriorly, apically, laterally, or inferiorly. Apical damage is not as common as the other three views. When damage is only to the anterior wall, the LAD coronary artery is usually involved. When damage is only to the inferior wall, the RCA is usually involved. When damage is to the lateral wall, the LAD or LCx arteries are usually involved.

Damage Changes in Specific Leads

The ECG shows specific changes in leads as ischemia becomes myocardial injury and the myocardial injury becomes a myocardial infarction. An ECG with ischemia will normally show a ST segment elevation and a tall, peaked T wave. As a reference point, **Figure 8-27** shows a normal ST segment as seen in Lead II.

reflective lead
A lead that faces an affected surface of an injured wall.

The affected wall can be viewed two ways. **Reflective leads** face the affected surface of the injured wall. Reciprocal leads can view the damage from the opposite wall of the damage and will provide an inverted view. Often, one of the reciprocal leads will provide a better view of the injury. **Figure 8-28** shows inferior wall damage with the reflecting leads and reciprocal lead views.

Recall from Chapter 6 that the anterior wall leads are viewed from the precordial leads V1, V2, V3, and V4; the lateral wall is viewed from Leads I and aVL and the precordial leads V5

Normal ST-T

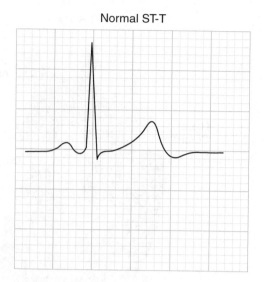

Figure 8-27 Normal ST segment

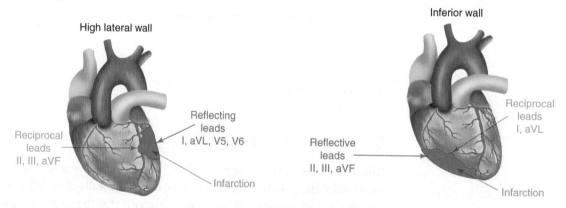

Figure 8-28 High lateral and inferior wall damage viewed by reflecting and reciprocal leads

and V6; and the inferior wall is viewed from Leads II, III, and aVF. The anterior wall reciprocal leads to V1, V2, V3, and V4 are the lateral Leads I and aVL and the precordial leads V5 and V6. The lateral wall reciprocal leads to Lead I and aVL are Leads II, III, or aVF. Inferior reciprocal leads include Lead I, III, aVF, and precordial leads V5 and V6. **Figure 8-29** shows the location of damage with an MI. **Table 8-2** summarizes which leads are reflective and reciprocal based on the location (heart wall) and the table also identified which artery is occluded. If the patient is complaining of cardiac pain and only the ST *depression* shows on the standard ECG, a second ECG may be requested using the posterior leads V7, V8, and V9.

Waveform Changes

As stated earlier, when the heart is denied oxygenated blood, the standard ECG will pick up the injury as changes in the ST segment, T wave, and if the blockage is severe or prolonged, changes will also be seen in the Q wave. It is important to note that not all ST segment elevations or depressions are AMIs. There are many causes of ST segment changes, including antiarrhythmic drugs, angina attacks, positive stress tests, hyperkalemia, and

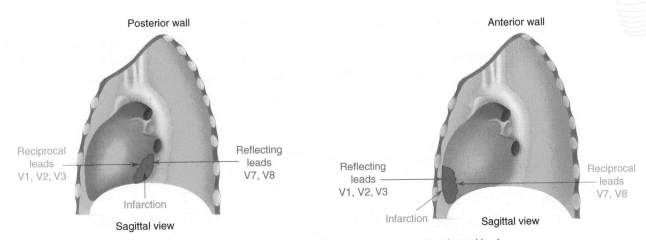

Figure 8-29 Sagittal view of posterior and anterior wall damage viewed by reflecting and reciprocal leads

Table 8-2 Myocardial Infarction Walls, Leads, and Arteries

Left Ventricle MI Injured Wall	Noted Changes in Standard ECG Leads (Reflective Leads)	Opposite-Wall View (Reciprocal Leads)	Involved Artery/Arteries
High lateral wall	I, aVL, V5, V6	II, III, aVF	LCx, LAD
Inferior wall	II, III, aVF	I, aVL	RCA
Posterior wall	V7, V8	V1, V2, V3	Posterior Descending RCA
Anterior wall	V1, V2, V3	V7, V8	LAD

hypokalemia. In some healthy people, ST segment abnormalities may be a normal variant. The following figures will identify abnormal waveforms that were identified as ischemia, injury, or infarcts. Ischemia waveform changes usually include ST segment elevation of at least 1 mm in limb leads and 2 mm in the precordial leads. The T wave may increase in size and may be tall and peaked or inverted. **Figure 8-30** shows how an abnormal ST segment may appear with acute ischemia or injury in leads V1, V2, V3, and V4 with an anterior wall injury.

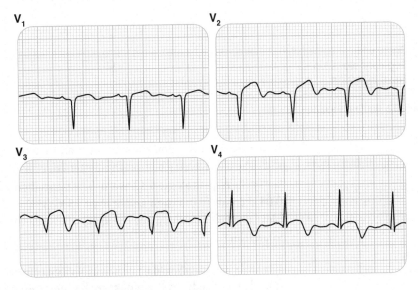

Figure 8-30 Anterior injury

The ischemia will continue if the blockage continues and is not medically recognized. As the blockage progresses, the myocardial cells are now showing signs of injury. The ST segment elevation is now visible in two or more contiguous leads and the T wave may be inverted or may be flattened. **Figure 8-31** shows how an abnormal ST segment may appear with acute ischemia or injury in Leads II, III, and aVF with an inferior wall injury.

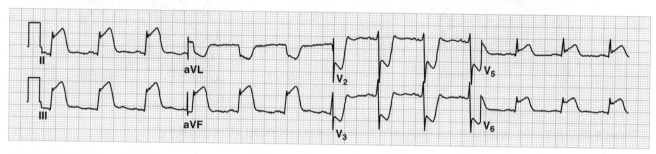

Figure 8-31 Inferior wall injury

When an acute myocardial infarction is evolving, the ECG tracing shows the ST segment appearing as a large, positive reflected, rounded T wave in Lead II, as shown in **Figure 8-32**. After approximately 24 hours, the ST segment decreases in size, and an inverted T wave may still be seen. A Q wave may develop. **Figure 8-33** shows a patient's ECG with an old inferior infarction.

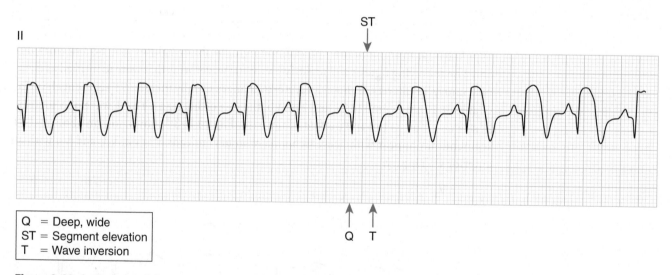

Q = Deep, wide
ST = Segment elevation
T = Wave inversion

Figure 8-32 Acute myocardial

pathological Q wave
A permanent, large, wide Q wave measuring over 0.04 seconds in duration and at least 25 percent to 35 percent of the amplitude of the entire QRS complex.

In the days, weeks, and months after an infarction, the ST segment will return to normal. The T wave may be upright, flattened, or inverted, and there may be a **pathological Q wave**. A pathological Q wave is a permanent, large, wide Q wave measuring over 0.04 seconds in duration and at least 25%–35% of the amplitude of the entire QRS complex. **Table 8-3** summarizes the signs of myocardial ischemia, injury, infarction, and post infarction.

Ischemia and injury due to blockage can be reversible when successful medical intervention clears or reduces the blockage. By the time the damage becomes an MI, the damage

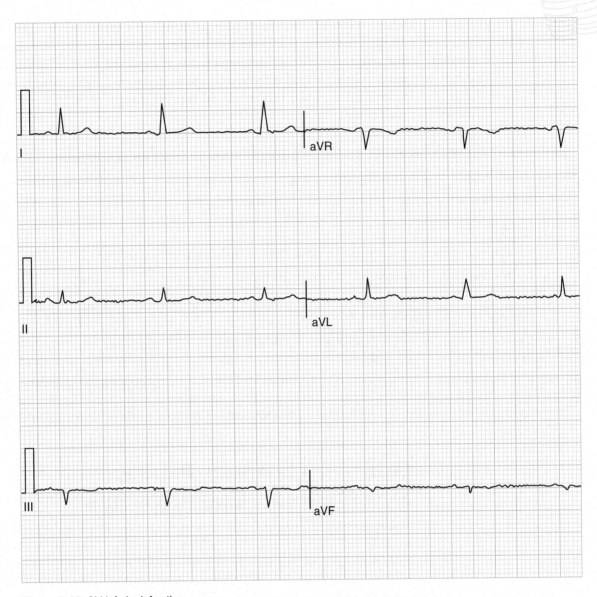

Figure 8-33 Old inferior infarction

Table 8-3 Signs of Myocardial Ischemia, Injury, and Infarction

	Waveform Changes
Ischemia	ST segment elevation—more than 1 mm in limb leads, 2 mm in precordial
	T wave increases in size; may be tall, peaked, inverted
Injury	ST segment elevation in two or more contiguous leads
	May see T wave inversion; may flatten
Infarction	ST segment elevation in two or more contiguous leads
	May see T wave inversion; may flatten
	Change in width and depth of the Q wave
Post-Infarction	ST segment returns to normal
	T wave may be upright, flattened, or inverted
	May see a pathologic Q wave

ablation
A medical procedure that uses high electrical energy to destroy abnormal electrical pathways in the heart.

is irreversible and considered permanent. When a person survives an MI, heart tissue has died and leaves scar tissue. Scar tissue in the heart can increase the risk of ventricular tachycardia. The two common forms of treatment are **ablation** and ventricular reconstruction. Ablation is the use of high electrical energy to destroy abnormal electrical pathways. Ventricular reconstruction requires surgery to remove scar tissue and dead heart tissue.

Quick Check 8-6

Fill in the blanks.

1. An acute myocardial infarction can be caused by blockage of one or more _____.
2. Most commonly, a myocardial infarction will occur in the _____ wall.
3. _____ leads face the affected surface of the injured wall, whereas _____ leads view damage from the opposite wall.
4. One of the first signs of ischemia or injury to a heart wall is ST segment _____ and an increased _____ wave.
5. A pathological _____ wave signifies _____ damage from an old infarction.

SUDDEN CARDIAC ARREST AND CARDIAC EMERGENCIES

This final section of the book will discuss emergency conditions and medications. Although the ECG technician does not have a license to practice medicine and cannot prescribe medications and cannot administer medications without specific instructions from a licensed practitioner, knowing what conditions might present and what medications should be on hand can save time and help the ECG technician become a vital part of an emergency team.

Sudden Cardiac Arrest

sudden cardiac arrest
Unexpected death due to a heart electrical system malfunction.

Sudden cardiac arrest causes an unexpected death due to a loss of heart function when the electrical system malfunctions. Sudden cardiac arrest, also referred to as sudden cardiac death (SCD), is the largest cause of natural deaths in the United States and occurs in men twice as often as women, and occurs primarily in adults between the ages of 35 and 45. Often there are no symptoms, but there are many risk factors, including suffering from a previous MI or coronary artery disease, or undetected congenital heart defects. Additionally, high cholesterol, obesity, diabetes, recreational drug abuse, an extremely low heart rate, and a family history of cardiovascular disease, especially abnormal heart rhythms, can be contributing factors to the loss of heart function and arrhythmias. If high-risk indicators are detected early enough, an ICD may be implanted.

Cardiac Compromise

cardiac compromise
Any cardiac issue.

Cardiac compromise refers to any cardiac issue. There are five primary issues that compromise the heart's ability to perform and can create an emergency situation. These issues include aneurysms, which weaken an arterial wall and can cause the vessel to rupture; coronary artery disease, which causes the coronary arteries to become narrow and can cause blockage of the oxygenated blood to the heart; electrical malfunctions, which can cause the heart's intrinsic rhythm to become irregular or absent; injury, especially blunt force injury; and mechanical malfunctions, such as failure of the heart to pump oxygenated blood efficiently and causing cardiopulmonary arrest. In many of these cardiopulmonary issues, a combination of cardiovascular, infectious, inflammatory, metabolic, neurological, or traumatic diseases or injuries took months (and perhaps years) to fester before the person recognized the need for treatment, or the person never sought medical intervention before coming to an emergency room.

Common Cardiac Compromises

(in alphabetical order)

- Aneurysms
- Coronary artery disease
- Electrical malfunctions of the heart
- Injury
- Mechanical malfunctions

The ECG technician can perform several tasks to assist a licensed practitioner if the patient shows signs of distress. In times of cardiac emergencies, the saying "Time is muscle" should be taken seriously, so knowing what to do and using both speed and compassion can save a patient's life. If a patient is alert and responsive, taking the medical history and getting the consent forms for treatment signed can save time. Taking good vital signs, especially the blood pressure, is also important. Patient observation, completing a clean ECG, and complete accurate documentation is vital. If a patient's condition worsens, knowing what the emergency protocol is, where the emergency equipment and defibrillator is located, how to turn on all the equipment, how to set up oxygen and an intravenous line (if protocol allows), and what blood tests may be ordered and how to complete the requisitions, as well as keeping an accurate count of the patient's degree of chest pain on a 1–10 scale will help you be an invaluable member of the team. ECG technicians should also know the contraindications to be aware of, such as hypotension and drugs taken within the past 24 hours; this will help in the care of a patient in cardiac distress. Above all, stay calm.

Emergency Medications

The licensed practitioner may use any one of the following drugs based upon their assessment of the cardiac compromise. **Table 8-4** identifies each drug's indications, route, dosage, and how it is supplied. The ECG technician should know the type of equipment, such as IV lines, syringes, needles, and personal protective equipment (PPE), including gloves, gowns, and masks, that needs to be available for emergency situations. Most facilities keep a crash cart loaded and ready for immediate use with these supplies. A **crash cart** is a cart, usually on wheels, which is stocked with emergency medications, supplies, IV solutions and tubing, ECG electrodes, a handheld ECG machine, and a defibrillator. The contents and drugs on the crash cart will differ by location. It may be the ECG technician's job to keep the crash cart properly stocked and everything currently dated (not expired). Completeness inspections should be frequent.

Table 8-4 Emergency Cardiac Medications

Medication	Typical Route and Dose	How Supplied	Indication
Epinephrine	IV, 1 mg	1 mg/10 mL (1:10,000) syringe	V-Fib, V-Tach, asystole, PEA, bradycardia
Atropine	IV, 0.5 mg- max 3 mg	1 mg/10 mL syringe	Bradycardia
Amiodarone	IV, 300 mg	150 mg/3 mL vial	V-Fib, V-Tach
Lidocaine	IV, 1–1.5 mg/kg	100 mg/5 mL syringe	V-Fib, V-Tach
Vasopressin	IV, 40 units	20 units/mL 1 mL vial	V-Fib, V-Tach, asystole
Adenosine	IV, 6 mg	6 mg/2 mL prefilled syringe	Supraventricular tachycardia
Dopamine	IV, 5–20 mcg/kg/min	400 mg/250 mL IV bag	Bradycardia
Nitroglycerin	Sublingually, 0.4 mg	0.4 mg spray or tab	Acute coronary syndromes

SUMMARY

- Four major classifications of arrhythmias include sinus, atrial, junctional, and ventricular arrhythmias.

- Compared to the normal sinus rhythm, sinus arrhythmias usually change in rate, including tachycardia (too fast) or bradycardia (too slow), or the R-R interval is irregular. All sinus rhythms originate from the SA node.

- In atrial arrhythmias, the AV node overrides the SA node by producing an ectopic beat. The most notable change from the normal sinus rhythm will occur in the P wave.

- Junctional beats occur when the impulse originates in the area between the AV node and the bundle of His. The most notable change from the normal sinus rhythm is in the P wave, which is normally recorded as P prime (P′).

- Premature junctional complexes occur as a single ectopic beat that originates in the AV junction and often have a heart rate of 40–60 bpm that is dependent upon the underlying rhythm.

- Accelerated junctional rhythms will have a heart rate of 60–100 bpm, but since this is coming from the AV node, this rate is considered fast.

- Ventricular arrhythmias are the most serious abnormal waveform because they originate in the lowest level of conduction, which are in the ventricles. Many ventricular arrhythmias are emergency situations, often found when a person experiences cardiac arrest. The ECG technician needs to be able to quickly identify and seek a licensed practitioner when observing ventricular arrhythmias.

- Ventricular tachycardia and premature ventricular complexes usually present with an underlying rhythm that is normal. Ventricular fibrillation has no regularity to the rhythm, and ventricular asystole presents as a flat line.

- Pulseless electrical activity (PEA) occurs when there is no palpable pulse, no blood pressure, and no cardiac output. Ventricular asystole is very similar to PEA, but the ECG tracing with ventricular asystole is usually a flat line, whereas the PEA tracing may show a sinus rhythm.

- Pacemakers measure the movement of electricity in the heart. Two types of pacemakers can be installed—TCP temporary pacemakers and permanent pacemakers. The pacemaker can pace a heart in the atria only, the ventricle only, or in dual mode, which is pacing both the atria and ventricles.

- The most common category of pacemaker is the synchronous pacemaker, also called a demand pacemaker. The subcategories of the synchronous pacemakers include a style that will create an impulse only when the patient's heart rhythm does not keep pace. The second style adjusts to patient activity and will only send an impulse if necessary (for example, in times of rest).

- Synchronous pacemakers and the implantable cardioverter defibrillators consist of a pulse generator, one or more flexible lead wires, and one or more electrodes. The pulse generator contains computer circuits and a battery. When the battery gets weak, the patient will need to have a procedure done to install a new pulse generator, but the leads and electrodes normally do not get replaced.

- Pacemakers can malfunction in three ways. They can fail to capture a paced chamber, capture the chamber but not record a waveform, or oversense or undersense the intrinsic P or R waves.

- When a heart is denied oxygenated blood due to a blockage in the coronary arteries, myocardial damage occurs. The damage occurs in three stages, including ischemia, injury, and an infarction. Ischemia and injury damage can be reversed if the blockage is removed, but with an infarction, necrosis of heart tissue cannot be reversed.

- Crash carts are used to keep emergency supplies and medications located in one place and moveable on location as needed.

Critical Thinking Challenge

8-1. Use Figure 8-34 to answer the following questions.

1. Identify the heart rate. _____

2. Identify the rhythm. _____

3. What type of waveform is this? _____

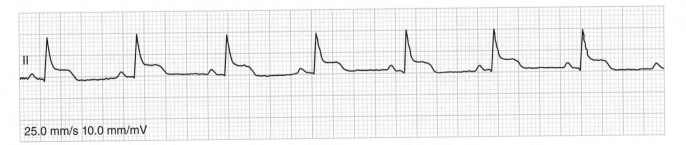

25.0 mm/s 10.0 mm/mV

Figure 8-34

8-2. Use Figure 8-35 to answer the following questions.

1. Identify the heart rate. _____

2. Identify the rhythm. _____

3. What type of waveform is this? _____

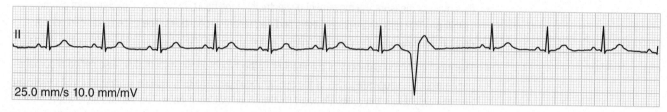

25.0 mm/s 10.0 mm/mV

Figure 8-35

8-3. Use Figure 8-36 to answer the following questions.

1. Identify the heart rate. _____

2. Identify the rhythm _____

3. What type of waveform is this? _____

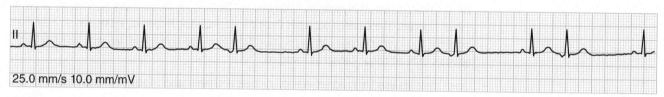

25.0 mm/s 10.0 mm/mV

Figure 8-36

Additional Activities

8-1. Match the level of heart damage with all waveform changes that usually occur. Each level of heart damage will have more than one waveform change, and each waveform change may be used more than once.

Heart Damage   **Waveform Changes**

1. Ischemia   _____

2. Injury   _____

3. Infarction   _____

4. Post infarction   _____

Waveform Changes

A. ST segment elevation is normal.

B. ST segment elevation in one lead, large with positive reflection.

C. ST segment elevation in two or more contiguous leads.

D. May see T wave inversion, may flatten.

E. T wave increases in size, may appear tall, peaked, or inverted.

F. T wave may appear rounded, flattened, or inverted.

G. May see changes in width and depth of Q wave.

H. May see pathologic Q wave.

8-2. Determine the pacemaker code from the following information:

- The chamber being paced is the right atrium.
- Sensing for intrinsic rate of ventricles.
- Inhibit pulse when intrinsic rate is more than 60 bpm.

Code is _____

8-3. The left ventricle injured walls are identified and numbered below. Match the injured wall to the reflective leads where the damage may be viewed *and* to the most likely involved artery or arteries.

Injured Wall

1. Anterior wall   _____

2. Inferior wall   _____

3. Lateral wall   _____

Choices:

Reflective Leads   **Artery**

A. I, aVL, V5, and V6   D. Left anterior descending coronary artery

B. II, III, aVF   E. Left circumflex coronary artery

C. V3 and V4   F. Right coronary artery

Chapter Eight Test

Part 1. Match the cardiac condition with the emergency medication usually administered. There may be more than one answer for each drug.

Emergency Medication

1. Adenosine _____

2. Amiodarone _____

3. Atropine _____

4. Dopamine _____

5. Epinephrine _____

6. Lidocaine _____

7. Nitroglycerin _____

8. Vasopressin _____

Cardiac Condition

A. Acute coronary syndrome

B. Asystole

C. Bradycardia

D. Supraventricular tachycardia

E. Ventricular fibrillation or ventricular tachycardia

F. Pulseless electrical activity

Part 2. Fill in the blanks.

1. An electrical impulse created within the heart is called a(n) _____ rhythm.

2. Two pacemaker spikes with no waveform between the spikes indicates a loss of

_____.

3. _____ is a medical procedure that destroys abnormal electrical pathways in the heart.

4–6. The three levels of myocardial injury caused by coronary artery blockage, listed from least to unrecoverable damage include _____, _____, and _____.

7. ICDs use a pulse _____ to track electrical activity.

BONUS

Use Figure 8-37 to answer the following questions.

1. Identify the heart rate. _____

2. Identify the rhythm. _____

3. What type of waveform is this? _____

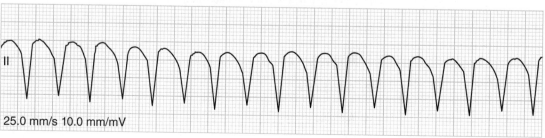

25.0 mm/s 10.0 mm/mV

Figure 8-37

Chapter Eight Quick Check Answers

Answer order is important except where noted otherwise (shown in parentheses).

When two correct answers are possible, both answers are given separated by the word "or."

8-1:

1. atrial tachycardia, 150

2. atrial fibrillation or A-Fib, 103

3. premature atrial complex or PAC, 70

4. normal sinus rhythm or NSR, 75

5. atrial flutter, 70

8-2:

1. junctional, 39

2. premature junctional complex or PJC, 71

3. junctional tachycardia, 125

4. accelerated junctional rhythm, 70

5. accelerated junctional rhythm, 67

8-3:

1. idioventricular rhythm, 35

2. ventricular fibrillation or V-Fib, 81

3. multifocal or multiform premature ventricular complex (PVCs), 67

4. ventricular asystole, atrial HR, 113

5. V-Tach or ventricular tachycardia, 171

8-4:

1. electricity, depolarize

2. bradycardia

3. generator, lead, electrodes

4. dual, spikes

5. atrial, ventricular

8-5:

1. complex, timer or clock

2. P, inhibits

3. flat line

4. ICD, electrical stimulus

5. high energy

8-6:

1. coronary arteries

2. left ventricular

3. reflective, reciprocal

4. elevation, T

5. Q, permanent

Appendices

The competency sheet is used to grade performance when completing an electrocardiogram (ECG) on a human subject in the correct order, in a timely manner, artifact free, and documented correctly. Various accrediting agencies may have different objectives.

Each item in the various categories has a point value, which when totaled will equal 100 percent. See the grading scale given in the sidebar. A competency is not "hidden" until the time of the test; rather, students should practice until they master every category. Competency testing is a timed event. Each patient procedure should be completed within 10 minutes, including the documentation.

Grading Scale

Total Points Available: 150. A percentage grade is given for every 5 percent on the chart that follows. For an exact score, divide your total points earned by 1.5. For example, if you earned 130 points, your score would be 87 percent (130/1.5 = 86.66, rounded up to the next whole number).

100 percent = 150 points

95 percent = 143 points

90 percent = 135 points

85 percent = 128 points

80 percent = 120 points

75 percent = 113 points

70 percent = 105 points

ECG Competency Assessment

Student Name _____

Date _____   **Score** _____   **Attempt #** _____

Time Start _____   **Time Stop** _____

	COMPLETED		Points awarded
	YES	NO	

Communication
(3 points each = 27 possible points; if *not necessary*, add 3 points)

Introduced self to patient _____ _____ _____

Verified patient identity and that consent form is signed _____ _____ _____

Entered demographic information into computer _____ _____ _____

Explained the procedure _____ _____ _____

Asked if patient had any questions _____ _____ _____

Asked patient if he or she needs assistance _____ _____ _____

   Assisted as necessary _____ _____ _____

Gave patient privacy to disrobe _____ _____ _____

Knocked on door before entering when patient disrobed _____ _____ _____

Standard Precautions
(5 points each = 10 possible points)

Washed hands _____ _____ _____

Verified room was ready—cleaned after previous patient _____ _____ _____

Supplies and Equipment
(3 points each = 9 possible points)

Turned on ECG machine and computer _____ _____ _____

Prepared supplies prior to calling the patient _____ _____ _____

Verified clean drapes were available in room _____ _____ _____

	COMPLETED		Points awarded
	YES	NO	

EXAM
(5 points each = 50 possible points, if *not necessary*, add 5 points)

Skin preparation completed ___ ___ ___

   Shaved IF necessary ___ ___ ___

Placed electrodes correctly—standard leads ___ ___ ___

Placed electrodes correctly—precordial leads ___ ___ ___

Checked for any nonsticking electrodes ___ ___ ___

   Applied alcohol; reapplied electrodes if necessary ___ ___ ___

Attached standard leads to electrodes ___ ___ ___

Attached precordial leads to electrodes ___ ___ ___

Asked if patient had any questions ___ ___ ___

   Reteach if necessary ___ ___ ___

Quality Control
(5 points each = 30 possible points; if *not necessary*, add 5 points)

Checked calibration ___ ___ ___

Checked for interference ___ ___ ___

   Corrected if necessary ___ ___ ___

Checked for artifacts before removing electrodes ___ ___ ___

   IF artifacts, were they corrected? ___ ___ ___

   IF artifacts, take new ECG after corrections ___ ___ ___

End of Test
(3 points each = 9 possible points)

Explained office procedure on obtaining the results ___ ___ ___

Removed electrodes from patient ___ ___ ___

Provided privacy to patient to redress ___ ___ ___

Documentation
(5 points each = 15 possible points)

Recorded ECG ___ ___ ___

Documented any test modifications (including reason) ___ ___ ___

Completed procedure within 10 minutes ___ ___ ___

Total Points Available = 150 points   Your Points = ___

Student Signature _____   Instructor Signature _____

Comments:

Supplies:

- **Watch**

  Always wear a watch that has a second hand. When working in a cardiology office, taking the blood pressure manually and taking the pulse correctly are of upmost importance, and you will use the second hand on the watch when completing these vitals.

- **Uniform**

  Obviously, a clean uniform is mandatory. Most schools require you to wear scrubs of a particular color. In many clinics, the staff all wear scrubs of the same color. Some clinics may require employees and students to iron their scrubs.

- **Name Tag**

  Never hide the fact that you are a student from a patient. Do not be offended if the patient requests an employee instead of a student to perform the ECG, because patients have the right to do so.

  Your name tag is important for legal reasons (see "Liability Insurance"). The patient has a right to know that you are a student.

- **Personal Grooming**

  If you have visible tattoos or sculptured nails, know the clinic guidelines before interviewing with the clinic for your externship. Often, clinics will have rules stating that tattoos must be covered, nails should be trimmed, clean, and without colorful polish, glitter, or items glued to the nail. Many clinics do not allow sculptured or long nails. Shoes are important! They need to be clean. If tennis shoes are allowed, they should be of a solid color. Socks should be a neutral color or match the color of the uniform or shoes.

- **Liability Insurance**

  Whenever you are working with people, they are entitled to receive the best-quality medical care, presented with dignity, respect, and confidentiality. Negligence, accidents, and mistakes do happen, and if they result in patient injury, you could be held personally responsible. Professional liability insurance can protect you against lawsuits. A school will often cover you as a student under their liability insurance, but realize that the coverage is to protect the school. You need your own insurance once you have graduated.

Other Considerations:

- **Personal Cell Phones**

  If there is one vice that almost every student has, it is bringing a cell phone (or other electronic gadget) to the clinic and using it during working hours. Don't do it! Personal cell phones are a liability to the employer and to you; they can cause interference with the electrocardiogram (ECG), and they also can put you at risk for potential lawsuits if you use them to record or take pictures of patients. Never take pictures when patients are in the area without specific written permission from the patients to be photographed. Implied consent is *not* acceptable. The Health Information Portability and Accountability Act (HIPAA) requires full disclosure. It is rude to be texting on employer time, and when you are an employee, this type of activity could prevent your advancement or continued employment because the abuse of personal cell phones is often documented on your evaluation.

- **HIPAA**

  At this point of your training, you may have only been practicing ECGs on mannequins. In the clinics, or with real people, always remember to start by identifying yourself and acknowledging the patient, and keep the following points in mind:

  - You cannot even acknowledge publicly or to anyone who is not part of the care team that a person came to the facility.

  - Confidentiality in every aspect—from the initial communication to obtaining personal information, obtaining demographic data, medical data, and even casual patient communication—is required by law. All communication and encounters should be held in the strictest confidence.

  - Any questions or concerns that you may have on procedures should be discussed only with the clinical coordinator or person you are reporting to. Speaking to other office personnel can be considered gossip, and you may be held accountable for breaching the HIPAA rules requiring confidentiality.

  - If obtaining a patient history, or if you are observing someone else obtaining a personal history, do not be judgmental in any way. In other words, do not make comments on what the patient has stated and be sure to document only what the patient has stated, without adding your opinion. Do not make gestures such as raising your eyebrows or shrugging your shoulders at comments made by the patient. Remember to use open-ended questioning techniques. Take your work seriously!

  - Patients are always entitled to dignity and respect. Be sure to properly drape both male and female patients appropriately for the ECG.

  - Never assume that the patient already knows the procedure. Be sure to explain in detail what the patient should remove, such as all metal objects, cell phones, belts, change from pockets, and necklaces, and tell the person only to disrobe from the waist up. Explain that the gown should open in the front. After explaining the procedure, ask the patient if he or she has any questions before you leave the room. Knock before entering when the patient is in the room.

Occupational Safety and Health Administration (OSHA)

- **Sanitizing Equipment**

  Most electrodes used today are disposable, one-time-use equipment. However, be sure that the other items, such as the bed and the leads, are sanitized regularly. Most facilities use disposable paper covers for the beds and pillows that need to be replaced after every patient, but the bed, pillow, and leads need to be sanitized between patients if any body fluids were left on the surface or came in contact with the equipment after patient use.

- **Hand Hygiene**

  Always wash your hands or use an alcohol-based hand rub before direct contact with patients. If you come in contact with any patient body fluids, be sure to wash your hands using antimicrobial soap and water. Always wash your hands after removing gloves.

- **Personal Protective Equipment (PPE)**

  Normally, the ECG is completed without needing any additional PPE such as gloves or gowns. The exception for when using PPE is required would be when the patient has uncontained body fluids or potentially infectious diseases. If this is the case, use gloves and a gown. If the patient has an airborne disease, wear a mask. If you have a cough that produces any excretions you should also wear a mask.

STANDARD PRECAUTIONS

Assume that every person is potentially infected or colonized with an organism that could be transmitted in the healthcare setting.

Hand Hygiene

Avoid unnecessary touching of surfaces in close proximity to the patient.

When hands are visibly dirty, contaminated with proteinaceous material, or visibly soiled with blood or body fluids, wash hands with soap and water.

If hands are not visibly soiled, or after removing visible material with soap and water, decontaminate hands with an alcohol-based hand rub. Alternatively, hands may be washed with an antimicrobial soap and water.

Perform hand hygiene:
> Before having direct contact with patients.
> After contact with blood, body fluids or excretions, mucous membranes, nonintact skin, or wound dressings.
> After contact with a patient's intact skin (e.g., when taking a pulse or blood pressure or lifting a patient).
> If hands will be moving from a contaminated-body site to a clean-body site during patient care.
> After contact with inanimate objects (including medical equipment) in the immediate vicinity of the patient.
> After removing gloves.

Personal protective equipment (PPE)

Wear PPE when the nature of the anticipated patient interaction indicates that contact with blood or body fluids may occur.

Before leaving the patient's room or cubicle, remove and discard PPE.

Gloves

Wear gloves when contact with blood or other potentially infectious materials, mucous membranes, nonintact skin, or potentially contaminated intact skin (e.g., of a patient incontinent of stool or urine) could occur.

Remove gloves after contact with a patient and/or the surrounding environment using proper technique to prevent hand contamination. Do not wear the same pair of gloves for the care of more than one patient.

Change gloves during patient care if the hands will move from a contaminated body-site (e.g., perineal area) to a clean body-site (e.g., face).

Gowns

Wear a gown to protect skin and prevent soiling or contamination of clothing during procedures and patient-care activities when contact with blood, body fluids, secretions, or excretions is anticipated.

Wear a gown for direct patient contact if the patient has uncontained secretions or excretions.

Remove gown and perform hand hygiene before leaving the patient's environment.

Mouth, nose, eye protection

Use PPE to protect the mucous membranes of the eyes, nose and mouth during procedures and patient-care activities that are likely to generate splashes or sprays of blood, body fluids, secretions and excretions.

During aerosol-generating procedures wear one of the following: a face shield that fully covers the front and sides of the face, a mask with attached shield, or a mask and goggles.

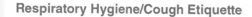

Respiratory Hygiene/Cough Etiquette

Educate healthcare personnel to contain respiratory secretions to prevent droplet and fomite transmission of respiratory pathogens, especially during seasonal outbreaks of viral respiratory tract infections.

Offer masks to coughing patients and other symptomatic persons (e.g., persons who accompany ill patients) upon entry into the facility.

Patient-care equipment and instruments/devices

Wear PPE (e.g., gloves, gown), according to the level of anticipated contamination, when handling patient-care equipment and instruments/devices that are visibly soiled or may have been in contact with blood or body fluids.

Care of the environment

Include multi-use electronic equipment in policies and procedures for preventing contamination and for cleaning and disinfection, especially those items that are used by patients, those used during delivery of patient care, and mobile devices that are moved in and out of patient rooms frequently (e.g., daily).

Textiles and laundry

Handle used textiles and fabrics with minimum agitation to avoid contamination of air, surfaces and persons.

The chapter in which the acronym first appears is listed in parentheses.

ABI	ankle brachial index (Chapter 5)		**dL**	deciliter (Chapter 2)
ABPI	ankle brachial pulse index (Chapter 5)		**eAG**	average glucose (Chapter 5)
ACE	angiotensin converting enzyme inhibitor (Chapter 4)		**ECG**	electrocardiogram (Chapter 5)
			ECT	electroconvulsive therapy (Chapter 7)
ADA	American Diabetes Association (Chapter 5)		**EMR**	electronic medical record (Chapter 6)
ADH	antidiuretic hormone (Chapter 2)		**EMT**	emergency medical technician (Chapter 5)
A-Fib	atrial fibrillation (Chapter 8)		**EPS**	electrophysiology study (Chapter 8)
AHA	American Heart Association (Chapter 6)		**F**	Fahrenheit (Chapter 2)
AMI	acute myocardial infarction (Chapter 8)		**FDA**	Food and Drug Administration (Chapter 4)
ANS	autonomic nervous system (Chapter 2)		**GABA**	glutamate and gamma-aminobutyric (Chapter 2)
ARB	angiotensin II receptor blocker (Chapter 4)		**HbA1C**	glycated hemoglobin blood test (Chapter 5)
AV	atrioventricular node (Chapter 1)		**HCTZ**	hydrochlorothiazide (Chapter 4)
aV	augmented leads (Chapter 6)		**HDL**	high-density lipoprotein (Chapter 2)
BNP	brain natriuretic peptide (Chapter 2)		**HIPAA**	Health Information Portability and Accountability Act (Chapter 5)
BP	blood pressure (Chapter 3)		**HR**	heart rate (Chapter 3)
bpm	beats per minute (Chapter 2)		**HRV**	heart rate variability (Chapter 5)
C	Celsius (Chapter 2)		**hs**	hour of sleep (Chapter 4)
CA	coronary arteries (Chapter 1)		**hsCRP**	high-sensitivity C-reactive protein (Chapter 5)
Ca	calcium (Chapter 2)		**HTN**	hypertension (Chapter 5)
CAD	coronary artery disease (Chapter 4)		**ICD**	implantable cardioverter defibrillator (Chapter 8)
Caps	capsules (Chapter 4)			
CCB	calcium channel blocker (Chapter 4)		**in**	inch (Chapter 2)
CDC	Centers for Disease Control (Chapter 5)		**IV**	intravenous (Chapter 8)
			IVR	idioventricular rhythm (Chapter 8)
CHF	congestive heart failure (Chapter 3)		**JVP**	jugular venous pressure (Chapter 5)
cm	centimeter (Chapter 1)		**K**	potassium (Chapter 2)
CNS	central nervous system (Chapter 2)		**kg**	kilogram (Chapter 8)
CO	cardiac output (Chapter 1)		**L**	liter (Chapter 3)
COPD	chronic obstructive pulmonary disease (Chapter 2)		**LA**	left arm (Chapter 1)
CPR	cardiopulmonary resuscitation (Chapter 8)		**LAD**	left anterior descending artery (Chapter 8)
CRP	C-reactive Protein (Chapter 5)		**LADA**	latent autoimmune diabetes in adults (Chapter 5)
CVA	cerebral vascular accident (Chapter 2)			

LCx	left circumflex coronary artery (Chapter 8)	**POTS**	postural orthostatic tachycardia syndrome (Chapter 2)
LDL	low density lipoprotein (Chapter 4)	**PP**	pulse pressure (Chapter 3)
LL	left leg (Chapter 1)	**P-P**	P to P wave (Chapter 7)
LMWH	low molecular-weight heparin (Chapter 4)	**PR**	conduction delay during depolarization (Chapter 7)
Lp(a)	lipoprotein (Chapter 5)	**PRI**	atrial depolarization (Chapter 7)
LV	left ventricle (Chapter 1)	**PRN**	when necessary (Chapter 4)
mA	milliamps (Chapter 8)	**PSNS**	parasympathetic nervous system (Chapter 2)
max	maximum (Chapter 8)	**PSVT**	paroxysmal supraventricular tachycardia (Chapter 8)
mcg	microgram (Chapter 8)		
Mg	magnesium (Chapter 3)	**PT**	prothrombine test (Chapter 4)
mg	milligram	**PVC**	premature ventricular complex (Chapter 4)
MI	myocardial infarction (Chapter 8)	**PVD**	peripheral vascular disease (Chapter 5)
min	minute (Chapter 4)		
min	minimum (Chapter 8)	**PVR**	peripheral vascular resistance (Chapter 3)
mL	milliliter (Chapter 1)		
mm Hg	millimeters of mercury (Chapter 3)	**QD**	once daily (Chapter 4)
ms	millisecond (Chapter 3)	**qid**	four times a day (Chapter 4)
mV	millivolt (Chapter 3)	**QRS**	rapid ventricular depolarization (Chapter 7)
Na	sodium (Chapter 2)		
NBME	National Board of Medical Examiners (Appendix E)	**QT**	depolarization through repolarization cycle (Chapter 7)
NIH	National Institute of Health (Chapter 5)	**RA**	right arm (Chapter 1)
NSAID	nonsteroidal anti-inflammatory drug (Chapter 4)	**RCA**	right coronary artery (Chapter 8)
		RL	right leg (Chapter 1)
NSR	normal sinus rhythm (Chapter 7)	**R-R**	R wave to R wave (Chapter 7)
OPQRST	Onset, Provocation, Quality, Radiation, Severity, Time (Chapter 5)	**RV**	right ventricle (Chapter 1)
OTC	over the counter (Chapter 4)	**SA**	sinoatrial node (Chapter 1)
P′	P prime (Chapter 8)	**SAMPLE**	Signs and symptoms, Allergies, Medications, Past medical history, Last oral intake, Events (Chapter 5)
PAC	premature atrial complex (Chapter 4)		
PAD	peripheral arterial disease (Chapter 5)		
PEA	pulseless electrical activity (Chapter 8)	**SCD**	sudden cardiac death (Chapter 8)
pg	picograms (Chapter 5)	**SNS**	sympathetic nervous system (Chapter 2)
pH	potential of hydrogen (Chapter 2)	**SOAP**	Subjective, Objective, Assessment, Plan (Chapter 5)
PJC	premature junctional complex (Chapter 8)	**SOB**	shortness of breath (Chapter 8)
PNS	peripheral nervous system (Chapter 2)	**SpO$_2$**	pulse oxygen saturation level (Chapter 5)

ST conduction delay between S and T waves (Chapter 7)

STAT immediately, emergency (Chapter 6)

SV Stroke volume (Chapter 3)

SVT supraventricular tachycardia (Chapter 8)

T3 triodothyronine hormone (Chapter 2)

T4 thyroxine hormone (Chapter 2)

Tab tablet (Chapter 4)

TCP transcutaneous pacemaker (Chapter 8)

TIA transit ischemic attack (Chapter 4)

tid three times a day (Chapter 4)

TP reference point for ST or PR segments (Chapter 7)

TPR total peripheral resistance (Chapter 2)

TSH thyroid stimulating hormone (Chapter 2)

V vector (Chapter 6)

VLDL very low density lipoprotein (Chapter 5)

V-tach ventricular tachycardia (Chapter 8)

WHO World Health Organization (Chapter 5)

WNL within normal limits (Chapter 5)

The following information is general, helpful information for most national exams. Please keep in mind that not all exams you take will follow this format.

Be sure to use the specific guidelines by the accrediting agency or exam qualification guidelines to know specific information for the exam that you are going to take. For instance, if you are preparing for the National Healthcareer Association (NHA) EKG Technician Certification Exam, you should familiarize yourself with their website, www.nhanow.com, which provides information about registering and preparing for the exam. This website also provides a detailed test plan outlining the skills that the exam assesses. This textbook was designed to help you gain those skills necessary to pass the NHA's EKG Technician Certification Exam.

NATIONAL EXAM CREATION

Most national medical exams have test creation teams from each specific field who have learned the proper strategies to create a fair, unbiased exam at the National Board of Medical Examiners (NBME), located in Philadelphia, PA. Educators and content experts from each specific exam will then write the exam using their knowledge and the test strategy guidelines they learned from the NBME. Test creators are usually selected for their expertise in the field and come from all parts of the United States. They develop new test questions and then meet, often at the NBME office, to review every new question written. Next, accepted questions will be put into a test bank replacing up to one-third of the previous test bank questions. This method allows the newest industry trends to be included in national exams. Using this method also makes it fair to all applicants, regardless of whether the test they take is calculated on a raw score or a weighted value score, or is a computerized test or a pencil-and-paper test.

NATIONAL EXAM SCORING

The majority of the written national exams are scored by one of two methods. The first method is called the raw score. The raw score calculates how many questions were correctly answered out of how many total questions were asked. A passing scale is then determined with a cutoff number representing passing or failing. The second method is called the weighted value score. In the weighted value score, several versions of the test are given at one time. All the tests are graded with a raw score but then compared to the total number of tests taken; and the total number of correctly answered questions of the total number of possible answers is computed. Then a scaled score is developed to determine the cutoff score, which represents passing or failing the exam. Most national tests require applicants to go to testing centers to take the computerized exam. A few agencies do still allow a paper-and-pencil exam to be taken. Either way, all exams are timed and given on a specific prescheduled day and time.

TEST-TAKING STRATEGIES

National exam material usually takes weeks to months to learn and study for. Studying the night before an exam, or "cramming," is probably one of the worst strategies (other than not studying at all) that a prospective exam taker can do. Using the following guidelines, along with this book, should help you maximize your score and pass the national exam the first time you sit for it. Remember that each time you must retake the exam, it will cost you an additional fee. Some organizations will allow you to sit for the exam only a certain number of times. The following test-taking strategies could increase your score by more than 25 percent.

From the beginning of the course and throughout the course:
If the class is not being given online, go to every class. Whether it is face-to-face or online, read the objectives and terms before the scheduled first day of the class. Before an exam, check to see if you can respond correctly to each objective that was covered for that exam. Complete all the Quick Check questions prior to the day of the exam. Complete the Critical Thinking Challenges, Review Activities, and

Chapter Test at the end of each chapter before taking a chapter exam. Review the chapter terminology. Take the time to review all your incorrect answers to the Quick Checks. Reread the material as necessary.

At the time of registration for the test:

It is very important to check and recheck the qualifications required to take the exam. The application should be complete; if a situation does not apply to you, do not leave the requested answer blank unless directed to do so; instead, insert "N/A." Answer every question truthfully.

Many national exams will ask you in the application if you want to allow your school access to your score. This is your choice, but many schools do need the information to compile statistics on their student success rates, so it is helpful for you to comply with this request.

Be sure to pay attention to the correct method of payment accepted and the total amount to submit. When an incorrect payment amount is submitted, often the application is denied, delayed, or returned to the sender. Once you have submitted the documentation and payment, a confirmation of the test date is usually emailed to you. Be on the lookout for it. Do not lose, delete, or fail to open the letter that the testing agency emails or sends because often the letter is required for admission to the testing center. Check your junk mailbox if you have not received the letter in a reasonable time.

Continue studying for the test during this time.

The night before the test:

Get a good night's sleep, even if you are not scheduled to take the test until the afternoon. Do *not* study the night before the exam, and do not eat foods or ingest drinks that are not part of your normal routine. If you are unfamiliar with the testing location, take a trial run to the location and time how long it takes to arrive. Don't wait until the day of the test to look for the testing location!

Test day

Arrive at the testing center early. You may not be able to enter until 15 minutes prior to your scheduled test time, but you will be relieved that you are there and are not rushing in at the last minute. It takes a few minutes to register and confirm your identity once you arrive. Be prepared with the correct paperwork (usually the acceptance letter and one or two picture IDs—often a school ID and a driver's license or state-issued ID). Also be prepared to submit a fingerprint for identity.

Do not plan on taking anything else into the testing center: no scrap paper, no cell phones, no books, no computers, no company—just you. Again, usually you may enter about 15 minutes prior to the scheduled test time. Plan on spending the entire allotted time. Do not rush through the test.

REMEMBER TO:

- Read each question completely. First, try to answer the question without looking at the choices.

- If you do not know the answer, take a guess—do not leave a question blank. Do not change answers unless you know for sure that the answer you entered was incorrect.

- If you happen to finish early, most tests allow you to go back. Do *not* change your answers if you are still unsure which answer is correct!

Many computerized tests will give you an unofficial test score as the last screen. Be sure you are looking for this. Some testing centers can print the screen with the unofficial test score; other centers cannot and will not be able to bring up your score once you have left the computer. If you finish early, be considerate of those test takers that are still working. Leave quietly!

After the test

Know what is required of you after you have completed the exam. Some accreditation agencies will list you as provisional until you submit proof of graduation; other agencies will not list you at all if paperwork is pending. Do not change addresses before you receive your certification in the mail. If you *must* move, try to use the new address on the application form so that your results will be sent to your new address.

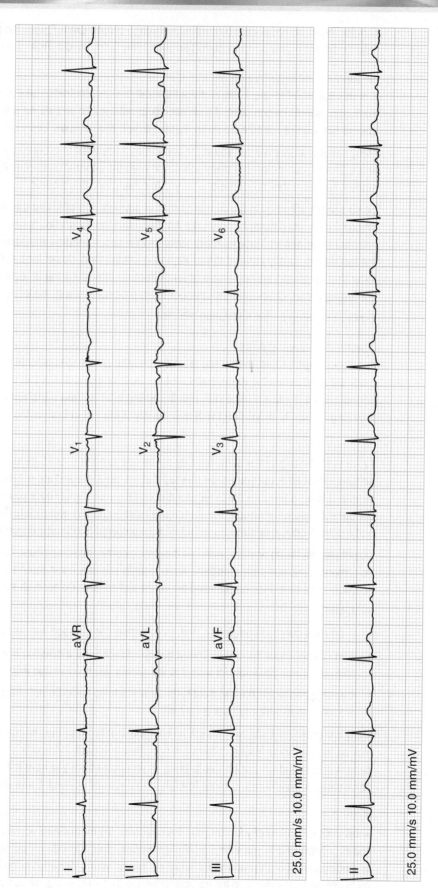

25.0 mm/s 10.0 mm/mV

25.0 mm/s 10.0 mm/mV

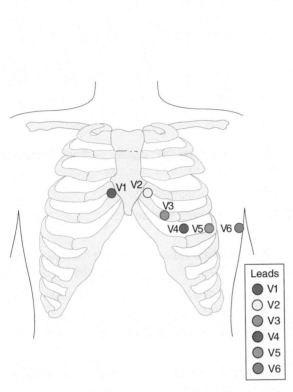

Leads

- ● V1
- ○ V2
- ● V3
- ● V4
- ● V5
- ● V6

Precordial Electrodes

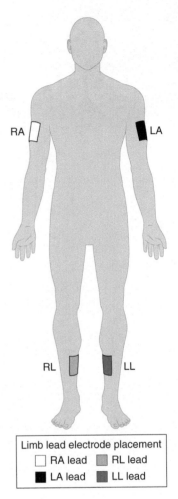

Limb lead electrode placement

- ☐ RA lead
- ■ LA lead
- ☐ RL lead
- ■ LL lead

Limb Lead Electrodes

References &
Suggested Readings

Abrams, J. (1995). The role of nitrates in coronary heart disease [Abstract]. *Archives of Internal Medicine, 155*(4), 357–364. Retrieved from http://www.ncbi.nlm.nih.gov/pubmed/7848018.

ACLS-ALGORITHMS.COM. *ACLS drugs* (n.d.). Retrieved from http://acls-algorithms.com/acls-drugs/.

ACLS MEDICAL TRAINING.COM (n.d.). *Crash carts*. Retrieved from https://www.aclsmedocaltraining.com/crash-carts/.

Advameg, Inc. Anticoagulant and antiplatelet drugs. In *Encyclopedia of Surgery*. Retrieved from http://www.surgeryencyclopedia.com/A-Ce/Anticoagulant-and-Antiplatelet-Drugs.html.

Advanced Cardiac Life Support (ACLS) Training Center (n.d.). *Crash cart supply and equipment checklist*. Retrieved from https://www.acls.net/acls-crash-cart.htm.

Alpaslan, M. (n.d.). *Calibration of the ECG*. Retrieved from http://www.metealpaslan.com/ecg/nekg4en.htm.

American Heart Association (n.d). *Cardiac medications at-a-glance*. Retrieved from http://www.heart.org/idc/groups/heart-public/@wcm/@hcm/cardiac_medications.

American Heart Association (n.d.). *What is metabolic syndrome?* Retrieved from http://www.heart.org/HEARTORG/Conditions/More/MetabolicSyndrome/.

American Heart Association (2014). *Blood pressure vs. heart rate*. Retrieved from http://www.heart.org/HEARTORG/Conditions/HighBloodPressure/AboutHighBloodPressure.

American Society of Hematology (2008). *Antithrombotic therapy*. Retrieved from http://www.hematology.org/About/History/50-Years/1523.aspx.

Ashley, E. A., & Niebauer, J. (2004). Chapter 3: Conquering the ECG. In *Cardiology explained*. Retrieved from http://www.ncbi.nlm.nih.gov/books/NBK2214/.

Astle, S. M. (2005). Restoring electrolyte balance. In *Modern Medicine*. Retrieved from http://www.modernmedicine.com/modern-medicine/content/restoring-electrolyte-balance.

Baranchuk, A., et al. (2009). *Electrocardiography pitfalls and artifacts: The 10 commandments*. Retrieved from http://ccn.aacnjournals.org/content/29/1/67.

Benson, R. (2005–2006). *Pacemaker nomenclature*. Retrieved from http://anesthesia.slu.edu/pdf/pacemaker.pdf.

Blesi, M., & Wise, B. A. (2012). *Medical assisting: Administrative and clinical competencies* (7th ed.). Clifton Park, NY: Cengage Learning.

Bouthillet, T. (2008). Contiguous and reciprocal lead charts. In *EMS 12-lead*. Retrieved from http://www.ems12lead.com/2008/12/19/contiguous-and-reciprocal-lead-charts/.

Boye, P., et al. (2011). Prediction of life-threatening arrhythmic events in patients with chronic myocardial infarction by contrast-enhanced CMR [Abbreviations and Acronyms]. *Journal of*

American College of Cardiology, 4(8). Retrieved from http://imaging.onlinejacc.org/article .aspx?articleid=1110358.

Buch, E., Boyer, N. G., & Belott, P. H. (2011). Pacemaker and defibrillator lead extraction. *Circulation, 123,* 378–380. Retrieved from http://circ.ahajournals.org/content/123/11/e378.full.

Cleveland Clinic (n.d.). *Sudden cardiac death (sudden cardiac arrest).* Retrieved from http://my .clevelandclinic.org/services/heart/disorders/arrhythmia/scd.

Cleveland Clinic (n.d.). *Types of arrhythmias.* Retrieved from http://my.clevelandclinic.org/services /heart/disorders/arrhythmia/types.

Cowley, M. (2008). *Electrodes, leads, & wires.* Retrieved from http://www.mikecowley.co.uk/leads.htm.

Curnew, G. P. (2001). 5 minutes on pacemakers—The ABCs of pacemakers: Who gets what kind, and why [Electronic version]. *Parkhurst Exchange, 19*(3). Retrieved from http://www.parkhurstexchange .com/clinical-reviews/apr11/pacemakers.

Ehrlich, A., & Schroeder, C. L. (2013). *Medical terminology for health professionals* (7th ed.). Clifton Park, NY: Cengage Learning.

Elshazly, M., & Nissen, S. (n.d.). *Cardiovascular emergencies.* Retrieved from http://www .clevelandclinicmeded.com/medicalpubs/diseasemanagement/cardiology/cardiovascular -emergencies/.

Emergency Nurses Association (2013). *Right-sided and posterior electrocardiograms (ECGs).* Retrieved from https://www.ena.org/practice-research/practice/documents/rightsideecg.pdf.

Ernst, Y. (2013). *Doing ECGs the right way: A reflection.* Retrieved from http://thebolus.org/doing-ecgs -the-right-way-a-reflection/.

Estes, M. E. Z. (2014). *Health assessment and physical examination* (5th ed.). Clifton Park, NY: Cengage Learning.

Fleisher, L. A., Frank, S. M., Sessler, D. I., Cheng, C., Matsukawa, T., & Vannier, C. A. (1996). Thermoregulation and heart rate variability [Abstract]. *Journal of Clinical Science, 90*(2), 97–103. Retrieved from http://www.ncbi.nlm.nih.gov/pubmed/8829887.

Food and Drug Administration Staff (2011). *Guidance for industry and food and drug administration staff: Class II special controls guidance document: Electrocardiograph electrodes.* Retrieved from http://www.fda.gov/MedicalDevices/DeviceRegulationandGuidance/GuidanceDocuments.

Francis, J. (2012). *EKG interpretation: What is pulse deficit?* Retrieved from https://cardiophile.org /what-is-pulse-deficit/.

Friedman, E. A. (2015). *Diuretics and heart failure.* Retrieved from http://emedicine.medscape.com /article/2145340-overview.

George, A., Arumugham, P. S., & Figueredo, V. M. (2010). aVR—The forgotten lead. *Experimental & Clinical Cardiology, 15*(2), e36–e44. Retrieved from http://www.ncbi.nlm.nih.gov/pmc/articles /PMC2898534/.

Grauer, K. (2013). *ECG interpretation review #74 (computerized ECG interpretation—peaked T waves—QS complexes—computer)* Retrieved from http://ecg-interpretation.blogspot .com/2013/09/ecg-interpretation-review-74.html.

Grauer, K. (2012). *ECG interpretation review #47 (normal variants-early repolarization-benign-ST elevation- pericarditis – ERP- STEMI).* Retrieved from http://ecg-interpretation.blogspot .com/2012/07/ecg-interpretation-review-47-normal.html.

Hanes, R. (2014). *Special patient considerations.* Retrieved from https://prezi.com/ntw5t_6fy77i /special-patient-considerations/.

Harrington, R. A., Chan T. C., & Brady, W. J. (2012). Electrocardiographic electrode misplacement, misconnection, and artifact. *Journal of Emergency Medicine [Electronic edition].* Retrieved from http://www.medscape.com/viewarticle/775860.

Heart Healthy Women.org (n.d.). *Ankle-Brachial index (ABI) test.* Retrieved from http://www.hearthealthyworman.org/tests-diagnosis/featured/ankle-brachial-index-abi-test.

Heart & Stroke Foundation (2011). Nitrates (nitroglycerin). Retrieved from http://www.heartandstroke.com/nitrates(nitroglycerin).

Hirsh, J., Anand, S. S., Halperin, J. L., & Fuster, V. (2001). Guide to anticoagulant therapy: Heparin. *Circuluation, 103,* 2994–3018. Retrieved from http://circ.ahajournals.org/content/103/24/2994.

Hurst, J. W. (2000). Images in cardiovascular medicine "switched" precordial leads. *Circulation, 101,* 2870–2871. Retrieved from http://circ.ahajournals.org/content/101/24/2870.full.

John Hopkins Medicine Health Library (n.d.). *Overview of pacemakers and implantable cardioverter defibrillators (ICDs).* Retrieved from http://www.hopkinsmedicine.org/healthlibrary/conditions/adult/cardiovascular_diseases/overview_of_pacemakers_and_implantable_cardioverter_defibrillators_icds_85,P00234/.

Kadish, A.H., et al. (2001). ACC/AHA clinical competence statement on electriocardiology and ambulatory electrocardiography. *Circulation, 104,* 3169–3178. Retrieved from http://circ.ahajournals.org/content/104/25/3169.full.

Kalsmith, B. M. (2009). Role of the brain natriuretic peptide in heart failure management. *Circulation: Heart Failure, 2,* 379. Retrieved from http://circheartfailure.ahajournals.org/content/2/4/379.extract.jpg.

Klabunde, R. E. (2015). Cardiac cycle. In *Cardiovascular physiology concepts.* Retrieved from http://www.cvphysiology.com/Heart%20Disease/HD002.htm.

Kligfield, P., et al. (2007). AHA/ACC/HRS scientific statement: Recommendations for the standardization and interpretation of the electrocardiogram. *Circulation, 115,* 1306–1324. Retrieved from http://circ.ahajournals.org/content/115/10/1306.full.

LaMonte, C. S., & Freiman, A. H. (1965). The electrocardiogram after mastectomy. *Circulation, 32,* 746–754. Retrieved from http://circ.ahajournals.org/content/32/5/746.full.pdf.

Lewis, K. M. (2010). *Multiple-lead ECGs: A practical analysis of arrhythmias.* Clifton Park, NY: Cengage Learning.

Lewis, K. M. (2010). *Sensible application of the ECG: A pocket guide.* Albany, NY: Delmar, Thomson Learning.

Lewis, K. M. (2001). *ECG: Practical applications pocket reference guide.* Clifton Park, NY: Cengage Learning.

Lewis, K. M., & Handel, K. A. (2000). *Sensible analysis of the 12-lead ECG.* Clifton Park, NY: Cengage Learning.

Lindh, W. Q., Pooler, M., Tamparo, C. D., Dahl, B. M., & Morris, J. (2014). *Comprehensive medical assisting* (5th ed.). Clifton Park, NY: Cengage Learning.

Mayo Clinic Staff (n.d.). High blood pressure (hypertension). Retrieved from http://www.mayoclinic.org/diseases-conditions/high-blood-pressure/in-depth/calcium-channel-blockers.

Mayo Clinic Staff (2013). *Ankle-brachial index.* Retrieved from http://www.mayoclinic.com/health/ankle-brachail-index/MY00074.

Mayo Clinic Staff (2013). *Tests and procedures: Pacemaker.* Retrieved from http://www.mayoclinic.org/tests-procedures/pacemaker/basics/results/prc-20014279.

MedlinePlus® (n.d.) *Fluid and electrolyte balance*. Retrieved from http://www.nlm.nih.gov /medlineplus/fluidandelectrolytebalance.html.

MedlinePlus®, U.S. National Library of Medicine, National Institute of Health (NIH) (n.d.). *Atrial fibrillation or flutter*. Retrieved from http://www.nlm.nih.gov/medlineplus/ency/article/000184.htm.

MedlinePlus®, U.S. National Library of Medicine, National Institute of Health (NIH) (n.d.). *Ventricular tachycardia*. Retrieved from http://www.nlm.nih.gov/medlineplus/ency/article/000187.htm.

MemorialCare Heart and Vascular Institute (n.d.). *Abnormal heart rhythms (arrhythmias)*. Retrieved from http://www.memorialcare.org/services/glossary/a/abnormal-heart-rhythms-arrhythmias.

Merck Manual for Health Care Professionals (n.d.). *Overview of arrhythmias*. Retrieved from http:// www.merckmanuals.com/professional/cardiovascular_disorders/arrhythmias_and _conduction_disorders.

Moisio, M. A. (2010). *Medical terminology for insurance and coding*. Clifton Park, NY: Cengage Learning.

Morris, F., & Brady, W. J. (2002). ABC of clinical electrocardiography: Acute myocardial infarction— Part 1. *BMJ, 324,* 831. Retrieved from http://www.ncbi.nim.nih.gov/pmc/articles/PMC1122768/.

Moukabary, T. (2007). Willem Einthoven (1860–1927), father of electrocardiography. *Cardiology Journal, 14*(3), 316–317. Retrieved from http://czasopisma.viamedica.pl/cj/article /view/21712/17316.

Muma, L. K. (n.d.). *Basics of EKG interpretation: A programmed study: Section three*. Retrieved from http://www.usfca.edu/fac-staff/ritter/threeekg.htm.

Muma, L. K. (n.d.). *Basics of EKG interpretation: A programmed study: Section four*. Retrieved from http://www.usfca.edu/fac-staff/ritter/fourekg.htm.

National Heart, Lung, and Blood Institute. (2011) *What is an arrhythmia?* Retrieved from http://www .nhlbi.nih.gov/health/health-topics/topics/arr/.

Olshansky, B., & Hayes, D. L. (2015). *Patient information: Pacemakers (beyond the basics)*. Retrieved from http://www.uptodate.com/contents/pacemakers-beyond-the-basics.

Oregon Health and Science University (OHSU) (n.d.). *Major cause of ST segment elevation*. Retrieved from https://sites.google.com/site/ohsuecg/home/major-causes-of-st-segment-elevation.

Oregon Health and Science University (OHSU) (n.d.). *Myocardial injury, ischemia, and infarction*. Retrieved from https://sites.google.com/site/ohsuecg/home/myocardial-injury-ischemia-and-infarction.

Oregon Health and Science University (OHSU) (n.d.). *Various morphologies of ST-T waves, as seen in lead V2*. Retrieved from https://sites.google.com/site/ohsuecg/home/various-morphologies -of-st-t-waves-as-seen-in-lead-v2.

Oregon Health and Science University (OHSU) Library (n.d.). *Lead misplacement*. Retrieved from https://sites.google.com/ohsuecg/home/lead-misplacement.

Pietrangelo, A. (n.d.). *What is ischemic cardiomyopathy?* Retrieved from http://www.healthline.com /health/ischemic-cardiomyopathy.

Reynolds, I. G. (2010). Emergency cardiac drugs: Essential facts for med-surg nurses. *American Nurses Today [Electronic Edition], 5*(7). Retrieved from http://www.americannursetoday.com /emergency-cardiac-drugs-essential-facts-for-med-surg-nurses/.

Rizzo, D. C. (2010). *Fundamentals of anatomy and physiology* (3rd ed.). Clifton Park, NY: Cengage Learning.

Rudiger, A., Schob, L., & Follath, F. (2003). Influence of electrode misplacement on the electrocardio- graphic signs of inferior myocardial ischemia. *American Journal of Emergency Medicine, 21*(7), 574–577. Retrieved from http://www.ncbi.nlm.nih.gov/pubmed/14655240?dopt=Abstract.

Schwinger, R. H., & Erdmann, E. (1992). Heart failure and electrolyte disturbances. *Methods and Findings in Experimental and Clinical Pharmacology, 14*(4), 315–325. Retrieved from http://www.ncbi.nlm.nih.gov/pubmed/1507935.

Scott, A. S., & Fong, E. (2014). *Body structures and functions* (12th ed.). Clifton Park, NY: Cengage Learning.

Scott & White Memorial Hospital—Health Library. (n.d.). *Pacemaker battery change.* Retrieved from http://www.sw.org/HealthLibrary?page=Pacemaker%20Battery%20Change.

Shea, M. J. (2012). Electrocardiography (ECG). *Merck manuals professional edition [Electronic].* Retrieved from http://www.merckmanuals.com/professional/cardiovascular-disorders/cardiovascular-tests-and-procedures/electrocardiography-ecg.

Society for Cardiological Science and Technology (2010). *Clinical guidelines by consensus recording a standard 12-lead electrocardiogram: An approved methodology.* Retrieved from http://www.scst.org.uk/resources/consensus_guideline_for_recording_a_12_lead_ecg_Rev_072010b.pdf.

Stanford Hospital and Clinics (n.d.). *Atrial flutter.* Retrieved from http://stanfordhospital.org/cardiovsdcularhealth/conditions/atrial-flutter.html.

Texas Heart® Institute (2014). *Calcium channel blockers.* Retrieved from http://www.texasheartinstitute.org/HIC/Topics/Meds/calcmeds.cfm.

Texas Heart® Institute (2014). *Categories of arrhythmias.* Retrieved from http://www.texasheart.org/HIC/Topics/Cond/arrhycat.cfm.

Texas Heart® Institute (2014). *Diuretics.* Retrieved from http://www.texasheart.org/HIC/Topics/Meds/diurmeds.cfm.

Texas Heart® Institute (2014). *Implantable cardioverter defibrillator (ICD).* Retrieved from http://www.texasheart.org/HIC/Topics/Proced/icdtopic.cfm.

Texas Heart® Institute (2014) *Pacemakers.* Retrieved from http://www.texasheart.org/HIC/Topics/Proced/pacemake.cfm.

Texas Heart® Institute (2013). *Nitrates.* Retrieved from http://www.texasheart.org/HIC/Topics/Meds/nitrmeds.cfm.

Turley, A. (n.d.). *Introduction to cardiac device function and troubleshooting.* Retrieved from http://bhrs.com/files/files/Physiologist%20-%20Presentations/11-Introduction%20to%20Cardiac%20Device%20Function%20and%20Troubleshooting.pdf.

Wallace, A. (2008). *Pacemakers for anesthesiologists made incredibly simple.* Retrieved from http://www.cardiacengineering.com/pacemakers-wallace.pdf.

WebMD (n.d.). *Angiotensin II receptor blockers (ARBs).* Retrieved from http://www.webmed.com/heart-disease/angiotensin-ii-receptor-blockers-arbs.

WebMD (n.d.). *Brain natriuretic peptide (BNP) test.* Retrieved from http://www.webmd.com/heart-disease/brain-natriuretic-peptide-bnp-test.

Wedro, B. (n.d.). *Heart rhythm disorders (abnormal heart rhythms).* Retrieved from http://www.medicinenet.com/script/main/art.asp?articlekey=84544.

World Health Organization (WHO) (2007). *Emergency drug guidelines.* Retrieved from http://www.who.int/selection_medicines/country_lists/kir_emergency_2007.pdf.

Glossary

The chapter where each term is first defined is shown in parentheses after the definition.

ablation A medical procedure that uses high electrical energy to destroy abnormal electrical pathways in the heart (Chapter 8)

accelerated junctional rhythm A rhythm between 60 and 100 beats per minute; originates in the atrioventricular (AV) junctional area and contains P′ waves (Chapter 8)

action potential A change in polarity of a cardiac cell, from negative charge to positive charge or from positive charge to negative charge (Chapter 3)

acute A sudden or recent event, usually an event of less than 24 hours' duration (Chapter 8)

agonal An irregular terminal rhythm that occurs when the heart rate drops below 20 beats per minute and the QRS pattern loses uniformity (Chapter 8)

afterload A force that interferes with systemic blood flow from the left ventricle, caused primarily by atrial vascular resistance (Chapter 3)

alveoli Tiny air sacs located in the lungs at the end of the bronchi, where oxygen and carbon dioxide is exchanged (Chapter 2)

amplitude The strength or magnitude of the action potential as shown on an ECG recording (Chapter 7)

anatomically contiguous Describes leads that provide a different angle view but are located on the same wall of the heart (Chapter 6)

ankle brachial index (ABI) A noninvasive test performed to obtain a ratio of the systolic blood pressure in the lower legs in comparison to the systolic blood pressure in the arms; also called ankle brachial pressure index (ABPI) (Chapter 5)

angina Heart pain caused by inadequate oxygen to the heart caused by blocked or constricted arteries and veins (Chapter 4)

angiotensin A hormone created in the liver as a protein responsible for regulating sodium and water balance in the body (Chapter 4)

antianginal A category of drugs used to reduce angina (Chapter 4)

antiarrhythmic An agent (drug) used to control or prevent arrhythmias (Chapter 4)

antihyperlipidemic A category of drugs used to lower cholesterol (Chapter 4)

antihypertensive A category of drugs used to lower blood pressure (Chapter 4)

antithrombotic A category of drugs used to prevent or treat blood clots (Chapter 4)

aorta The largest blood vessel in the body (Chapter 1)

aortic valve A valve located between the left ventricle and the ascending aorta and prevents the backflow of blood into the left ventricle; also called aortic semilunar valve (Chapter 1)

arrhythmia Heartbeat rhythms caused by alterations in time, quality, force, or sequence (Chapter 4)

artery A blood vessel that is traveling away from the heart and is full of oxygen. The exception to oxygenated blood traveling away from the heart is found in the pulmonary artery, which carries deoxygenated blood to the lungs (Chapter 1)

arterioles The smallest arteries, which control systemic blood flow and total peripheral resistance by contracting or relaxing (Chapter 1)

artifact An unusual waveform that appears on the ECG but is not caused by the heart; rather, it originates from outside interference, technician or machine error, or patient movement (Chapter 7)

asynchronous pacemaker A pacemaker that generates a continuous current at a preset rate (Chapter 8)

atrial arrhythmias The atrioventricular (AV) node overrides the sinoatrial (SA) node impulses, and the AV node becomes the heart's pacemaker (Chapter 8)

atrial fibrillation (A-Fib) Electrical impulses that are not regular, causing the heart to contract in a disorganized pattern (Chapter 8)

atrial flutter The atria become very irritable due to a rapid reoccurring ectopic impulse, causing the heart to beat at 250–350 beats per minute (Chapter 8)

atrial kick An atrial contraction that forces the remaining blood (not previously drained from the atria to the ventricles) to enter the ventricles before the atrioventricular (AV) valves close (Chapter 3)

atrial tachycardia The atrioventricular (AV) node overrides the sinoatrial (SA) node impulses and the AV node becomes the heart's pacemaker. Heart rate is over 100 beats per minute (Chapter 8)

atrioventricular (AV) node The heart's secondary pacemaker; also part of the conduction system where electrical impulses are generated; located in the lower right atrium (Chapter 1)

atrium One of the upper chambers of the heart; primarily functions as a reservoir for incoming blood; the plural form is atria (Chapter 1)

augmented leads Unipolar limb leads identified as aVR, aVL, and aVF; leads are shown from the frontal view and are amplified by the ECG machine by 50 percent over the standard limb leads so that they are readable on an ECG strip (Chapter 6)

automaticity A unique characteristic of myocardial cells to spontaneously create electricity without outside stimulation or internal stimulation by the nervous system (Chapter 3)

autonomic nervous system (ANS) The ANS's chief function is to act as a control system in the body through brain activity and nerve endings; also called involuntary nervous system or visceral nervous system (Chapter 2)

beats per minute (bpm) The number of heartbeats in 1 minute; used to calculate heart rate on a rhythm strip (Chapter 7)

bicuspid valve A valve that separates the left atrium from the left ventricle; prevents backflow of blood into the left atrium during ventricular systole; also called mitral valve (Chapter 1)

bioavailability The rate a drug is absorbed or the degree at which a drug is absorbed into the body (Chapter 4)

biphasic Waveforms with two distinct phases: one phase is above and one phase is below the isoelectric line (Chapter 7)

bipolar lead Electrical voltage in a lead that has both a positive and a negative pole; the Limb leads I, II, and II are all bipolar, shown from the frontal view (Chapter 6)

bradycardia A consistent heart rate slower than 60 beats per minute (Chapter 7)

bronchi A subdivision of the trachea that brings air into the lungs (Chapter 2)

bundle branches Two electrical conduction pathways that sends impulses to the ventricles by connecting the bundle of His to the Purkinje network (Chapter 3)

bundle of His An electrical conduction pathway that connects the upper and lower chambers of the heart (Chapter 3)

capillary A very thin and fragile blood vessel; the smallest blood vessel in the body (Chapter 1)

cardiac compromise Any cardiac issue (Chapter 8)

cardiac cycle The time it takes for the heart to complete one cycle from ventricular contraction to ventricular relaxation (Chapter 3)

cardiac output (CO) A measure of pulmonary blood volume pumped by the left ventricle in 1 minute (Chapter 1)

cardiomegaly An enlarged heart (Chapter 4)

cardioversion A process of using chemical (antiarrhythmic drugs) or timed electrical (shock) procedures to restore a normal sinus rhythm (NSR) (Chapter 8)

central nervous system (CNS) The master controller, made up of the brain and the spinal cord (Chapter 2)

cerebral vascular accident (CVA) A stroke, blood flow to the brain is blocked or greatly reduced, either by blood clots or plaque buildup, or by blood vessel hemorrhage (Chapter 2)

chorda tendinea Fibrous connective tissue that attaches the tips of the mitral and tricuspid valves to the papillary muscles of the ventricles, thus preventing the atrioventricular (AV) valves from being pushed backward into the atria during ventricular contractions; the plural form is chordae tendineae (Chapter 1)

chronic obstructive pulmonary disease (COPD) A progressive lung disease which, over time, prevents normal breathing due to damage of the alveoli or thickening of the bronchi (Chapter 2)

conductivity The unique ability of myocardial cells to transmit and receive electrical impulses to and from other myocardial cells (Chapter 3)

compensatory pause On an ECG, the duration is twice the distance between two R-R intervals that have the underlying rhythm disturbance caused by a premature ventricular complex (PVC) (Chapter 8)

contractility The ability of the myocardial cells to shorten and contract before recovering from a ventricular contraction (Chapter 3)

coronary arteries (CA) Originating off the aorta, these arteries wrap around and are imbedded in the heart muscle to supply rich, oxygenated blood to the atria and ventricles (Chapter 1)

coronary sinus The collection site for deoxygenated blood from the heart that will be drained into the right atrium (Chapter 1)

coronary sulcus A depression (resembling a valley) surrounding the external surface of the heart muscle; separates the atria from the ventricles (Chapter 1)

crash cart A cart that is usually on wheels and stocked with emergency medications, supplies, intravenous (IV) solutions and tubing, ECG electrodes, a handheld ECG machine, and a defibrillator (Chapter 8)

deflection The amount of deviation from the isoelectric line, determined by the lead placement (Chapter 7)

depolarization Sodium ions cross the cell membrane, causing a reversal of intracellular membrane charges from negative to positive (Chapter 3)

diaphoresis Excessive sweating (Chapter 2)

diaphragm The muscle that separates the thoracic cavity from the abdomen; its main purpose is to control breathing (Chapter 2)

diastole The resting phase of a heart muscle, when the chambers fill with blood (Chapter 3)

differential diagnosis Tests or procedures used by health care professionals to find potential causes for conditions with similar symptoms (Chapter 6)

dysautonomia Conditions, malfunctions, or diseases of the autonomic nervous system (ANS) (Chapter 2)

dyspnea Shortness of breath (Chapter 2)

dysrhythmia Regularly occurring abnormal, faulty, or disordered rhythms (Chapter 4)

ectopic beat A heartbeat that originates outside the sinoatrial (SA) node (Chapter 8)

electrocardiogram (ECG) A noninvasive diagnostic test performed on a patient in which electrodes are placed on the body to measure the electrical activity of the heart (Chapter 5)

electrode A small, self-adhesive pad used to amplify electrical current from a patient; contains a layer of conductive gel and an area to attach a lead wire to an ECG machine (Chapter 6)

electrolytes Compounds that are soluble in water and form free ions, which then conduct electricity (Chapter 2)

electrophysiology study (EPS) A study performed on an implanted cardioverter defibrillator (ICD) to determine if the ICD is working correctly (Chapter 8)

end diastolic volume The volume of blood in the left ventricle when the ventricle is filled to capacity; typical adult level is 120 mL (Chapter 3)

end systolic volume The volume of blood that remains in the left ventricle after a contraction; typical adult level is 50 mL (Chapter 3)

endocardium tissue The innermost layer of the heart wall, lines the chambers and the heart valves (Chapter 1)

epicardium tissue The smooth outer layer of the heart wall where the coronary arteries are located; also called visceral pericardium (Chapter 1)

escape beat A junctional beat that originates in the bundle of His, or a ventricular rhythm that takes over supraventricular pacing (Chapter 8)

excitability A cardiac cell's unique ability to respond to electrical stimulus; also called irritability (Chapter 3)

extracellular Located outside a cell membrane (Chapter 3)

fibrillation Electrical signals that produce a quiver (not a contraction) in the heart muscles of the atria or ventricles (Chapter 4)

fibrin A protein that forms a mesh to keep platelets together (Chapter 4)

gain control An adjustment that can be made to the standard ECG tracing which will increase or reduce the ECG graphic image (Chapter 7)

glycation Having too much glucose in the blood, which causes the glucose to bind to hemoglobin (Chapter 5)

great coronary vein A blood vessel that carries waste from the heart muscle to the coronary sinus (Chapter 1)

ground lead A lead that carries no current (Chapter 6)

Health Information Portability and Accountability Act (HIPAA) (1996) A federal law that established national standards in several areas, including the quality, efficiency, effectiveness, and cost of health care; and in protecting patient rights, safety, security, access, confidentiality, and disclosure of identifiable health information by all types of media; and established notification standards, penalties, and enforcement activities for noncompliance by every member of all areas in the health care industry (Chapter 5)

heart disease A structural or functional abnormality of the heart or cardiovascular system (Chapter 4)

heart failure A condition when the heart can no longer function normally and the pumping action of the heart muscle is greatly reduced, causing insufficient systemic blood flow (Chapter 4)

heart rate The number of times the heart beats in 1 minute (Chapter 3)

heart rate variability (HRV) Heartbeat fluctuations or very specific patterns in beat-to-beat intervals that usually can predict a condition before any symptoms appear (Chapter 5)

heart rhythm A measurable, regularly recurring, impulse of the heart (Chapter 7)

His-Purkinje system Consists of the bundle of His, the left- and right-bundle branches, and the Purkinje fibers; is located surrounding the ventricles (Chapter 1)

homeostasis The process of stabilizing the body's internal environment so that all the body's organs work optimally (Chapter 2)

hyperkalemia High blood potassium (Chapter 2)

hypertension High blood pressure (Chapter 2)

hypertrophy Abnormal thickening of the walls and structures of the heart (Chapter 4)

idioventricular rhythm (IVR) An impulse originating in the ventricles, produces a rhythm of 20–40 beats per minute (Chapter 8)

implantable cardioverter defibrillator (ICD) A device implanted into patients who need two levels of heart stimulus; one level is designed to correct ventricular tachycardia, and a stronger level of "shock" is designed to correct ventricular fibrillation (Chapter 8)

implied consent Nonverbal consent, often used in emergency medical care if a patient is unable to provide informed consent but the patient's actions (such as seeking medical care) suggest that medical intervention is desired (Chapter 6)

infarct Localized dead tissue area where a hemorrhagic event occurred (Chapter 2)

inferior vena cava A vein that drains deoxygenated blood from the body below the heart into the right atrium (Chapter 1)

informed consent The legal doctrine that gives people the right to make decisions about their medical treatment by being informed of the medical procedure, the risks involved, the benefit of the procedure, possible alternatives, and consequences of choosing not to have a procedure (Chapter 6)

insulin resistance The human body's inability to utilize insulin produced in the pancreas, which then causes too much glucose to build up in the blood (Chapter 5)

interval On an ECG image, the period of time between two waves that complete an event and includes time where no electrical activity is being recorded on the ECG (Chapter 7)

internodal pathways Four pathways that provide a route for electrical impulses to travel; three pathways travel from the sinoatrial (SA) node to the atrioventricular (AV) node, and the fourth path carries the impulse from the SA node to the left atrium (Chapter 3)

intracellular Located within cell membrane (Chapter 3)

intrinsic rhythm A heart rhythm created by a person's own heart rather than by an artificial means (Chapter 8)

irregularly irregular rhythm A cardiac rhythm with no R-R pattern or similarity between the PR or QRS intervals (Chapter 7)

ischemia A decrease in oxygenated blood flow to the heart muscle (Chapter 8)

isoelectric line No electrical activity is occurring in the heart at a point in time; appears as a flat line on the ECG tracing; also called baseline (Chapter 7)

jugular venous pressure (JVP) The observation and measurement of the jugular vein in the neck to determine venous blood pressure and volume (Chapter 5)

junctional arrhythmias Instances that occur when the sinoatrial (SA) node either fails to conduct an impulse or there is a blockage of the impulse so the impulse originates in the atrioventricular (AV) node (Chapter 8)

junctional rhythm A pacemaker impulse created in the bundle of His (Chapter 8)

junctional tachycardia A junctional rhythm with a rate of 100–140 beats per minute (Chapter 8)

leads Insulated conductor wires that are attached to electrodes and measure voltage changes from different views or angles of the heart, as determined by the placement of the electrodes on the body (Chapter 6)

loss of capture On the ECG, two pacemaker spikes with no waveforms between the spikes (Chapter 8)

metabolic syndrome A group of symptoms or risk factors including abdominal obesity, high blood pressure, high triglycerides, high fasting blood glucose level, and low high-density lipoprotein (HDL) cholesterol level, which, when combined, can be the underlying cause of many cardiovascular diseases, including heart attacks and strokes (Chapter 2)

metabolism The body's process of using water, oxygen, ions, and other components of blood to grow, heal, and create energy (Chapter 2)

morphology The structural appearance of a wave or waveform (Chapter 7)

myocardial infarction (MI) An occlusion of the coronary arteries that prevents oxygenated blood from circulating within the heart, causing permanent heart muscle tissue damage (Chapter 8)

myocardium tissue The thickest layer of muscle tissue in the heart wall (Chapter 1)

necrosis Tissue death (Chapter 8)

nephrons Areas in the kidney where urine is produced (Chapter 2)

neurons Basic nerve cells that carry signals along electrochemical waves for communication (Chapter 2)

neurotransmitters Chemicals that transmit signals to the adrenal glands (Chapter 2)

noninvasive Patient tests or procedures that do not penetrate the skin and body orifices are not entered (Chapter 5)

normal sinus rhythm (NSR) On an ECG, a group of characteristics that include a heart rate between 60 and 100 beats per minute, regular and uniform P waves before every QRS complex, a PR interval between 0.12 and 0.20 seconds, and a QRS complex of less than 0.12 seconds (Chapter 7)

normal wave progression A concept associated with comparison of the precordial views of the ECG; V1–V6 show an amplitude change in each precordial lead, with V1 showing a small R wave and a large S wave, progressing through V6, which shows a large R wave and a small S wave (Chapter 7)

obstructive sleep apnea A sleep disorder where the airway becomes blocked or collapses, preventing oxygen from reaching the lungs (Chapter 2)

open-ended questioning An interview technique used to obtain information that allows and encourages more response from an individual than a simple yes or no answer (Chapter 5)

OPQRST A mnemonic acronym meaning Onset, Provocation, Quality, Radiation, Severity, and Time; the OPQRST assessment is used primarily for cardiac events (Chapter 5)

P prime (P') A term used to represent a P wave that originated from anywhere other than from the sinoatrial (SA) node (Chapter 8)

pace To follow or track a heartbeat or rhythm (Chapter 8)

pacemaker A device that measures the movement of electricity in the heart; designed to provide an electrical stimulus in the event that the heart does not provide a normal heartbeat (Chapter 8)

pacemaker spikes Marks that appear on an ECG signifying the patient has a pacemaker (Chapter 8)

pacing electrode Single or multiple leads that can be unipolar or bipolar, and can provide the electrical stimulus in a pacemaker (Chapter 8)

papillary muscle A muscle that holds the tricuspid and mitral valves in place along the heart wall (Chapter 1)

parasympathetic nervous system (PSNS) The function of the PSNS is to conserve energy, which is done through sleep, resting, or lack of potential threats; often referred to as the heart's rest and digest response to outside stimuli or the lack of any stimuli (Chapter 2)

pathological Q wave A permanent, large, wide Q wave measuring over 0.04 seconds in duration and at least 25 percent to 35 percent of the amplitude of the entire QRS complex (Chapter 8)

peripheral nervous system (PNS) Consists of 12 pairs of cranial nerves and 31 pairs of spinal nerves that utilizes three specialized types of nerve cells (autonomic, sensory, and somatic) to communicate from the central nervous system (CNS) to the body (Chapter 2)

peripheral vascular resistance Arterial opposition to blood flow; can be measured by a blood pressure reading (Chapter 3)

pH (potential of hydrogen) A measure of the amount of acidity and alkalinity in the body (Chapter 2)

pharmacodynamics The study of how drugs act in living organisms (Chapter 4)

pharmacokinetics. The study of how the body metabolizes a drug and how the body distributes or excretes drugs (Chapter 4)

pharmacogenetics The study of how drugs interrelate based on genetics (Chapter 4)

platelets A type of blood cell that can create a mass of thrombin (Chapter 4)

polarization A process where a cell is at rest, the intracellular membrane is negatively charged (Chapter 3)

polymorphic Waveforms with changing polarity (Chapter 8)

precordial leads Chest leads that view the heart from a horizontal plane (Chapter 6)

preload At the end of diastole, the amount of blood in the left ventricle and the pressure used to stretch the muscle fibers (Chapter 3)

premature atrial complex (PAC) Heart rhythm disturbances; an extra beat originating in the atrium; also called premature atrial contraction (Chapter 4)

premature junctional complex (PJC) Heart rhythm disturbances; occur when there is one or more ectopic beats originating in ventricles (Chapter 8)

premature ventricular complex (PVC) Heart rhythm disturbances; an extra beat originating in the ventricles; also called premature ventricular contraction (Chapter 4)

primary hypertension High blood pressure that has no identifiable cause and is believed to develop over time; also referred to as essential or idiopathic hypertension (Chapter 5)

primary prevention drug A drug prescribed before a cardiovascular event, such as before a stroke or myocardial infarction (MI) (Chapter 4)

pulmonary artery A blood vessel that carries deoxygenated blood to the lungs from the right ventricle (Chapter 1)

pulmonary circulation The process that takes place when deoxygenated blood leaves the heart to gather oxygen in the lungs and then returns to the heart as oxygenated blood (Chapter 1)

pulmonic valve A valve located between the right ventricle and the pulmonary arteries; also called pulmonary semilunar valve (Chapter 1)

pulse oximeter A device used to measure arterial blood oxygen saturation and the heart rate in a noninvasive manner (Chapter 5)

pulse pressure The difference between diastolic blood pressure and systolic blood pressure (Chapter 3)

pulseless electrical activity (PEA) A condition where the heart muscle cannot contract, even though electrical activity appears on the ECG (Chapter 8)

Purkinje network A group of network fibers that serve as the third pacemaker of the heart; generates electrical impulses at a rate of 20–40 beats per minute (Chapter 3)

reciprocal Lead views that can be interchangeable; used especially when acute injury is suspected but it is not showing on standard ECG lead views (Chapter 6)

reflective lead A lead that faces an affected surface of an injured wall (Chapter 8)

refractory period A time during the repolarization phase when cardiac cells cannot receive additional electrical impulses (Chapter 3)

regularly irregular rhythm A heart rhythm that deviates from a normal rhythm on a regular basis and usually occurs as a patterned event (Chapter 7)

renin A secretion created in the kidneys that produces angiotensin II, which is a powerful arterial and venous constrictor (Chapter 2)

retrograde An impulse that goes backward in the conduction path (Chapter 8)

rhabdomyolysis A rare muscle injury that can lead to kidney failure or death (Chapter 4)

repolarization A process where electrolytes cross cell membranes back to the original polarity, thus returning the heart to a resting state and leaving the extracellular charge positive and the intracellular charge negative (Chapter 3)

resting state A cardiac cell is considered to be in a resting state when it is not contracting; also called resting membrane potential or polarized state (Chapter 3)

SAMPLE A mnemonic acronym meaning Signs and symptoms, Allergies, Medications, Past medical history or injuries or illnesses, Last oral intake, and Events that led up to the current illness or injury (Chapter 5)

secondary hypertension A sudden increase in blood pressure caused by an underlying condition (Chapter 5)

secondary prevention drug A drug prescribed to limit heart disease from further damaging the heart or to reduce symptoms (Chapter 4)

segment On the ECG strip, a time period with no electrical activity occurring between waves; if normal, looks like a flat line (Chapter 7)

septum A dividing wall in the heart made of thick muscle which separates the right side of the heart from the left side of the heart (Chapter 1)

sinoatrial (SA) node The first site in the heart where electrical impulses are generated; often referred to as the "heart's pacemaker"; located in the upper right atrium (Chapter 1)

sinus arrhythmia An electrical impulse that begins in the SA node and changes the heart rate with a person's respirations (Chapter 8)

sinus bradycardia A heartbeat with a normal rhythm but beating too slowly, at less than 60 beats per minute (Chapter 4)

sinus rhythm A rhythm that follows all the rules for a normal sinus rhythm (NSR) *except* that the heart rate is too fast or too slow (Chapter 7)

sinus tachycardia A heartbeat with a normal rhythm but beating too fast (at more than 100 beats per minute) (Chapter 4)

SOAP A mnemonic acronym meaning Subjective, Objective, Assessment, and Plan (Chapter 5)

somatic tremor A muscle movement that shows up on an ECG as an artifact; can be either voluntary or involuntary muscle movement (Chapter 7)

sphygmomanometer A device used to measure arterial blood pressure in a noninvasive manner (Chapter 5)

Starling's Law of the Heart The degree of the stretch of the heart muscle; is directly related to the force of the blood being ejected from the ventricles (Chapter 3)

stroke volume The amount of blood ejected by the ventricles with each contraction (Chapter 3)

sudden cardiac arrest Unexpected death due to a heart electrical system malfunction (Chapter 8)

superior vena cava A vein that drains deoxygenated blood from the upper body into the right atrium; also called precava (Chapter 1)

supraventricular Originating above the atrioventricular (AV) node (Chapter 4)

supraventricular arrhythmias Arrhythmias that originate above the ventricles (Chapter 8)

supraventricular tachycardia (SVT) Occurs when the electrical system above the ventricles sends abnormal impulses that interfere with sinoatrial (SA) node impulses, creating a very fast heart rate that begins and ends suddenly (Chapter 8)

sympathetic nervous system (SNS) A system that regulates the rate and force of a contraction through stimulation; often referred to as the heart's "fight-or-flight" response because the heart can respond by increasing the strength and rate of contractions very quickly in response to stress and other stimuli (Chapter 2)

synchronous pacemaker One type of this device sets the heart rate at a preprogrammed pace, and the second type changes the heart rate according to patient activity; also called a demand pacemaker (Chapter 8)

syncope A condition when a person becomes lightheaded or faints (Chapter 4)

systemic circulation The blood flow from the heart to the body *except* to the lungs; the process of oxygenated blood leaving the heart through the aorta and completing a loop throughout the body via the arteries and veins (Chapter 1)

systole The contraction phase of a heart muscle (Chapter 3)

tachycardia A consistent heart rate over 100 beats per minute (Chapter 7)

terminal rhythm A continuous rhythm that cannot reverse to a normal rhythm without medical intervention (Chapter 8)

thermoregulation Regulation of the body's core temperature (Chapter 2)

thrombosis A condition in which a blood clot has become dislodged from the vessel wall and is now circulating within the bloodstream (Chapter 4)

thrombus A blood clot that is attached to the vessel wall where it formed (Chapter 4)

total peripheral resistance (TPR) A change in blood pressure measured as blood completes the cycle from arterial blood leaving the heart to venous blood returning to the heart (Chapter 1)

trachea A tube that brings air to and from the lungs (Chapter 2)

transcutaneous pacemaker (TCP) An external pacemaker with two parts that include electrodes that are placed in a special pad attached to the skin, and a power source (Chapter 8)

tricuspid valve A valve located between the right atrium and right ventricle which prevents the backflow of blood into the right atrium during ventricular systole (Chapter 1)

underlying rhythm A review of an overall rhythm on the ECG when an abnormality is not included in the rhythm; for example, a review of the ECG without including an ectopic beat to see if it is otherwise a normal rhythm (Chapter 8)

unipolar lead A lead that records electrical voltage in only one direction (from one pole); the augmented limb leads and all precordial leads are unipolar (Chapter 6)

vagus nerve The primary nerve providing communication between the brain and the heart (Chapter 2)

vasoconstriction A process where blood vessels constrict, reducing in diameter, which causes the blood pressure, vascular resistance, and body temperature to increase while blood flow and heart rate are decreased; opposite of vasodilation (Chapter 1)

vasodilatation Blood vessels widen, increasing in diameter. Vasodilation is the opposite of vasoconstriction so blood pressure, vascular resistance, and body temperature are decreased and blood flow and heart rate increases (Chapter 1)

vasodilators Medications that reduce the heart's workload by relaxing and dilating the blood vessels, which allows them to hold more blood, therefore increasing the flow of oxygen-rich blood to the heart; also called nitrates (Chapter 4)

vector (V) A graphical record that is made up of lines showing the direction of electrical forces (Chapter 6)

vein A blood vessel that carries deoxygenated blood back to the heart, except for the four pulmonary veins, which carry oxygenated blood from the lungs to the left atrium (Chapter 1)

ventricles The lower chambers of the heart (Chapter 1)

ventricular asystole The absence of any ventricular activity (Chapter 8)

ventricular fibrillation (V-Fib) chaotic indistinguishable waves caused by multiple ectopic and reentry patterns originating from many different areas in the ventricular walls (Chapter 8)

ventricular tachycardia (V-Tach) A high ventricular heart rate of 150–250 beats a minute (Chapter 8)

venules The smallest veins (Chapter 1)

voltage An amount of electrical stimulus or the difference in action potential created by cardiac cell movement within the heart (Chapter 7)

wave Electrical activity within the walls of the heart leading up to a ventricular contraction (Chapter 7)

waveform Electrical movement in either an upward or downward direction from the baseline of an ECG (Chapter 7)

within normal limits (WNL) A range of numbers given to medical tests or procedures that show the results to be within a medically selected normal healthy range for a specific population of people (e.g., children, adults, geriatric, etc.) (Chapter 5)

Index

E